T0074171

NUTRITION AND HEALTH SERIES

Adrianne Bendich, PhD, FACN, SERIES EDITOR

For further volumes:
http://www.springer.com/series/7659

Ted Wilson Ph.D. • Norman J. Temple Ph.D.
Editors

Beverage Impacts on Health and Nutrition

Second Edition

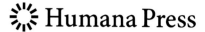 Humana Press

Editors
Ted Wilson Ph.D.
Department of Biology
Winona State University
Winona, MN, USA

Norman J. Temple Ph.D.
Centre for Science
Athabasca University
Athabasca, AB, Canada

ISBN 978-3-319-23671-1   ISBN 978-3-319-23672-8   (eBook)
DOI 10.1007/978-3-319-23672-8

Library of Congress Control Number: 2015960840

Springer Cham Heidelberg New York Dordrecht London

Printed on acid-free paper

Springer International Publishing AG Switzerland is part of Springer Science+Business Media (www.springer.com)

In a stream we often fish for trout, but in nutrition we try to fish for the truth. These chapters are the flies we use to fish for the truth of healthier lives. I hope my sons Jack and Dirk can use this information on our path to catching big fish.

Ted Wilson

"To Joseph, my adorable grandson"
Norman J. Temple

Foreword

The roles of beverage consumption and hydration in health are two of the most important, underestimated, and poorly communicated aspects in all of nutrition. While diverse beverages provide multiple health-promoting properties, perhaps the most important is hydration. All beverages hydrate.

The simple fact is that humans are basically water. The human body contains between 60 and 70 % water, and even a decrease of 1 or 2 % in hydration status can cause a significant decline in performance. It is no wonder that the US Military carefully studies hydration in pilots. Think of a jet pilot going at supersonic speeds making a slight error and flying a 20 million dollar jet into the side of a mountain!

Proper hydration is also critical to sports performance at all levels. Olympic athletes whose races are often decided by one one-hundredth of a second clearly understand the importance of proper hydration. It is also important for the average fitness enthusiast and should be important to everyone. Proper hydration is critically important to virtually every chemical reaction in the body and perhaps, most importantly, vital to the control of body temperature. In cases of natural disasters such as earthquakes, flooding, or even disease outbreaks, water is first rushed in since people can only go for a day or two without water without significant health problems, whereas they can often go up to 30 days without food before expiring.

Despite all of the important health considerations related to beverage consumption and hydration, when it comes to the area of nutrition, we often ignore this vital aspect. For example, the Dietary Guidelines for Americans pays scant attention to hydration as a component of sound nutritional practices. Little attention is devoted in the medical community or general public except during heat waves when people are urged to drink more fluids.

With this as background, the excellent volume edited by Wilson and Temple, *Beverage Impacts on Nutrition and Health*, is an important addition to the nutrition and health literature. This volume contains an enormous body of evidence-based information on diverse aspects of beverages and health. It covers an exceptionally broad scope of beverages all the way from alcoholic beverages to tea and coffee, sports drinks, and milk and many others—all in one volume. This is a welcome addition to the health and nutrition literature and should be on the bookshelf of every physician or other healthcare worker, athletic trainer, and nutrition professional.

Boston, MA, USA   James M. Rippe

Preface

Mountains are climbed because they have always been there, but books are usually written because they are not there. The first edition of *Beverage Impacts on Health and Nutrition* was published in 2004, and much has changed since then in our understanding of how beverages impact our health. Consumer beverage preferences and habits change as do their meaning in our lives. What has not changed since 2004—or, indeed, since the dawn of time—is that beverages represent an important part of our nutrition and that understanding their impact on our lives is critical for the good nutrition needed for a long and healthy life.

This second edition of this book is intended as a reference or classroom text source for health professionals, dietitians, physicians, university researchers, students, and beverage industry researchers and marketers. In a single book, it provides objective reviews on a wide range of global health issues associated with beverages. The book discusses how the history of beverages sets the stage for how and why we in the twenty-first century consume what we consume. Specific chapters update the reader about coffee, tea, alcohol, cranberry juice, citrus juices, cow's milk, soy milk, and our first beverage breast milk. The chapters then discuss recent beverage developments regarding satiety, diabetes, older adults, and athletes. Chapters then provide important reviews on controversial topics including energy drinks, bottled water, soft drink marketing, the nutritional effects of sugar, high-fructose corn syrup, and the effect of color on taste perception. The final chapters examine beverage labeling requirement legality, beverage ingredient formulations, and how beverage trends are important in determining what we are likely to consume in the future.

This second edition of this book reminds us of the rapid pace of development in the world of beverages in recent years. As a result, there is an impressive range of beverages now being marketed for reasons of taste and palatability, use in the diet, ability to improve health and well-being, and, of course, manufacturer profitability.

This speaks volumes to human ingenuity in the beverage industry and volumes to the quality of the research summarized in the chapters contained in this book. The book as a whole is greater than the sum of its component chapters.

Winona, MN, USA   Ted Wilson
Athabasca, AB, Canada   Norman J. Temple

Series Editor Page

The great success of the *Nutrition and Health* series is the result of the consistent overriding mission of providing health professionals with texts that are essential because each includes: (1) a synthesis of the state of the science; (2) timely, in-depth reviews by the leading researchers and clinicians in their respective fields; (3) extensive, up-to-date fully annotated reference lists; (4) a detailed index; (5) relevant tables and figures; (6) identification of paradigm shifts and the consequences; (7) virtually no overlap of information between chapters, but targeted, interchapter referrals; (8) suggestions of areas for future research; and (9) balanced, data-driven answers to patient as well as health professional questions which are based upon the totality of evidence rather than the findings of any single study.

The series volumes are not the outcome of a symposium. Rather, each editor has the potential to examine a chosen area with a broad perspective, both in subject matter and in the choice of chapter authors. The international perspective, especially with regard to public health initiatives, is emphasized where appropriate. The editors, whose trainings are both research and practice oriented, have the opportunity to develop a primary objective for their book, define the scope and focus, and then invite the leading authorities from around the world to be part of their initiative. The authors are encouraged to provide an overview of the field, discuss their own research, and relate the research findings to potential human health consequences. Because each book is developed de novo, the chapters are coordinated so that the resulting volume imparts greater knowledge than the sum of the information contained in the individual chapters.

Beverage Impacts on Health and Nutrition, Second Edition, edited by Ted Wilson, Ph.D., and Norman J. Temple, Ph.D., is a timely addition to the *Nutrition and Health* series. The editors have significant expertise in the role of beverages as critical nutritional strategies to aid in the growth and development of children and maintenance of hydration in adults and those with certain diseases and conditions that exacerbate the loss of fluids. They have invited the leaders in the field to develop the 24 relevant, practice-oriented chapters in this unique and clinically valuable volume. The volume contains chapters with differing perspectives, thus permitting health professionals an in-depth understanding of the bases for both possible concerns and recommendations. Dr. Ted Wilson, Ph.D., is professor of biology at Winona State University in Winona, Minnesota. His research examines how diet affects human nutritional physiology and whether food/dietary supplement health claims can be supported by measurable physiological changes. He has studied many foods and dietary supplements including pistachios, low-carbohydrate diets, cranberries, cranberry juice, apple juice, grape juice, wine, resveratrol, creatine phosphate, soy phytoestrogens, eggplant, coffee, tea, and energy drinks. He has examined the associations between these dietary factors and the development of heart failure, diabetes, and obesity. Diet-induced changes that have been studied include physiological evaluations of plasma lipid profiles, antioxidants, vasodilation, nitric oxide, platelet aggregation, and glycemic and insulinemic responses using in vivo and in vitro models. With Dr. N. Temple he edited the first edition of *Beverages in Nutrition and Health* (Humana Press, 2004), the three editions of *Nutritional Health: Strategies for Disease Prevention* (Springer/Humana Press, 2012), and *Nutrition Guide for Physicians* (Springer/Humana Press, 2010). He also enjoys teaching courses such as nutrition, cardiovascular physiology, cell signal transduction, and cell biology. When not in the laboratory, he enjoys family time, the outdoors, and farming. Norman J. Temple, Ph.D., is professor of nutrition at Athabasca University in Alberta, Canada. He has published 80 papers, mainly in the area of nutrition in relation to health. He has also published 12 books. Together with Denis Burkitt he coedited *Western Diseases: Their Dietary Prevention and Reversibility* (Humana Press, 1994). This continued and extended Burkitt's pioneering work on the role of dietary fiber in chronic diseases of lifestyle. The editors have contributed several volumes to the *Nutrition and Health* book series in addition to the current volume. Dr. Temple coedited *Nutrition Guide for Physicians* (2010) and the three editions of *Nutritional Health: Strategies for Disease Prevention* (2012). He also coedited *Excessive Medical Spending: Facing the Challenge* (2007). He conducts collaborative research in Cape Town on the role of the changing diet in South Africa on the pattern of diseases in that country, including obesity, diabetes, and heart disease.

This book fulfills an unmet need for nutritionists, dieticians, sports and exercise physiologists, pediatric and adult diabetologists and gastroenterologists, residents and fellows, pediatricians, gerontologists, nurses, and general practitioners who treat patients with questions concerning the right beverages for themselves and their families because this comprehensive volume provides data-driven advice concerning the implementation of nutritional interventions that include fluid intakes. The volume is also of value to professors of related fields and graduate and medical students who require objective, comprehensive reviews concerning topics such as sweetened beverages, alcoholic beverages, dairy- and soy-based drinks, and other topics that are of great interest to the public.

The first two chapters of the volume are broad introductions to beverages. Chapter 1, written by the volume's coeditors, provides a comprehensive overview of the volume's contents and a short description of each chapter. Chapter 2, also coauthored by one of the editors, presents a historical perspective on the use of key beverages in man's development. Ancient civilization's descriptions of the various animal milks that were consumed are reviewed. There is an important analysis of the role of fermented beverages, including wine, in different religions and in trade between nations early in history. Chocolate drinks, drinks containing kola, coffee, and tea are also examined. The importance of beverages in ceremonies of rites of passage and in providing hospitality is noted. Of interest is the discussion of the human conflicts that have arisen and are still under way in some parts of the world with regard to access to water. The final discussion of the preparation and delivery of beverages during space flight completes the historic perspective.

Part II contains six chapters that each examine a particular beverage and the active ingredients that are associated with the benefits and/or harm of the beverage. The comprehensive chapter on coffee describes the role of caffeine and the many phenolic compounds found in coffee products. The review of the literature includes the survey and intervention studies linking moderate coffee consumption with lowered risk of total mortality, cardiovascular disease, diabetes, heart disease, stroke, and a number of cancers in different organs. In the chapter on tea, there is an in-depth discussion of the three major types of tea (black, green, and oolong), brewing styles, and proposed mechanisms of action of the major catechins. The helpful tables and figures contain useful reviews of the literature. The chapter on alcoholic beverages, written by a coeditor of this volume, describes the harmful effects of overconsumption as well as the benefits associated with moderate, regular intake, especially of wine. The next chapter examines the nonalcoholic components of wine and posits the potential for these components to beneficially affect the microbiome and reduce the chronic inflammation associated with major chronic diseases with an emphasis on atherosclerotic cardiovascular disease. Chapter 7 looks at the clinical intervention data that show a significant reduction in both occurrence and recurrence of urinary tract infections with consistent intakes of cranberry juice. There is a review of the process of identifying proanthocyanidins as the active agent and a discussion of the other nutrients found in cranberries. The last chapter in this part examines the data linking orange juice and grapefruit juice and related products made from these fruits with reduction in chronic inflammation seen in infections, diabetes, cardiovascular disease, osteoporosis, obesity, and certain cancers. The chapter includes a review of the effects of grapefruit juice on the metabolism of certain drugs.

The next three parts, each containing three related chapters, examine the importance of different groups of beverages including milks, satiety and energy balance drinks, and sports drinks. Part III reviews the health effects of milk from three sources: dairy, soy, and human breast milk/infant formula. The three chapters present detailed information concerning the nutritional and phytochemical composition of the milks and infant formula. Each chapter reviews the clinical survey data associating the milks with reduced risk of certain chronic diseases. Chapter 9 reviews the data linking higher intakes of cow's milk with lowered risk of cardiovascular disease, hypertension and stroke, osteoporosis, breast and certain other cancers, weight control, diabetes, and kidney stones. Chapter 10 asks if soy or other grain-based milks can substitute for cow's milk and suggests that there are insufficient data to currently make a decision. Citing a number of positive attributes found in soy milk, including the abundance of phytochemicals, and the importance of having this choice for individuals who suffer from cow's milk allergies and intolerance, the authors indicate that further studies are certainly needed. The last chapter in this part reviews the beneficial aspects of human milk for term infants in both developed and developing nations. There is also an in-depth discussion of the components of the three major protein-based infant formulas and their appropriate use.

Three chapters examine the role of beverages in satiety and energy balance, their use in individuals with the metabolic syndrome or diabetes, and beverage use for nutritional supplementation in older adults. Chapter 12 provides data that indicate the weak satiation effect of beverages and the potential for the caloric content of beverages to be added rather than substituted for calories in solid foods. The distinction is made between satiation of thirst and hunger signals in the body. The chapter on effects of beverages in the diabetic patient reviews the potential value of fruit/vegetable juices, alcoholic beverages, milks, and sugar-sweetened and artificially sweetened beverages and suggests that issues with carbohydrate intakes from these beverages can be moderated to fit into the total recommended daily caloric intake. Chapter 14 provides guidance concerning the use of supplemental caloric and/or protein drinks for older adults who are malnourished and do not consume sufficient calories from solid foods. In this population, supplemental beverages have been shown to decrease mortality.

Chapters 15–17 review the composition of sports drinks, energy drinks, and bottled waters. Chapter 15 presents a balanced review of the data concerning sports drinks compared to cool water consumed by athletes. Sports drinks often contain sugar, electrolytes, and flavoring ingredients to add to palatability. Pre-exercise hydration as well as during exercise and postexercise is examined, and the physiological changes are discussed and tabulated. Carbohydrate sources, including glucose, sucrose, fructose, and maltodextrin, are compared. Isotonic drinks and sources of electrolytes are also reviewed. Chapter 16 looks at the historic development of the category called bottled water and provides the regulatory definitions for purified water, mineral water, and artesian water used in the USA, Canada, and the European Union. The chapter includes a discussion of the rationales used in consuming bottled compared to tap water.

The next parts of this comprehensive volume are devoted to the marketing of carbonated soft drinks and a number of the critical factors that make these beverages so appealing to the public. The final chapter looks into the future and the potential refinements to beverages that are becoming available to food technologists and supported by scientific studies. Chapters 18 and 19 examine the current patterns of carbonated beverage marketing and intake and potential effects on health outcomes and suggest that sugar-sweetened beverages may have adverse effects on certain health outcomes. Chapter 20 presents an opposing view based upon the chemistry of the sugars and the experimental and clinical evidence that does not support these adverse effects. The inclusion of chapters that examine the literature and arrive at different conclusions is of great value to the health professional and advanced student as these chapters provide a strong rationale for further discussion and evaluation of the literature.

Part VII contains three chapters that examine a number of characteristics of beverages as well as the regulatory environment that beverage manufacturers, mainly in the USA, must conform with to maintain their legal status. Chapter 21 reviews the critical role of beverage color. Beverage color is used by consumers from a very young age to anticipate the flavor of the beverage. The chapter describes the importance of cultural differences in perceptions of the flavor of a beverage based upon its color. The importance of maintaining the expected color of a beverage even when growing conditions change is described using orange juice as an example. There is also a description of the effects of the container in which the beverage is held and how the container's color can alter the perceived color of the beverage. Chapter 22 concentrates on the secondary ingredients that are often found in manufactured beverages. Ingredients that are often added to nonalcoholic beverages include organic acids, fatty acids, starches, gums, salts, sweeteners, flavors, and colors. The chapter identifies some of the more common additives used in nonalcoholic beverages and provides an explanation of their functions. Chapter 23 reviews the current FDA regulations that cover the numerous types of beverages discussed in this volume. There is also a discussion of certain legal actions that have been taken when beverage labels contain unsubstantiated claims. The chapter contains relevant references to the FDA's Code of Federal Regulations that are of great value to the health professional and educator who is interested in the legal basis of beverage labeling and labels. The final book chapter, authored by the volume's editors, examines current trends in the development of beverages and suggests that there will be many changes in the future to the types of beverages we consume, the ingredients in beverages, the way we access beverages, the effects of economic development on the types of beverages consumed, and the effects of environmental changes on the quality and quantity of certain beverages. Examples included in this unique chapter consist of the development of apps that point to new beverages; the growth of the use of natural, noncaloric sweeteners in carbonated and other beverages; the growth of the smoothies and juice bar businesses; and the changes in the Chinese beverage marketplace with increased wealth from rice wine to burgundy and other more expensive grape-based wines. Lastly, there is an insightful discussion of the potential consequences of the severe drought seen in California that may portend the increased reliance on bottled water and other bottled beverages.

The above description of the volume's 24 chapters attests to the depth of information provided by the 40 well-recognized and respected chapter authors. Each chapter includes complete definitions of terms with the abbreviations fully defined for the reader and consistent use of terms between chapters. The volume includes over 40 detailed tables and informative figures; an extensive, detailed index; and more than 1200 up-to-date references that provide the reader with excellent sources of worthwhile information. Thus, the volume provides a broad base of knowledge concerning the multifaceted role of beverages in both health and disease.

In conclusion, this book, edited by Ted Wilson, Ph.D., and Norman J. Temple, Ph.D., provides health professionals in many areas of research and practice with the most up-to-date, well-referenced volume on the importance of beverages in maintaining the hydration of healthy individuals and patients and, in many cases, enhancing the nutritional status of malnourished patients. Individual chapters review the historical uses and current literature concerning the health consequences of coffee and tea and the alcoholic and nonalcoholic components of wine. The volume chapters carefully document the critical value of examining the totality of the scientific literature especially when undertaking medical nutrition evaluations. Unique chapters examine the controversies concerning the nutritional requirements and health effects for supplemental beverages, sugar-sweetened beverages, bottled water, fruit juices, infant formulas, bovine milk versus plant milks including soy and rice, and other liquids, especially for specific population groups such as infants and children, pregnant women, obese patients, patients with chronic diseases, and older adults. This volume serves the reader as the benchmark in this complex area of interrelationships between the essential nutrients found in solid foods and those often contained in beverages including vitamins, minerals, and fiber. Practice-based nutritionists are provided data-driven recommendations concerning specific treatments required to optimize the beverage intakes of diabetic patients, obese patients, and others with medical needs. Because of the broad range of topics included in this comprehensive volume, medial and graduate students, nurses, dieticians, regulatory affairs personnel, as well as practitioners can better understand the complexities of these interactions. Unique chapters also examine the importance of behavioral modification and the use of quality standards to improve beverage contents. In conclusion, the editors are applauded for their efforts to develop the most authoritative resource in the field to date, and this excellent text is a very welcome addition to the *Nutrition and Health* series.

Morristown, NJ, USA   Adrianne Bendich
                                                                         Series Editor

About the Series Editor

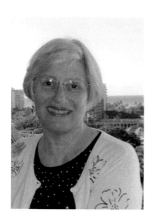

Dr. Adrianne Bendich, Ph.D., F.A.S.N., F.A.C.N., has served as the "Nutrition and Health" series editor for 20 years and has provided leadership and guidance to more than 200 editors who have developed the 70+ well-respected and highly recommended volumes in the series.

In addition to the second edition of this book, edited by Ted Wilson, Ph.D., and Norman J. Temple, Ph.D., major new editions published in 2012–2015 and expected to be published shortly include:

1. *Preventive Nutrition*: *The Comprehensive Guide for Health Professionals, Fifth Edition*, edited by Adrianne Bendich, Ph.D., and Richard J. Deckelbaum, M.D., 2015
2. *Nutrition in Cystic Fibrosis*: *A Guide for Clinicians*, edited by Elizabeth H. Yen, M.D. and Amanda R. Leonard, M.P.H, R.D., C.D.E., 2015
3. *Glutamine in Clinical Nutrition*, edited by Rajkumar Rajendram, Victor R. Preedy and Vinood B. Patel, 2015
4. *Nutrition and Bone Health, Second Edition*, edited by Michael F. Holick and Jeri W. Nieves, 2015

5. *Branched Chain Amino Acids in Clinical Nutrition, Volume 2*, edited by Rajkumar Rajendram, Victor R. Preedy and Vinood B. Patel, 2015
6. *Branched Chain Amino Acids in Clinical Nutrition, Volume 1*, edited by Rajkumar Rajendram, Victor R. Preedy and Vinood B. Patel, 2015
7. *Fructose, High Fructose Corn Syrup, Sucrose and Health*, edited by James M. Rippe, 2014
8. *Handbook of Clinical Nutrition and Aging, Third Edition*, edited by Connie Watkins Bales, Julie L. Locher and Edward Saltzman, 2014
9. *Nutrition and Pediatric Pulmonary Disease*, edited by Dr. Youngran Chung and Dr. Robert Dumont, 2014
10. *Integrative Weight Management*, edited by Dr. Gerald E. Mullin, Dr. Lawrence J. Cheskin and Dr. Laura E. Matarese, 2014
11. *Nutrition in Kidney Disease, Second Edition*, edited by Dr. Laura D. Byham-Gray, Dr. Jerrilynn D. Burrowes and Dr. Glenn M. Chertow, 2014
12. *Handbook of Food Fortification and Health, Volume I*, edited by Dr. Victor R. Preedy, Dr. Rajaventhan Srirajaskanthan, Dr. Vinood B. Patel, 2013
13. *Handbook of Food Fortification and Health, Volume II*, edited by Dr. Victor R. Preedy, Dr. Rajaventhan Srirajaskanthan, Dr. Vinood B. Patel, 2013
14. *Diet Quality: An Evidence-Based Approach, Volume I*, edited by Dr. Victor R. Preedy, Dr. Lan-Ahn Hunter and Dr. Vinood B. Patel, 2013
15. *Diet Quality: An Evidence-Based Approach, Volume II*, edited by Dr. Victor R. Preedy, Dr. Lan-Ahn Hunter and Dr. Vinood B. Patel, 2013
16. *The Handbook of Clinical Nutrition and Stroke*, edited by Mandy L. Corrigan, M.P.H, R.D., Arlene A. Escuro, M.S., R.D., and Donald F. Kirby, M.D., F.A.C.P., F.A.C.N., F.A.C.G., 2013
17. *Nutrition in Infancy, Volume I*, edited by Dr. Ronald Ross Watson, Dr. George Grimble, Dr. Victor Preedy and Dr. Sherma Zibadi, 2013
18. *Nutrition in Infancy, Volume II*, edited by Dr. Ronald Ross Watson, Dr. George Grimble, Dr. Victor Preedy and Dr. Sherma Zibadi, 2013
19. *Carotenoids and Human Health*, edited by Dr. Sherry A. Tanumihardjo, 2013
20. *Bioactive Dietary Factors and Plant Extracts in Dermatology*, edited by Dr. Ronald Ross Watson and Dr. Sherma Zibadi, 2013
21. *Omega 6/3 Fatty Acids*, edited by Dr. Fabien De Meester, Dr. Ronald Ross Watson and Dr. Sherma Zibadi, 2013
22. *Nutrition in Pediatric Pulmonary Disease*, edited by Dr. Robert Dumont and Dr. Youngran Chung, 2013
23. *Magnesium and Health*, edited by Dr. Ronald Ross Watson and Dr. Victor R. Preedy, 2012.
24. *Alcohol, Nutrition and Health Consequences*, edited by Dr. Ronald Ross Watson, Dr. Victor R. Preedy, and Dr. Sherma Zibadi, 2012
25. *Nutritional Health, Strategies for Disease Prevention, Third Edition*, edited by Norman J. Temple, Ted Wilson, and David R. Jacobs, Jr., 2012
26. *Chocolate in Health and Nutrition*, edited by Dr. Ronald Ross Watson, Dr. Victor R. Preedy, and Dr. Sherma Zibadi, 2012
27. *Iron Physiology and Pathophysiology in Humans*, edited by Dr. Gregory J. Anderson and Dr. Gordon D. McLaren, 2012

Earlier books include *Vitamin D, Second Edition*, edited by Dr. Michael Holick; *Dietary Components and Immune Function*, edited by Dr. Ronald Ross Watson, Dr. Sherma Zibadi, and Dr. Victor R. Preedy; *Bioactive Compounds and Cancer*, edited by Dr. John A. Milner and Dr. Donato F. Romagnolo; *Modern Dietary Fat Intakes in Disease Promotion*, edited by Dr. Fabien De Meester, Dr. Sherma Zibadi, and Dr. Ronald Ross Watson; *Iron Deficiency and Overload*, edited by Dr. Shlomo Yehuda and Dr. David Mostofsky; *Nutrition Guide for Physicians*, edited by Dr. Edward Wilson, Dr. George A. Bray, Dr. Norman Temple, and Dr. Mary Struble; *Nutrition and Metabolism*, edited by Dr. Christos Mantzoros and *Fluid and Electrolytes in Pediatrics*, edited by Leonard Feld and Dr. Frederick Kaskel. Recent volumes include *Handbook of Drug-Nutrient Interactions*, edited by Dr. Joseph Boullata and Dr. Vincent Armenti; *Probiotics in Pediatric Medicine*, edited by Dr. Sonia Michail and Dr. Philip Sherman; *Handbook of Nutrition and Pregnancy*, edited by Dr. Carol Lammi-Keefe, Dr. Sarah Couch, and Dr. Elliot Philipson; *Nutrition and Rheumatic Disease*, edited by Dr. Laura Coleman; *Nutrition and Kidney Disease*, edited by Dr. Laura Byham-Gray, Dr. Jerrilynn Burrowes, and Dr. Glenn Chertow; *Nutrition and Health in Developing Countries*, edited by Dr. Richard Semba and Dr. Martin Bloem; *Calcium in Human Health*, edited by Dr. Robert Heaney and Dr. Connie Weaver; and *Nutrition and Bone Health*, edited by Dr. Michael Holick and Dr. Bess Dawson-Hughes.

Dr. Bendich is president of Consultants in Consumer Healthcare LLC and is the editor of ten books including *Preventive Nutrition: The Comprehensive Guide for Health Professionals, Fifth Edition*, coedited with Dr. Richard Deckelbaum (www.springer.com/series/7659). Dr. Bendich serves on the Editorial Boards of the *Journal of Nutrition in Gerontology and Geriatrics* and *Antioxidants* and has served as associate editor for *Nutrition* the International Journal, served on the Editorial Board of the *Journal of Women's Health and Gender-Based Medicine*, and served on the Board of Directors of the American College of Nutrition.

Dr. Bendich was director of Medical Affairs at GlaxoSmithKline (GSK) Consumer Healthcare and provided medical leadership for many well-known brands including TUMS and Os-Cal. Dr. Bendich had primary responsibility for GSK's support for the Women's Health Initiative (WHI) intervention study. Prior to joining GSK, Dr. Bendich was at Roche Vitamins Inc. and was involved with the groundbreaking clinical studies showing that folic acid-containing multivitamins significantly reduced major classes of birth defects. Dr. Bendich has coauthored over 100 major clinical research studies in the area of preventive nutrition. She is recognized as a leading authority on antioxidants, nutrition and immunity, pregnancy outcomes, vitamin safety, and the cost-effectiveness of vitamin/mineral supplementation.

Dr. Bendich received the Roche Research Award, is a *Tribute to Women and Industry* awardee, and was a recipient of the Burroughs Wellcome Visiting Professorship in Basic Medical Sciences. Dr. Bendich was given the Council for Responsible Nutrition (CRN) Apple Award in recognition of her many contributions to the scientific understanding of dietary supplements. In 2012, she was recognized for her contributions to the field of clinical nutrition by the American Society for Nutrition and was elected a fellow of ASN. Dr. Bendich is adjunct professor at Rutgers University. She is listed in Who's Who in American Women.

Volume Editor Biographies

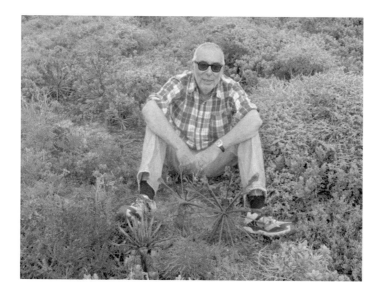

Norman J. Temple, Ph.D., is a professor of nutrition at Athabasca University in Alberta, Canada. He has published 80 papers, mainly in the area of nutrition in relation to health. He has also published 12 books. Together with Denis Burkitt, he coedited *Western Diseases: Their Dietary Prevention and Reversibility* (1994). This continued and extended Burkitt's pioneering work on the role of dietary fiber in chronic diseases of lifestyle. He coedited *Nutrition Guide for Physicians* (2010) and *Nutritional Health: Strategies for Disease Prevention* (2012; now in its third edition). He also coedited *Excessive Medical Spending: Facing the Challenge* (2007). He conducts collaborative research in Cape Town on the role of the changing diet in South Africa on the pattern of diseases in that country, such as obesity, diabetes, and heart disease.

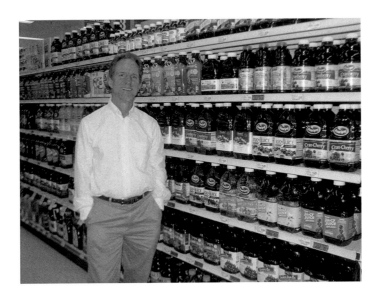

Dr. Ted Wilson, Ph.D., is a professor of biology at Winona State University in Winona, Minnesota. His research examines how diet affects human nutritional physiology and whether food/dietary supplement health claims can be supported by measurable physiological changes. He has studied many foods, dietary supplements, and disease conditions including pistachios, low-carbohydrate diets, cranberries, cranberry juice, apple juice, grape juice, wine, resveratrol, creatine phosphate, soy phytoestrogens, eggplants, coffee, tea, energy drinks, heart failure prognosis, diabetes, and obesity. Diet-induced changes have included physiological evaluations of plasma lipid profile, antioxidants, vasodilation, nitric oxide, platelet aggregation, and glycemic and insulinemic responses using in vivo and in vitro models. With Dr. N. Temple, he edited the first edition of *Beverages in Nutrition and Health* (Humana Press, 2004), *Nutritional Health: Strategies for Disease Prevention* (Humana Press, 2001 first, 2006 second, and 2012 third editions), and *Nutrition Guide for Physicians* (Humana/Springer Press Inc, 2010). He also enjoys teaching courses in nutrition, cardiovascular physiology, cell signal transduction, and cell biology. When not in the laboratory, he enjoys family time, the outdoors, and farming.

Acknowledgments

The editors, Ted Wilson and Norman Temple, wish to thank our series editor, Dr. Adrianne Bendich. We appreciate your enthusiastic support going back to 2001 of our first edition of *Nutritional Health: Strategies for Disease Prevention*, the first edition of this present book as well as the many other books in between. Thanks for the countless times you have shared a breakfast, lunch, dinner, or chat on the phone with us. The benefits of your enthusiasm for our work and the work of the many other fine authors in this Nutrition Series have been immeasurable. Your improvement in our understanding how to move the science of nutrition into the future has been priceless.

The editors have endless gratitude for the endless patience and encouragement given to us and the authors of the chapters in this book by the delightful Portia Wong, our developmental editor at Springer Science+Business Media, who managed the final preparation and corrections of the manuscript. We also thank Samantha Lonuzzi, our publishing editor at Springer, who helped with the morass of details needed to get this book to press. Our understanding of how beverages impact our daily lives is only improved when people have access to unbiased information; you both made this possible for everyone.

Contents

Part I Introduction to Beverages

1   How Beverages Impact Health and Nutrition.............................. 3
Ted Wilson, Norman J. Temple

2   A Brief History of Human Beverage Consumption:
Prehistory to the Present.. 11
Ted Wilson, Louis E. Grivetti

Part II Health Effects of Coffee, Tea, Wine, Alcohol, and Juices

3   Coffee Consumption and Its Impact on Health 29
Lodovica Cavalli, Alessandra Tavani

4   Health Benefits of Tea Consumption...................................... 49
Takuji Suzuki, Noriyuki Miyoshi, Sumio Hayakawa,
Shinjiro Imai, Mamoru Isemura, Yoriyuki Nakamura

5   What Are the Health Implications of Alcohol Consumption?.............. 69
Norman J. Temple

6   Nonalcoholic Components of Wine and Atherosclerotic
Cardiovascular Disease 83
Abigail J. O'Connor, Georges M. Halpern, Rosemary L. Walzem

7   Cranberry Juice: Effects on Health 101
Diane L. McKay, Ted Wilson

8   Citrus Juices Health Benefits.. 115
Paul F. Cancalon

Part III Health Effects of Milk: Dairy, Soy and Breast

9   **Effect of Cow's Milk on Human Health** 131
Laura A.G. Armas, Cary P. Frye, Robert P. Heaney

10 **Are Soy-Milk Products Viable Alternatives to Cow's Milk?** 151
Jayne V. Woodside, Sarah Brennan, Marie Cantwell

11 **Human Milk and Infant Formula: Nutritional Content and Health
Benefits**.. 163
James K. Friel, Wafaa A. Qasem

**Part IV Beverage Health Effects on Energy Balance, Diabetes,
and in Older Adults**

12 **Beverages, Satiation, Satiety, and Energy Balance**................................ 181
James H. Hollis

13 **Beverage Considerations for Persons with Metabolic
Syndrome and Diabetes Mellitus**.. 193
Margaret A. Maher, Lisa Kobs

14 **Oral Nutritional Supplementation Using Beverages for
Older Adults** 207
Shelley R. McDonald

Part V Health Effects of Sports Drinks, Energy Drinks and Water

15 **Sports Beverages for Optimizing Physical Performance** 225
Ronald J. Maughan, Susan M. Shirreffs

16 **Energy Drinks: The Elixirs of Our Time**... 243
Frances R. Ragsdale

17 **The Nutritional Value of Bottled Water**.. 259
Norman J. Temple, Kathryn Alp

Part VI Marketing of Soft Drinks and Effects of Beverage Sweeteners

18 **Marketing of Soft Drinks to Children and Adolescents:
Why We Need Government Policies**... 269
Norman J. Temple, Kathryn Alp

19 **Sugar in Beverages: Effects on Human Health**..................................... 277
Norman J. Temple, Kathryn Alp

20 **High-Fructose Corn Syrup Use in Beverages: Composition,
Manufacturing, Properties, Consumption, and Health Effects**........... 285
John S. White, Theresa A. Nicklas

**Part VII Beverage Mechanics: Color, Taste, Labeling,
             and Ingredient Function**

21 The Crucial Role of Color in the Perception of Beverages 305
     Charles Spence

22 Functions of Common Beverage Ingredients 317
     Heather N. Nelson, Kelli L. Rush, Ted Wilson

23 Labeling Requirements for Beverages in the USA 331
     Leslie T. Krasny

Part VIII What Is the Future of What We Will Chose to Drink?

24 Beverage Trends Affect Future Nutritional Health Impact 351
     Ted Wilson, Rachel Dahl, Norman Temple

Index... 359

Contributors

Kathryn Alp Centre for Science, Athabasca University, Athabasca, AB, Canada

Laura A.G. Armas, M.D., M.S. Creighton University, Omaha, NE, USA

Sarah Brennan, Ph.D. Centre for Public Health, Institute of Clinical Science B, Queens University Belfast, Belfast, Northern Ireland

Paul F. Cancalon Florida Department of Citrus, CREC, Lake Alfred, FL, USA

Marie Cantwell, Ph.D. Centre for Public Health, Institute of Clinical Science B, Queens University Belfast, Belfast, Northern Ireland

Lodovica Cavalli, Psy.D. Department of Epidemiology, Istituto di Ricerche Farmacologiche "Mario Negri", Institute for Pharmacological Research, Milan, Italy

Rachel Dahl Department of Biology, Winona State University, Winona, MN, USA

James K. Friel, Ph.D. Department of Human Nutritional Sciences, Faculty of Agricultural and Food Sciences, University of Manitoba, Winnipeg, MB, Canada

Cary P. Frye International Dairy Foods Association, Washington, DC, USA

Louis E. Grivetti, Ph.D. Department of Nutrition, University of California-Davis, Davis, CA, USA

Georges M. Halpern Department of Biomedical Sciences, City University of Hong Kong, Hong Kong, China

Sumio Hayakawa Department of Cellular and Molecular Medicine, Medical Research Institute, Tokyo Medical and Dental University, Tokyo, Japan

Robert P. Heaney, M.D. Creighton University, Omaha, NE, USA

James H. Hollis, Ph.D. Department of Food Science and Human Nutrition, Iowa State University, Ames, IA, USA

Shinjiro Imai Graduate School of Nutritional and Environmental Sciences, University of Shizuoka, Shizuoka, Japan

Mamoru Isemura Graduate School of Nutritional and Environmental Sciences, University of Shizuoka, Shizuoka, Japan

Lisa Kobs, M.S., R.D. Biology and Nutrition, University of Wisconsin – La Crosse, La Crosse, WI, USA

Leslie T. Krasny, M.A., J.D. Keller and Heckman LLP, Three Embarcadero Center, San Francisco, CA, USA

Margaret A. Maher, Ph.D., R.D. Biology and Nutrition, University of Wisconsin – La Crosse, La Crosse, WI, USA

Ronald J. Maughan, Ph.D. School of Sport, Exercise and Health Sciences, Loughborough University, Loughborough, UK

Shelley R. McDonald, D.O., Ph.D. Department of Medicine, Duke University Medical Center, Durham, NC, USA

Diane L. McKay, Ph.D. Friedman School of Nutrition Science and Policy, Jean Mayer USDA Human Nutrition Research Center on Aging, Tufts University, Boston, MA, USA

Noriyuki Miyoshi Graduate School of Nutritional and Environmental Sciences, University of Shizuoka, Shizuoka, Japan

Yoriyuki Nakamura Graduate School of Nutritional and Environmental Sciences, University of Shizuoka, Shizuoka, Japan

Heather N. Nelson Department of Biology, Winona State University, Winona, MN, USA

Theresa A. Nicklas, Dr. P.H. Department of Pediatrics, Children's Nutrition Research Center, Baylor College of Medicine, Houston, TX, USA

Abigail J. O'Connor Nutrition Graduate Program, Department of Nutrition and Food Science, Texas A&M University, College Station, TX, USA

Wafaa A. Qasem, M.D. Department of Human Nutritional Sciences, Faculty of Agricultural and Food Sciences, University of Manitoba, Winnipeg, MB, Canada

Frances R. Ragsdale, Ph.D. Department of Biology, Winona State University, Winona, MN, USA

Kelli L. Rush Department of Biology, Winona State University, Winona, MN, USA

Susan M. Shirreffs, Ph.D. Research and Development, GSK, AS1, Middlesex, UK

Charles Spence Crossmodal Research Laboratory, Department of Experimental Psychology, Oxford University, Oxford, UK

Takuji Suzuki Faculty of Education, Art and Science, Yamagata University, Yamagata, Japan

Alessandra Tavani, Sci.D. Department of Epidemiology, Istituto di Ricerche Farmacologiche "Mario Negri", Institute for Pharmacological Research, Milan, Italy

Norman J. Temple Centre for Science, Athabasca University, Athabasca, AB, Canada

Rosemary L. Walzem, R.D., Ph.D. Nutrition Graduate Program, Department of Poultry Science, Texas A&M University, College Station, TX, USA

John S. White, Ph.D. White Technical Research, Argenta, IL, USA

Ted Wilson, Ph.D. Department of Biology, Winona State University, Winona, MN, USA

Jayne V. Woodside, Ph.D. Centre for Public Health, Institute of Clinical Science B, Queens University Belfast, Belfast, Northern Ireland

Part I
Introduction to Beverages

Chapter 1
How Beverages Impact Health and Nutrition

Ted Wilson and Norman J. Temple

Keywords Beverage • Drink • Coffee • Tea • Alcohol • Wine • Juice • Milk • Satiety • Diabetes • Nutritional supplement • Athlete • Energy drink • Soft drink • Sugar • High-fructose corn syrup • Taste perception • Labeling requirements • Ingredient label

Key Points

1. Coffee, tea, alcohol, and wine when consumed in moderation can improve our nutritional health.
2. Phenolic compounds in cranberry and citrus juices provide benefits for urinary tract infections and cognitive function, respectively, and cardiovascular disease collectively.
3. Cow milk is known to promote improvements in cardiovascular disease risk and improved weight management, and soy and other plant milks may also be beneficial.
4. Beverages do not create the same satiety when compared to isocaloric foods, but can still be consumed in moderation by persons with metabolic syndrome and diabetes.
5. Specialized beverages for nutritional supplementation in older persons, sports drinks for athletes, energy drinks, and bottled water continue to become more popular.
6. Soft drink marketing, beverage sugar content, and high-fructose corn syrup use continue to be controversial with consumers and clinicians.

T. Wilson, Ph.D. (✉)
Department of Biology, Winona State University, 232 Pasteur Hall, Winona, MN 54603, USA
e-mail: twilson@winona.edu

N.J. Temple
Centre for Science, Athabasca University, Athabasca, AB, Canada

© Springer International Publishing Switzerland 2016   3
T. Wilson, N.J. Temple (eds.), *Beverage Impacts on Health and Nutrition*,
Nutrition and Health, DOI 10.1007/978-3-319-23672-8_1

7. Color is important in creating our taste perception.
8. Labeling requirement considerations are important with respect to health claims and the ingredients commonly found in beverages.

Introduction

Good nutrition remains the single most cost-effective way to improve the health and well-being of the greatest number of individuals on our planet. Over seven billion people on the planet will drink some sort of beverage today as part of their daily nutritional requirements leading to tens of billions of servings per day. Beverages are of many types, including water, coffee, tea, fruit juice, alcohol (beer, wine, hard liquor), milk, soda, energy drinks, or any combination of ingredients found in water. Human life occurs bathed in a sea of fluids; indeed, as a fetus we begin to drink even before birth. Beverage consumption starts immediately after we are born, usually with breast milk, and continues until death.

Characterizing how the ingredients mixed with the water impact our short- and long-term nutritional health is controversial and generally poorly understood. This book describes the discoveries regarding how different beverages impact our basic nutrition and our risk of disease. This book also helps us understand the potential value of these beverages for the promotion of optimal human health and well-being.

Ancient Beverages: Historical Overview

How does our use of beverages in ancient history influence the evolution of our nutrition, culture, and economic system today? The history of the human use of beverages sets the stage for how they impact our lives today, a topic discussed in the chapter by Wilson and Grivetti. In the last few decades, there has been an explosion in the number of beverage choices available. This has been made possible by using such industrial processes as carbonation, processing to add ingredients such as high-fructose corn syrup, vitamins, and minerals, and the development of new processing and preservation methods. Add to that intensive marketing by beverage manufacturers and new government labeling regulations and the nutritional playing field becomes very complicated relative to the former simplicity around beverages like coffee and tea.

Overview of Major Beverages

Drinking a cup of coffee or tea is how billions of people around the world start every day. Indeed, tea is the most popular beverage in the world (after water). How do the caffeine and phenolic compounds in coffee and tea affect our health? With respect to coffee, Cavalli and Tavani discuss the general lack of negative health associations and newly discovered potential benefits with respect to cancer, heart disease, diabetes, and even improved cognitive function. Similarly, Isemura's group in Japan provides us with new insights on how epigallocatechin gallate (EGCG) and other catechins from tea protect against cancer and heart disease. If we are ever to develop the ultimate dietary supplement—one that is cheap, safe, and effective against a range of diseases—then tea may well be a source of some of its ingredients.

Alcoholic fermentation was one of the first agro-industrial activities to employ human hands; alcohol (wine) has been a part of our diet for several thousand years. Temple discusses our new understanding of how a moderate intake of alcohol decreases the risk of cardiovascular disease, as well as of elevated blood pressure, dementia, and perhaps even type 2 diabetes. His chapter also looks at the close association between alcohol and risk of cancer, as well as of accidents, violence, and suicide. The mechanisms by which substances in wine may have specific health benefits that are distinct from those of alcohol are evaluated by O'Connor, Halpern, and Walzem. Cardioprotective effects of wine appear to occur in spite of poor absorption and rapid metabolism. New ways to interpret these findings include analysis of the microbiome, gene expression, and metabolomics; these are fields of study that are attracting much research interest.

Juices have an important impact on health as they have a significant caloric content, while their phenolic compounds may have distinct nutritional effects. When the pilgrims came to Plymouth, Massachusetts, they managed to survive only because they ate ascorbate-rich cranberries. Since that time, cranberry juice phenolic compounds have become associated with protection from urinary tract infections and cardioprotective effects. These and other new findings are discussed in the chapter by McKay and Wilson. Citrus juices remain some of the most popular juices in our diet. Cancalon reviews why they improve cognitive function and cardiovascular health and help reduce chronic inflammatory diseases. He also dispels some of the concerns regarding whether consumption of citrus juices leads to an increase in body weight.

A variety of milks and milk products have been in the diet of many human cultures for millennia; their dietary importance varies during the human life cycle. Armas, Fry, and Heaney review the evidence that milk can provide protection from osteoporosis, obesity, and heart disease. They also discuss many of the myths that have emerged in regard to milk consumption as well as the causes and effects of the slow reduction in national milk consumption in the USA. Because many people choose to avoid dairy products, substitutes are needed. There is suggestive evidence that soy may help prevent breast cancer and coronary heart disease. Woodside, Brennan, and Cantwell discuss the health qualities of the most commonly consumed substitute, soy milk, as well as of other up-and-coming products such as almond milk.

Overwhelming evidence points to breast milk as being the best source of nutrition for infants up to at least the age of 6 months. Why, then, does formula continue its popularity in all cultures? Freil and Qasam discuss the role played by commercial forces in the marketing of neonate/infant formula. Human milk is not the same drink a few days postpartum as it is after 3 months and is different again after 1 year. Milk is responsive to the infant and its nutrient content can change within a single feeding. Hopefully, this chapter will help increase the popularity of breastfeeding for almost all infants.

Overview of Beverage Effects on Satiety, Metabolic Syndrome, and Diabetes

Beverages represent the source of about one fifth or more of the average American's caloric intake; this has been implicated in many disease processes. The evidence for association has not always supported the claims, and some of the evidence has seemingly been ignored. Not all caloric intake is alike; the chapter by Hollis examines how the macronutrients present in beverages impact satiety differently from those in solid foods and how this may be important in regulating human caloric intake. Caloric overconsumption is tightly correlated with obesity, metabolic syndrome, and type 2 diabetes. The chapter by Maher and Kobs reviews the evidence regarding which beverages are most appropriate for persons with these conditions.

Overview of Beverages for Older Persons and Athletes

Nutritional support beverages have potential value for helping older persons meet the challenges they face when their diet fails to meet their nutritional needs. As explained in the chapter by McDonald, these beverages can help older persons achieve their required intake of vitamins and minerals and help them to maintain or even gain needed body weight. Understanding how to use these support beverages may help counter the nutritional deficiencies that plague many elderly persons and put them at risk for different diseases.

A wide range of beverages designed to improve physiological performance are ubiquitous at every gym and sporting event. How do they work? Do they really help? Maughan and Shirreffs summarize the optimal composition of these beverages with respect to carbohydrate composition, electrolyte profile, and osmolarity. The chapter also considers the question of ideal delivery time.

Overview of Energy Drinks and Bottled Water

Energy drinks continue to grow increasingly popular globally and represent a multibillion dollar commercial enterprise. Do they help stimulate cognitive function and speed our thinking? Are they a health risk that should be banned? One particular challenge for understanding their health effects is their vague legal definition. How the hype and reality of energy drinks impacts nutritional health is evaluated in the chapter by Ragsdale. These drinks were just becoming popular with youth and young professionals when the first edition of this book was published in 2004, but many of these consumers are now reaching middle age and carrying their youthful drink preferences or health consequences with them.

Was it really necessary for Americans to consume 9.2 billion gallons of bottled water in 2011? Our transition to living in an urbanized, and sometimes affluent, culture has created new opportunities for the marketing of safe water. This has led millions of people to consume bottled water, a beverage that can often cost considerably more than gasoline. Temple and Alp discuss some of the surprising facts regarding the quality and content of these products, as well as the reasons for why they are so commonly consumed.

Overview of Beverage Sugar, Marketing, and High-Fructose Corn Syrup

The chapters by Temple and Alp discuss sugar-sweetened beverages. The first chapter looks at the likely impact on health of consuming these beverages. A great deal of evidence has accrued in this area over the past decade. Every soft drink consumed is a missed opportunity to consume energy accompanied by a nutritious matrix of food constituents. The second chapter examines the marketing of these beverages. How does marketing affect soft drink consumption patterns of children and young adults? These chapters also consider the thorny issue of setting guidelines for the consumption of these beverages and of appropriate government policy.

Few beverage ingredients have been demonized by the popular media in the manner that high-fructose corn syrup (HFCS) has been treated. The data clearly demonstrate that calories from HFCS are the same as most other calories in the diet. The chapter by White and Nicklas clarifies the HFCS myths and realities with regard to its safety, composition, and manufacturing for use in beverages.

Overview of Beverage Color and Taste Perception

What makes a beverage taste and look the way it does? The chapter by Spence demonstrates that what you see "is" often what we tend to taste. Because color and scent are important in the lives of the herbal plants themselves, one may suspect that these phytochemicals may be indicators of plant nutritional value to the human brain. Color and scent relate closely to taste and flavors that represent the qualities of color and appearance that are very important for determining our perception of beverage taste, and it seems our brain perceives beverage color as predictive of beverage nutritional quality. Color and scent relate closely to taste and flavors. The color of a beverage is very important for determining our perception of the taste of the beverage. It seems that our brain perceives beverage color as predictive of the nutritional quality of the beverage.

Overview of Beverage Regulation and Ingredient Functions

Regulation of beverage content and marketing practice has been a part of American life for nearly a century since the establishment of the US Food and Drug Administration and the original "snake oil laws" of the 1920s. The fast-growing popularity of using beverage health claims on a label as part of a marketing strategy has created a resurgence of concern and interest in the area of beverage label regulation. The chapter by Krasny provides an update of the status of these laws and regulations with regard to how beverages can be legally marketed in the USA. One wonders about what balance of regulation and cooperation, coupled with information from the research into the many aspects of the nutrition of beverages and solid foods presented in this book, might produce both a healthy economy and a healthy consumer base.

The ingredient label on a beverage can be very simple (100 % coffee) or it can represent a complicated list of 50 or more plants, plant extracts, flavors, and chemicals. How is the consumer to truly know what they drink if they cannot navigate the ingredient label? How is the clinician supposed to advise the consumer if they are not fluent regarding the basic functions of the ingredients on a beverage label? The role of many common ingredients is discussed in the chapter by Nelson, Rush, and Wilson.

Conclusion

What is often forgotten by nutritionists is the reality that trends are important for determining what beverages the consumer "chooses" to drink. At the end of the day, endless nagging by a physician, the National Institutes of Health, or the World Health Organization cannot "force" a consumer to change their beverages habits. Peers and their perceived habits have a tremendous influence on the beverages that a consumer "chooses" to consume. Trends represent how the beverage consumption habits of people evolve, a topic explored in the final chapter of this book.

The reader needs to bear in mind that government, academia, industry, and consumers play different roles for determining the nutritional health of our society, but none can ever be too far out of step with the others. Consumers cannot consume beverages that are not available. Government cannot regulate so strongly that industry is not profitable. Industry cannot sell beverages that no one will buy. Consumers are showing a greater tendency to read ingredient labels, evaluate potential beverage nutritional quality online, and make purchasing choices based on their perceptions of the nutritional value and safety of beverages. An important role is also played by journalists and the media. They often take all scientific statements as new truths, not conveying to the consumer that the latest scientific "discovery" may really be misleading (as it is one small part of a complex story).

In recent decades, researchers have made considerable progress in our understanding of possible associations between beverages and the chronic disease. This book provides a better understanding of how to optimize beverage consumption for enhancing the health of the population. The book also helps the reader to understand how current and probable future innovations in the beverage industry have the potential to affect our health in both positive and negative ways. At risk of stating the obvious, beverage nutrition research is very much an ongoing activity whose evolution is towards better understanding the content of this *second edition* of *Beverage Impacts on Health and Nutrition*.

Chapter 2
A Brief History of Human Beverage Consumption: Prehistory to the Present

Ted Wilson and Louis E. Grivetti

Keywords Water • Milk • Fermentation • Wine • Cacao • Coffee • Kola • Tea • Culture • Religion • War • Olympics • Space flight

Key Points

1. Written descriptions of the importance of water as a beverage date back to 1500 BCE.
2. Stone Age rock art depictions of milk consumption date to over 4000 BCE.
3. Trade routes for fermented beverages were established over 4000 BCE, and more recent route for trade in tea, coffee, and cacao remains important to this day.
4. Beverages have had a major impact on the development of our cultures, religions, and the successes of war.
5. Beverage choices were important for athletes in the original Olympic Games of Greece, important for success in present-day sporting events, and will be critical for development of space travel to other planets today.

The humans arise after periods of fitful sleep. They climb down from tree-top lairs and amble towards nearby water holes. Alert to the potential presence of predators, they kneel, brush algal scum from the pond surfaces, fill their cupped hands, and take their first drinks of the day…

T. Wilson, Ph.D. (✉)
Department of Biology, Winona State University, Winona, MN 54603, USA
e-mail: ewilson@winona.edu

L.E. Grivetti, Ph.D.
Department of Nutrition, University of California-Davis, Davis, CA 95616-8500, USA
e-mail: legrivetti@ucdavis.edu

© Springer International Publishing Switzerland 2016   11
T. Wilson, N.J. Temple (eds.), *Beverage Impacts on Health and Nutrition*,
Nutrition and Health, DOI 10.1007/978-3-319-23672-8_2

Two million years later…

The humans arise after periods of fitful sleep. They dress and walk across the dirt floors of their huts. They grasp crude pottery cups, walk outside and meet others at the village cisterns. They fill their cups with polluted water, and take their first drinks of the day…

Six thousand years later…

The humans arise after periods of restful sleep. They dress and walk across their spotless, upscale kitchens. They prepare their favorite morning beverages. They sit on breakfast nook stools with mugs filled with steaming goodness, and take their first drinks of the day…

Introduction

How did humans learn to drink? Are drinking preferences instinctive? How did humans learn which beverages were safe to drink? Did earliest humans watch and imitate the drinking behavior of animals? How would early humans know whether or not a pond of standing water was suitable to drink? At the dawn of human history life spans were short, and illness that followed drinking polluted water would be associated with bacteria or toxins. Then, as now, aesthetics and a well-developed sense of smell, taste, color, and appearance determine our beverage selection as well as our place in natural selection. For a review of how color alters taste perception, see the chapter in this book by Spence.

How does one drink? Earliest humans had no cups or ways to store water, so by necessity they frequented water holes or other sources of standing or running water. It is presumed that earliest humans channeled rain runoff, drank snow melt, and consumed rainfall collected from the crotch of trees or natural depressions. Simple observations on the timing and quality of rainfall and the probability of water at any specific geographical location would have served ancient humans well. Slowly, through observation and trial-and-error, early humans learned to predict sources of water even in subsurface deposits beneath the sands of dry stream beds and also learned which fruits and succulents/cacti in arid lands offered refreshing, life-supporting fluids to drink. Norman and Alp provide a more detailed discussion of modern-day bottled water as a beverage.

There has existed since remote antiquity a world of different beverages: freshwater, fresh plant juices, fresh animal fluids (whether blood, milk, sometimes urine), fermented plant and animal products, and various mixtures. Some beverages are primarily water, but others came to be prepared from a myriad of fresh or dried barks, flowers, pods, resins/saps, roots, and resins. The chapters by Isemura examine tea more specifically, and the chapter by Cavallie and Tavani examines coffee in this regard. Some beverages are drunk to satisfy thirst, some provide simple pleasures, and some are drunk for cultural and religious significance, while still others for their medicinal value.

When did the first person put their fruit in a cup, smash it into a pulp, and drink it fresh in their cave as "the world's first fruit smoothie" or how long did it take to determine that a fruit smoothie could become alcohol after a week or so? For modern reviews on specific fruit and vegetable juice effects on health and nutrition, see the chapters by Cancalon for citrus juices or McKay and Wilson for the review of cranberry juice. Temple discusses the effects of alcohol in the diet, and O'Connor and Walzem review the effects of fermentation (wine) more specifically.

The purpose of this introductory chapter is not to review all of the impacts that beverage have had on human health and nutrition but to discuss how widespread these impacts have been and to demonstrate how beverages influence various aspects of our health, our culture, and the economics of our society.

Water

Water is the oldest beverage and one of the first to be medicinally characterized with respect to impact on health. For reviews on the topic of water, see the chapter by Temple and Alp. The Charaka-Samhita document [1] is the oldest known Asian medical text (c. 1500 BCE). The text presents a classification of common beverages for physicians and addresses their presumed medical properties and attributes:

> Water (*jala*), by nature has six qualities: cold, pure, wholesome, palatability, clean, light. When water falls to earth, it depends for its properties on the containing soil. Water in white soil is astringent. Water in pale soil is bitter. Water in brown soil is alkaline. Water in hilly areas is pungent. Water in black soil is sweet. Water derived from rain, hailstone, and snow has unmanifested *rasa* (taste); Fresh rainwater of the rainy season is heavy, blocks body channels, and is sweet;…. Rivers with water polluted with soil, feces, insects, snakes, and rats, and carrying rain water aggravate all *dosas*. [1]

The Origins of Milking

For millions of years breast milk has, for us and our ancestors, been the first beverage (see the chapter by Freil and Qasem). Replacement with animal milk carried tremendous implications and potential nutritional advantages. The first irrefutable evidence for milking domesticated livestock, and by implication human use of milk and the manufacture of dairy products, dates to approximately 4000 BCE and is based upon Stone Age rock art produced in the central Sahara region of Africa [2]. By 1500 BCE milk use was widely distributed, and in India many of the qualities of milk had already been described in the Charaka-Samhita [1].

> Cow milk has ten properties: sweet, cold, soft, fatty, viscous, smooth, slimy, heavy, dull, and clear. Buffalo milk is heavier and colder than that from cow; useful to cure sleeplessness and excessive digestive power. Camel milk is rough, hot, slightly saline, light, and prescribed for hardness in the bowels, works against worms… Milk from one-hooved animals [donkey; horse] is hot, slightly sour, saline, rough, light, promotes strength, stability, alleviates *vata* in extremities. Goat milk is astringent….

The chapter by Armas, Frye, and Heaney reviews the modern health implications of cow's milk consumption.

Different cultures have widely diverging views regarding the suitability of animal milks as human foods or beverages. For some, it is a question of identification: since animal milks are for the young of specific animals, it is wrong to mix these foods since the consumer may take on characteristics of the animal. For others, it is an issue of ethics: taking milk from cows, ewes, or mares deprives the young of these species, causes them harm, and therefore breaks the tenet of ahimsa (i.e., nonviolence towards animals). Some also reject processed milk because of a belief that the process of pasteurization "devitalizes" the milk. This practice, however, is not without danger given the difficulties of maintaining cleanliness within the environmental setting of traditional dairies or even modern ones [3]. More recently, milk substitutes of vegetable origin have become popular. The chapter by Woodside reviews the use of soy, almond, and other alternative milks.

Fermented Beverages

General

Fermentation can be used to produce both plant- and animal-based beverages. As with many issues in the area of diet and health, the story is complex, and this is especially the case with the fermentation product alcohol. The moral and ethical considerations of overindulgence with alcohol have been touted since antiquity. Sages in ancient Egyptian, for example, admonished young men not to overindulge and to be respectful of their elders who became intoxicated. Alcoholic beverages also have multiple health-related harms and benefits. The benefits extend well beyond the so-called French paradox. The chapters by Temple, O'Connor, and Waltzem review the modern interpretations of the effects of alcohol, in general, and of wine, in particular, on nutritional health.

Wine and the Start of Trade and Commerce

The earliest evidence for the preparation/manufacture of fermented beverages predates writing (i.e., c. 3200 BCE). During recent decades excavations in northwestern Iran at Godin Tepe provided the first unequivocal evidence for the presence of wine. Analysis of residues at the bottom of large jars retrieved there reveals the presence of tartaric acid, a characteristic chemical signature confirming that the vases once contained juice from *Vitis vinifera* [4, 5]. Based upon this ancient Iranian evidence, trade in fermented beverages developed during the late Stone Age or early

Copper Age (Chalcolithic), perhaps around 4000 BCE. Increased demand and production created a prosperous wine trade promulgating the establishment of many Roman trade routes. Wrecks from the Roman era on the southern coast of France have provided partially intact amphorae that still contained traces of red pigment presumed to have been wine [5, 6].

Social Implications of Fermented Beverages

Throughout the ages, social attitudes towards fermented beverages—especially wine—have taken two distinctly divergent forms: good and evil. Attempts to address these divergent views in the USA lead to the temperance movement, the Volstead Act of 1919, and a temporary ban on alcohol sales.

Athenaeus, the third-century Greek social commentator born in the Egyptian delta city of Naucratis, provided numerous, positive examples whereby moderate use of fermented beverages improved the human condition. Athenaeus wrote that wine possessed the power to forge friendships and that drinking wine warmed and fused the human soul [7]. He also noted that wine drinking improved creativity, whereby poets received their muse, and if writers wished to produce anything of quality, they—by definition—should drink wine and should, likewise, avoid drinking water [7].

The dark side of wine use, drinking to intoxication and resulting alcoholism, can also be traced to remote antiquity. Egyptian tomb art depicts elegantly dressed, bejeweled beautiful women turning their heads to vomit because of excessive drinking, while tombs also depict other guests who have passed out due to intoxication and show the drunkards being carried out of the banquet halls, born on the shoulders of their comrades [8]. The ancient Egyptian scribe named Ani condemned intoxication: "Boast not that you can drink a jug of beer. You speak, and an unintelligible utterance issues from your mouth…you are found lying on the ground and you are like a child" [9]. Enough said about the historical (prehistorical?) aspects of how alcohol consumption affects the human condition.

Historic Nonalcoholic Beverages

Several beverages, specifically coffee and tea, have been lauded through the centuries for their flavor, effects, medicinal, recreational, and social roles. These beverages have also impacted the current status of trade and culture in the world today.

Cacao

Chocolate was prepared in liquid form as beverages until the mid-1830s when it became possible, technically, to remove cocoa fat and collect the solids. The original introduction of chocolate to Europe during the sixteenth century, therefore, was only in beverage form. Chocolate appeared for the first time in Europe in 1544, when introduced to the Spanish court by Mayan nobles who greeted Prince Philip [10]. The Mayan word, cacao, entered scientific nomenclature in 1753 when Linnaeus published his taxonomic system and coined the genus and species, *Theobroma cacao*, terms translated as the "food of the gods" [11]. Countless children make a daily choice at the lunch line to have either regular or chocolate milk. Countless nutritionists at the USDA, NIH, and elsewhere will ponder the nutritional and economic significance of the choices of these children.

Coffee

From earliest times, coffee has been a medicinal drug and social beverage. The origins of coffee are lost to legend, as some tales identify an Ethiopian goat shepherd as the first person to notice the effects that natural coffee beans had on his goats, while other stories advance the claim of Arab traders or Christian monks as the first people to prepare coffee as a beverage. Still other legends relate that the angel Gabrielle presented coffee to the Prophet Mohammed in order to replace wine. Whatever the origin, Muslim traders ultimately were responsible for the geographical spread of coffee throughout the Islamic world; others then spread the beverage globally [12].

Coffee, historically, has been used as a medicine to treat eye disorders, gout, and even scurvy [12]. By the early 1900s, scientific investigations on coffee had identified caffeine as being responsible for its stimulant effects. During the 1970s, the use of coffee/caffeine as an ergogenic aid became popular after a large body of literature indicated that caffeine improves endurance performance [13]. The effect of caffeine on sports performance is so pronounced that the International Olympic Committee has set maximum blood levels for athletes [14, 15].

This subject is reviewed in other chapters: coffee on health (Cavalli and Tavani), use of caffeine in sports drinks (Maughan and Shirreffs), and energy drinks (Ragsdale).

Kola

Cola nitida and *C. acuminata* trees of Africa produce kola nuts that are both chewed and prepared as beverages for their stimulant properties. Muslim physicians of the twelfth century reported that kola powder prepared as a beverage treated colic and stomach ache. Subsequent writers stated that kola reduces thirst pangs, and when mixed with milk cured headache, relieved fatigue, and improved the appetite [16]. The modern use of kola as a flavoring for beverages dates to the 1870s when mixtures of kola, sugar, and vanilla were served as tonics for invalids.

In 1886, John S. Pemberton invented the beverage, Coca-Cola, which initially was prepared using a combination of coca (i.e., cocaine: *Erythroxylum coca*) and kola and was dispensed, initially, as a drugstore remedy to cure headaches and hangovers [16]. Coca-Cola has since become one of the most widely distributed soft-drink products on our planet, and the Coca-Cola Company has become one of the largest corporate entities on the planet. Some children have even come to associate the Coca-Cola Company for the portrayal of Santa Claus in a red robe with a bottle of Coca-Cola. The impact of these drinks on energy balance and health is reviewed in the chapters by Hollis and by Temple and Alp.

It is no secret that sweetness is an important characteristic that determines the palatability of a beverage. The effect of sugar in beverages is described in the chapter by Temple and Alp. The use of high fructose corn syrup is described more specifically in the chapter by White and Nicklas.

Tea

The eight-century Chinese author, Lu Yu, produced one of the important texts on the properties of tea and how to serve the beverage [17]. His *Cha Ching* (Classic of Tea) considers a range of issues on how to make the best tea: "On the question of what water to use I would suggest that tea made from mountain streams is best, river water is all right, but well-water tea is quite inferior… Water from the slow-flowing streams, the stone-lined pools or milk-pure springs is the best of mountain water." [17]

Tea has long been touted for its healthful properties and according to some scholars may be the second most commonly drunk beverage on our planet after water [18]. The medicinal roles of tea today in the twenty-first century include use to alleviate the common cold and various infections, and tea may have a role in preventing or fighting cancer of the esophagus, lung, and stomach [19–21]. Up-to-date reviews of the effects of various types of tea can be found in the chapter by Isemura.

Beverages Impacts on the Development of Culture

Why are certain beverages associated particular certain cultural events, festivals, or seasons? How are beverages used in these events? How do these traditions continue to impact us today?

Art, Dance, Literature, Song, and Theater

Depiction of beverages in art is legion, from the tomb art of Ancient Egypt to depictions of drinking in Aztec and Mayan codices, painted before the conquest of Mexico. Most art galleries throughout the world present lithographs, mosaics, paintings, and prints that depict people dining, eating, and drinking. From Michaelangelo's masterpiece, *The Last Supper*, to Salvador Dali's *The Wines of Gala*, beverages are depicted as an integral part of human life and culture.

Beverages have been an integral and often fatal part of the creative spirit in the arts and literature. Jack London, Ernest Hemingway, and F. Scott Fitzgerald are all examples of great authors who consumed large amounts of alcohol, had alcohol as a theme in many of their greatest works, and had problems with alcoholism. In the late 1800s the art world was influenced by the greenish drink absinthe produced from Algerian wormwood with Edgar Degas using it as the subject of his *L'Absinthe* (1876). More recently, the phrase "Red Bull gives you wings" has become an anthem for the energy drinks consumed by young people around the world, a topic discussed in greater length in the chapter by Ragsdale.

Beverages and the Rites of Passage and Other Rituals

Beverages form part of the life cycle of humans and are integrated into birth, rites of passage, coming of age, marriage, and death. The birth of children worldwide is celebrated by offering beverages to guests who come to visit and inspect the newborn and to offer pleasantries and good wishes to the new parents: freshwater in some cultures, freshly brewed coffee or tea in others, and sometimes fermented beverages, whether beer or wines such as champagne, in other societies. Other beverage-related initiations worthy of note include the smashing of a bottle of champagne during the launching of ships, the three-martini "power lunch" that once served as the central point for business discussions and sealing deals, and blessings of holy water sprayed over assembled worshipers.

Beverages and Hospitality

Social activities require hospitality; beverages play important roles in cementing bonds of hospitality between individuals and nations. This can be summed up in the words: "Let's drink to it." Individuals invited into homes are served a multitude of beverages depending upon the country, geographical region, and period of time in history. In Egypt guests are served a range of beverages, sometimes specially brewed coffee (accompanied with a glass of water) and in other instances juices from fresh fruits or sugarcane. In Mongolia the tradition is an offering of hot tea to visitors (Wilson, field notes). Beverages are also important on a larger diplomatic scale, where toasts of rice wine were the social highlights of President Nixon's initial visit to the People's Republic of China, and of course toasts with vodka are central to diplomatic missions to Russia. While innocent to some, the guise of hospitality, alcohol, and sensitivity to alcoholism was often used to procure favorable treaties, often resulting in a complete loss of land rights for indigenous peoples. The disputes over treaties signed 150 years ago in the guise of "hospitality" remain in the courts of Australia, Canada, and the USA to this day.

Beverage Impact on Religions

Judaism

In Judaism, almond milk (*mizo*) drunk to break the fast of Yom Kippur is symbolic of purity. Wine is central to Jewish religious traditions. The Torah (Books of Moses) and other Old Testament books contain more than 230 references to wine [22]. The beverage is respected throughout Judaism for its religious, medical, and social uses yet is surrounded by specific ethical and moral behavior codes, with specific admonitions regarding intoxication that date to the earliest Jewish texts [22]. Of special interest to Maimonides was the role of wine in matters of human reproduction and cohabitation:

"Of greater benefit than any food or medicine for (male erection) is wine. There is no substitute for it in this respect, because the blood that is produced (by wine) is warm and moist and rejoices the soul, and strongly incites to sexual intercourse because of its special characteristic.... This is especially so if one takes some (wine) after the meal, and when one leaves the bath, for its effect in this regard is far greater than anything else." [23]

Christianity

Within Christianity, wine and bread are symbolic of the blood and body of Christ [24, 25]. Sacramental wine is viewed by many Mediterranean faithful as having curative properties; it may be poured over the body of Catholic believers thought to be possessed. Among Greek Orthodox faithful, wine is used to cleanse and wash the body of the deceased and to make an offering linking the deceased with Christ's resurrection [26]. Vines, grapes, and wine have served as symbolic icons throughout the centuries of Christian art.

Despite the dual attitude towards wine expressed historically throughout Christian literature, early Christian physicians recommended wine for therapeutic properties. Early Christians (nonphysicians) took ethical-moral viewpoints in regard to wine. One of these, Gregory of Nyssa (later St. Gregory), a religious scholar of the fourth century, wrote that wine, taken to excess, was the drug of madness, that it poisoned the soul, led to the destruction of the mind and the ruin of nature, and was "the danger of youth, the disgrace of old age, and the shame of women" [27].

Tradition holds that Mary, the mother of Jesus, gave birth inside a cave located within the precinct of Bethlehem in ancient Palestine. The story is commonly related that when Mary initiated breastfeeding, some of her milk spilled onto the floor of the cave and turned the stones white. For at least a millennium, this site has been called the Milk Grotto and receives tens of thousands of visitors yearly.

Islam

Despite Koranic and Hadithic injunctions against wine, Muslim physicians of the Middle Ages extolled the merits and healthful properties of this beverage. Specifically prohibited to believers is wine: "O believers, wine and arrow-shuffling, idols and diving-arrows are an abomination, some of Satan's work" [28]. While the specific Arabic term used in the Koran is khmer, the prohibition generally has been extended to include alcoholic beverages in general. Ibn Sina of Afsana (937–1037) is perhaps the preeminent Muslim physician of the Middle Ages. He wrote extensively on beverages, especially the medical-dietary role of wine: "To take wine after a meal is very unsatisfactory, for it is rapidly digested and enters the blood quickly and carries food on into the blood before it is properly digested." [29] He added: "To give wine to youths is like adding fire to a fire already prepared with matchwood. Young adults should take it in moderation." [29]

Finally, young students attending traditional Islamic schools throughout the Middle East and elsewhere transcribe passages of the Koran with chalk onto slate tablets using chalk onto smoothed boards. When the daily lessons are concluded and the passages memorized, the words are erased, and the chalk dust is commonly eaten as a form of religious pica. Across the Sahel states of Western Africa, other students use vegetable inks and cloth; at the conclusion of the lesson, the holy words are removed with damp clothes; the cloth containing the vegetable inks are soaked and rinsed; and the fluid is caught in a small bowl and subsequently drunk [30]. We are what we eat and drink; sometimes this is very true in terms of chalk or ink.

Beverages, Social Conflict, and War

Access to water has always been critical in warfare. Since antiquity, generals have sent detachments in advance of the main body of troops to secure and protect water holes and lakes. Conversely, the pattern has also been to deny advancing armies access to water; when an army is in retreat, the common practice has been to defile local wells by tossing bodies of animals or soldiers into the water to make it putrid. Not unexpectedly, technological inventions of water purification tablets (e.g., hala-zone during World War II) became an advantage, thereby making once putrid, unsafe waters safe.

There are numerous military references to the importance of water. For example, Sun Tzu wrote his classic on tactics and deception, *The Art of War*, c. 500 BCE. He noted the following: "When soldiers stand leaning on their spears, they are faint from want of food. If those who are sent to draw water begin by drinking themselves, the army is suffering from thirst." [31]

A classic of eastern Roman military tactics and logistics was written by Publius Flavius Vegetius Renatus during the fifth century CE. His critical observations included the following: "Neither should the army use bad or marsh water, for bad drinking water, like poison, causes disease in the drinkers." He added: "Shortages of grain, wine-vinegar, wine and salt should be prevented at all times." [32] Access to potable water continues to vex soldiers and commanders on all sides of conflicts in the Middle East today.

Indeed, deprivation of access to beverage luxuries has also brought nations to war. America's War of Independence was in part precipitated by British Stamp Taxes on the colonial luxury of tea. This ultimately led to the Boston Tea Party of 1765 and the events that brought independence to what became the USA.

Every summer armies of tourists travel to many countries of the world where they purchase beverages of unknown origin and composition from street vendors. This is especially problematic in countries with poor standards of hygiene. What may be advertised as fruit juice, sugarcane juice, and even potable water may contain water contaminated with a host of potential disease-causing organisms. When vendors sell chunks of ice, they hack off chips from the block—chips that fall onto the filthy street—and the vendors may then wipe the chips "clean" with their unwashed hands and then sell the chips to beverage vendors to cool the products they are selling to the occupying army (Grivetti, field notes, 1964–1967; 1969; 1979; 1993). The best advice, of course, would be for tourists and visitors to rehydrate with bottled beverages (without ice) and to never consume drinks prepared by street vendors [33].

Athletics, Sports, and Hydration

Although descriptions of training regimens of ancient athletes have been documented for centuries, accounts of foods and beverages used by ancient, elite athletes are rare. Epictetus, a philosopher of the first to second century CE, provided a challenge to athletes who wanted to win at the Olympic Games: "If you do, you will have to obey instructions, eat according to regulations, keep away from desserts, exercise on a fixed schedule at definite hours, in both heat and cold; you must not drink cold water nor can you have a drink of wine whenever you want." [34]

Turning to elite athletes of the modern era, we have more reliable information on food and beverage use. Data are available on 42 of the 49 nations that competed at the Berlin Olympic Games held in 1936. Strong coffee was part of the training regimen of only seven countries: Argentina, Australia/New Zealand, Brazil, Estonia, Greece, India, and Italy. Ironically, coffee was not a significant component of the diet of athletes from countries where coffee is commonly consumed, specifically Austria, Mexico, Peru, Switzerland, Turkey, or the USA. Milk in quantities greater than 2 L/day was consumed by athletes who represented Afghanistan, Bermuda, Brazil, Finland, Holland, Iceland, India, Norway, South Africa, and the USA. Whiskey in undefined quantities was a dietary component of Canadian athletes, while wine in undefined quantities appeared on the training regimen of French and Italian athletes. Chinese athletes drank limited quantities of milk and drank iced tea and orange juice, while Japanese athletes did not drink tea at all [35, 36]. More recently, the Atlanta Olympic Games of 1996 were managed by ARAMARK Corporation of Philadelphia, who provided milk (70,000 pounds) and bottled water (550,000 gallons) to American and visiting athletes [37].

Fluid-replacement beverages were developed in the 1960s, beginning with Gatorade. Currently, numerous sports beverages are marketed in the USA, among them All Sport and Powerade. The chapter in this book by Maughan and Shirreffs provides a description of how modern-day sports drinks are formulated to improve the performance of our modern athletes. The USA has also seen a growth in beverages marketed to maintain specific weights or to help us lose weight, a topic that becomes more important as healthy young athletes become more elderly observers of athletes. Some healthy young athletes will also become less active and overweight adults who will become less active as they grow older before developing metabolic syndrome and diabetes; beverage recommendations for these persons are described in greater detail in the chapter by Maher and Kobbs. Beverage nutritional support for the elderly is discussed in the chapter by McDonald, Bales, and Buhr.

It is perhaps appropriate to also note how beverages are used at the conclusion of certain sporting events, where the traditional beverage of victors in the Indianapolis 500 is milk and winners of the Tour de France drink champagne, then shake the bottle, and spray their fans with a champagne "mist." And who does not delight in (or is repelled by) the US pattern accorded NFL coaches who win the Super Bowl of being drenched in a cascade of ice-chilled Gatorade.

Beverages and Space Flight

Several key problems must be overcome before embarking upon periods of extended space flight, for example, the mission to Mars. In addition to the well-known problems of calcium metabolism and bone loss, potential radiation, and food-energy balance, water balance is perhaps the most critical: one may survive for several months on limited food supplies but only days without water.

Early estimates and calculations for water needs of astronauts were conducted in the 1960s, when decisions were made to produce closed systems that recycled wastewater from human urine and exhaled air for drinking, cooking, and washing needs. The estimated daily water requirement for drinking and cooking needs was 5000 mL/day for each astronaut [38].

Beverages developed and served to the early Mercury program astronauts were "Spartan" and not especially fine tasting, whereas Gemini program astronauts (1965–1966) fared substantially better. Food product developers realized it was impractical to associate specific consumables with "earthbound" concepts of breakfast, lunch, and dinner. Accordingly, astronauts were presented with 3-day menu cycles for each 24-h period. This included a range of beverages: cocoa, grapefruit drink, orange drink, orange-grapefruit drink, and tea [39, 40]. Indeed, the need to create a flavorful drink in space from recycled water led to the development of the orange drink beverage Tang®, now popular with more earthbound consumers.

Astronauts associated with the Skylab program experienced substantial improvements in both variety and presentation. Skylab astronauts could select from cocoa, cocoa-flavored liquid instant breakfast, coffee (black), grape drink, grapefruit (soluble crystal form), lemonade, and orange (soluble crystal form) [41]. The value for daily water needs by Skylab and some Shuttle crew astronauts has been established at 2000–2500 mL/day, with intakes increased depending upon activity level [42]. Still, there remains a key question: in the centuries to come, what beverages will be consumed once colonies are established on the Moon and Mars?

Beverages chosen for human consumption have progressed over the water scooped from a pond or river to a variety of complicated formulations. Modern beverages contain a myriad of chemical ingredients that all have very specific functions with respect to the appearance, taste, shelf-life, and nutritional qualities of what we drink today. The chapter by Nelson, Rush, and Wilson reviews those items commonly observed on a beverage ingredient label and their purpose. The chapter by Krasny describes the precise legal requirements of proper beverage labeling in the USA.

Conclusion

Beverages, whether from animal, plant, or natural sources, have served humans well through the millennia. Historically, water was identified as one of the four great elements: air, earth, fire, and water. Water and related companion beverages have been the focus of development and ultimately scientific scrutiny for centuries, dating well before the invention of writing. Water is such a simple compound, just three atoms— two hydrogens and an oxygen—but without water, humans could not exist.

Three hundred years from today…

The humans arise after periods of restful sleep, dress, and walk across their spotless living quarters. In their ergogenic-fitted workspace, they grind coffee beans grown hydroponically from recycled waste water. They nestle into their ergogenic chairs, molded to accommodate their bodies, and gaze outward through thick, meteoroid-resistant tempered windows and view the on-going construction taking place on the red dusty landscape of the Martian surface, and take their first drink of the day…

References

1. Charaka-Samhita. Agnivesa's treatise refined and annotated by Caraka and redacted by Drdhabala, vol. 1. Sutrasthana to Indriyasthana. Sharma P, editor. Delhi, India: Chaukambha Orientalia; 1981.
2. Simoons FJ. The antiquity of dairying in Asia and Africa. Geogr Rev. 1971;61:431–9.
3. Reed BA, Grivetti LE. Controlling on-farm inventories of bulk-tank raw milk. An opportunity to protect public health. J Dairy Sci. 2001;83:1–4.
4. Badler V. The archaeological evidence for winemaking, distribution, and consumption at Proto-Historic Godin Tepe, Iran. In: McGovern PE, Fleming SJ, Katz SH, editors. The origins and ancient history of wine. Langhorne: Gordon and Breach; 1995. p. 45–56.
5. Formenti F, Duthel JM. The analysis of wine and other organics inside amphoras of the Roman Period. In: McGovern PE, Fleming SJ, Katz SH, editors. The origins and ancient history of wine. Langhorne: Gordon and Breach; 1995. p. 79–85.
6. Grivetti LE. Wine: the food with two faces. In: McGovern PE, Fleming SJ, Katz SH, editors. The origins and ancient history of wine. Langhorne: Gordon and Breach; 1995. p. 9–22.
7. Athenaeus. The Deipnosophists (trans: Gulick CB), 7 vols. New York: G. P. PutnamŌs Sons; 1927–1941.
8. Darby WJ, Ghalioungui P, Grivetti LE. Food. The gift of Osiris, 2 vols. London: Academic; 1977.
9. Erman A. The literature of the ancient Egyptians (trans: Blackman AM). London: Methuen; 1927.
10. Coe SD, Coe MD. The true history of chocolate. London: Thames and Hudson; 1996.
11. Dillinger TL, Barriga P, Escárcega S, Jimenez M, Lowe DS, Grivetti LE. Food of the gods: cure for humanity? A cultural history of the medicinal and ritual use of chocolate. J Nutr. 2000;130(August supplement):2057S–72.
12. Topik SC. Coffee. In: Kiple KF, Ornelas KC, editors. The Cambridge world history of food, vol. 1. Cambridge: Cambridge University Press; 2000. p. 641–53.
13. Costill DL, Dalsky G, Find W. Effects of caffeine ingestion on metabolism and exercise performance. Med Sci Sports Exerc. 1978;10:155–8.
14. Williams MH. The use of nutritional ergogenic aids in sports. Is it an ethical issue? Int J Sport Nutr. 1994;4:120–31.
15. Applegate EA, Grivetti LE. Search for the competitive edge. A history of dietary fads and supplements. J Nutr. 1997;127 suppl 9:869S–73S.
16. Abaka E. Kola nut. In: Kiple KF, Ornelas KC, editors. The Cambridge world history of food, vol. 1. Cambridge: Cambridge University Press; 2000. p. 684–92.
17. Yu Lu. Classic of tea (trans: Carpenter FR). Boston: Little, Brown, and Company; 8th Century CE/1974.
18. Weisburger JH, Comer J. Tea. In: Kiple KF, Ornelas KC, editors. The Cambridge world history of food, vol. 1. Cambridge: Cambridge University Press; 2000. p. 712–20.
19. Katiyar SK, Mukhtar H. Tea consumption and cancer. World Rev Nutr Diet. 1996;79:154–84.
20. Weisburger JH. Tea and health. A historical perspective. Cancer Lett. 1997;114:315–7.
21. Yang CS, Lee MJ, Chen I, Yang GY. Polyphenols as inhibitors of carcinogenesis. Environ Health Perspect. 1997;4:971–6.
22. Goodrick EW, Kohlenberger 3rd JR. The new complete concordance (the complete English concordance to the New International version). Grand Rapids: Zonderuan; 1981.
23. Maimonides. Treatise on cohabitation. In: Treatises on poisons, hemorrhoids, cohabitation. Maimonides' medical writings (trans: Rosner F). Haifa: The Maimonides Research Institute; 1984.
24. Child H, Colles D. Cing and milk use in southern Asia. Anthropos. 1970;65:547–93.
25. Murray R. Symbols of church and kingdom. A study in early Syriac tradition. Cambridge: Cambridge University Press; 1975.

26. Danforth LM. The death rituals of rural Greece. Princeton: Princeton University Press; 1982.
27. Keenan ME. St. Gregory of Nyssa and the medical profession. Bull Hist Med. 1944;15:150–61.
28. Koran. The Koran interpreted (trans: Arberry AJ). New York: The Macmillan Company; 1955.
29. Ibn Sina. Avicenna's poem on medicine (trans: Krueger HC). Springfield: Charles C. Thomas; 1963.
30. Garrett S. Personal Communication. Kennesaw State University, Marietta, Georgia.
31. de Saxe M. My reveries upon the art of war. In: Roots of strategy. The 5 greatest military classics of all time (trans: Phillips TR). Harrisburg: Stackpole Books; 1985. p. 177–300.
32. Publius Flavius Vegetius Renatus. Epitoma Rei Militaris (Epitome of Military Science) (trans: Milner NP) (Translated Texts for Historians), vol. 16. Liverpool: Liverpool University Press; 5th Century CE/1993.
33. Simopoulos AP, Bhat RV. Street foods. World Rev Nutr Diet. 2000;86:1–175.
34. Philostratus Flavius. Concerning gymnastics (trans: Woody T). Ann Arbor: American Physical Education Association; 1936.
35. Schenk P. Die Verpflegung von 4700 Wettkšmpfern aus 42 Nationen im Olympischen Dorf wšrend der XI. Olympischen Spiele 1936 zu Berlin. Munch Med Wochenschr. 1936;83:1535–9.
36. Schenk P. Bericht Ÿber die Verpflegung der im ÒOlympischen DorfÓ untergebrachten Teilnehmer an den XI. Olympischen Spielen 1936 zu Berlin. Die Ernaehrung. 1937;2:1–24.
37. Grivetti LE, Applegate EA. From Olympia to Atlanta. A cultural-historical perspective on diet and athletic training. J Nutr. 1997;127(Suppl):860s–8.
38. Taylor AA, Finkelstein F, Hayes RE. Food for space travel. Examination of current capabilities and future needs. Washington, DC: Air Research and Development Command; 1960.
39. Klicka MV, Hollender HA, Lachance PA. Development of space foods. 4th International Congress of Dietetics, Stockholm, Sweden, 15 July, 1965. Ekonomiforestandarinnors Tidskrift. 1966;1:3–12.
40. Klicka MV, Hollender HA, Lachance PA. Foods for astronauts. J Am Dent Assoc. 1967;51:238–45.
41. Heidelbaugh ND, Smith Jr MC, Rambaut PC, Lutwak L, Huber CS, Stadler CR, Rouse BM. Clinical nutrition applications of space food technology. J Am Dent Assoc. 1973;62:383–9.
42. Lane HW, Leach C, Smith SM. Fluid and electrolyte homeostasis. In: Lane HW, Schoeller DA, editors. Nutrition in spaceflight and weightlessness models. Boca Raton: CRC; 2000. p. 119–39.

Part II
Health Effects of Coffee, Tea, Wine, Alcohol, and Juices

Chapter 3
Coffee Consumption and Its Impact on Health

Lodovica Cavalli and Alessandra Tavani

Keywords Coffee • Caffeine • Cancer • Cardiovascular disease

Key Points

1. Coffee contains many bioactive chemicals, including caffeine, diterpenes, minerals, acids and esters, and phenolic compounds, many of which are antioxidants.
2. A moderate intake of coffee slightly decreases total mortality, although the causality of this association is debated.
3. Coffee slightly increases blood pressure, decreases the incidence of diabetes, and may slightly decrease the risk of cardiovascular disease, including stroke. However, the possibility cannot be excluded that reverse causation is to some extent responsible for these observations. In non-/occasional drinkers, coffee in the first hour after ingestion may trigger acute myocardial infarction and stroke.
4. Coffee does not increase total cancer risk, but it decreases the incidence of oral and pharyngeal, liver, and endometrial cancers, while the relation with bladder cancer is still debated.
5. Coffee is not related to osteoporosis and may decrease risk of cognitive impairment and Parkinson's disease, although the causality is still debated.
6. Coffee drinking should be reduced in caffeine low metabolizers, and in patients with cirrhosis, gastritis and ulcer. Coffee drinking should be minimized in children, pregnant and lactating women.

L. Cavalli, Psy.D. • A. Tavani, Sci.D. (✉)
Department of Epidemiology, Istituto di Ricerche Farmacologiche "Mario Negri", Institute for Pharmacological Research, Via Giuseppe La Masa 19, 20156 Milan, Italy
e-mail: alessandra.tavani@marionegri.it

© Springer International Publishing Switzerland 2016
T. Wilson, N.J. Temple (eds.), *Beverage Impacts on Health and Nutrition*,
Nutrition and Health, DOI 10.1007/978-3-319-23672-8_3

Introduction

Coffee is the second most common beverage in the world after tea, and any effect of coffee is an important issue of nutritional health. Coffee contains about 2000 chemicals in addition to caffeine, the best known component of the beverage. These include many bioactive compounds with potential effects on health. The amount of caffeine and other components of coffee in the final beverage is variable and depends on type of coffee powder, brewing method, beverage preparation, and cup size [1]. This variation complicates our understanding of coffee's health effects. Coffee consumption was often associated with unfavorable effects on health, but some of these were not confirmed by more recent epidemiological evidence. This chapter discusses the known benefits and a few confirmed risks associated with coffee intake, trying to distinguish those possibly related to caffeine from those possibly related to other constituents of coffee.

Caffeine

Caffeine (1,3,7-trimethylxanthine) is an alkaloid present in a few beverages and foods apart from coffee. It acts as a competitive antagonist on the adenosine receptors A_1 and A_{2A} and has a wide variety of physiological effects (Table 3.1). In the central nervous system, it is a mild stimulant, reducing tiredness and reaction time [2], increasing alertness and energy, elevating mood, and inducing anxiety and insomnia. In the respiratory system, caffeine acts on the respiration center and induces bronchodilation. In the cardiovascular system, it increases heart rate and slightly increases blood pressure in the short term. Urinary system effects include a mild diuresis. Gastrointestinal tract action includes increased gastric secretion of HCl and pepsin, gastrointestinal motility, and biliary acids' secretion. Caffeine has

Table 3.1 Main physiological effects of caffeine

Body system	Pharmacological action of caffeine
Central nervous system	• Reduction of tiredness, reaction time
	• Increase of alertness, energy, mood, anxiety, insomnia
Respiratory system	• Stimulation of respiration center
	• Bronchodilation
Cardiovascular system	• Short-term slight increase of blood pressure
	• Increase of heart rate
Urinary system	• Mild diuresis
Gastrointestinal tract	• In the stomach: increased HCl and pepsin secretion
	• Increase of gastrointestinal motility
	• Increase of biliary acids' secretion
Adipose tissue	• Stimulation of lipolysis

a thermogenic effect and stimulates lipolysis in the adipose tissue. Caffeine potentiates the bioavailability and the analgesic effects of aspirin and nonsteroidal anti-inflammatory drugs. Tolerance and a mild dependence to the effects of caffeine appear already after 3–4 cups of coffee, and withdrawal syndrome includes weak sedation, headache, irritability, and sleepiness.

There are specific gene variants associated with caffeine metabolism, two of which are in the cytochrome P450 1A1 and 1A2 (*CYP1A1–CYP1A2*) gene region. As CYP1A2 is the main enzyme metabolizing caffeine, it greatly influences the caffeine body levels after ingestion, physiological effect intensity and duration, and, consequently, the amount of coffee consumption.

Caffeine potentially interacts with several drugs, mainly those active in the central nervous system. However, for most drugs, there are no clinically relevant interactions, except for very high consumption, such as 10 cups of coffee. The only potentially dangerous interaction of caffeine at relatively low doses is that with ephedra/ephedrine. While these substances are banned from being added to dietary supplements in the USA and some other countries, they are still added to some weight-loss products and nasal decongestants in a few countries. Another important interaction may be that of high intake of caffeine (i.e., that contained in energy drinks) and alcohol [3], a topic discussed in greater details in the chapter on energy drinks by Ragsdale.

Other Chemicals Contained in Coffee

The list of chemicals contained in coffee is far from being defined, and some substances are contained in some varieties of seeds and not in others. However, there are some basic chemical characteristics common to all types of coffee after roasting (Table 3.2), such as carbohydrates, nitrogenous compounds (including amino acids, proteins, caffeine, and trigonelline), lipids (including diterpenes, i.e., cafestol and kahweol), minerals (mainly potassium), acids and esters (including aliphatic and chlorogenic acids), and melanoidins. Many chemicals are antioxidants (mainly phenolic compounds such as chlorogenic, caffeic, ferulic, and coumaric acids), and coffee is one of the most important source of dietary antioxidants in many populations, including those with a high intake of fruit and vegetables [1].

Total Mortality

The association of coffee drinking at baseline with subsequent total and cause-specific mortality was considered in the National Institutes of Health (NIH)-AARP Diet and Health Study among approximately 400,000 men and women [4]. During about 13 years of follow-up, 33,731 men and 18,784 women died. After adjustment for tobacco smoking status and other potential confounders, the hazard ratios (HR)

Table 3.2 Chemical composition of roasted *Coffea arabica* and *Coffea robusta*

Compound	Approximate concentration (g/100 g of coffee powder)[a]	
	Coffea arabica	*Coffea robusta*
Carbohydrates/fibers	38.0	41.5
Nitrogenous compounds		
Amino acids/proteins	10.0	10.0
Caffeine	1.3	2.4
Trigonelline	1.0	0.7
Lipids		
Terpenes	17.0	11.0
Minerals, total	4.5	4.7
Potassium	1.8	1.9
Acids and esters		
Chlorogenic acids	2.7	3.1
Aliphatic acids	2.4	2.5
Melanoidins	23.0	23.0

[a]Concentrations depend on climate, soil composition, agricultural characteristics, methods of analyses, and roasting temperature [1]

for death among male coffee drinkers compared with nondrinkers were 0.94 (95 % confidence intervals, CI, 0.90–0.99) for 1 cup/day, 0.90 (95 % CI 0.86–0.93) for 2–3 cups, 0.88 (95 % CI 0.84–0.93) for 4–5 cups, and 0.90 (95 % CI 0.85–0.96) for 6 or more cups/day; the corresponding HRs among female drinkers were 0.95 (95 % CI 0.90–1.01), 0.87 (95 % CI 0.83–0.92), 0.84 (95 % CI 0.79–0.90), and 0.85 (95 % CI 0.78–0.93), with a significant trend in risk with dose.

The relationship between coffee consumption and all-cause mortality was studied in 24 other prospective cohort studies [5]. Among these, 20 found an inverse or null association, one of US Seventh-day Adventists found a significant direct association, and three found a significant increased risk only in men [5]. A recent meta-analysis pooled the results of 23 cohort studies and found an overall relative risk (RR) of all-cause mortality for the study-specific highest versus lowest (defined as ≤1 cup/day) coffee drinking categories of 0.88 (95 % CI 0.84–0.93). As smoking is an important determinant of mortality and is associated with drinking coffee, studies not adjusting for tobacco smoking have been considered separately to obtain information on the potential distorting effect of tobacco. The pooled RR for the highest coffee intake compared with low drinking from the 4 studies with RRs not adjusted for tobacco smoking was 0.91 (95 % CI 0.81–1.01). The corresponding RR for the 19 studies adjusting for tobacco smoking was 0.87 (95 % CI 0.82–0.93), similar in men and women. The pooled RR for an increment of 1 cup/day of coffee was 0.97 (95 % CI 0.96–0.98), obtained by pooling the RRs of the 17 smoking-adjusting studies that reported the RR for at least three categories of coffee consumption [5]. Compared with low drinking (≤1 cup/day), the pooled RRs were 0.91 (95 % CI 0.88–0.94) for moderate drinking (>1 to ≤3 cups/day) and 0.87 (95 % CI 0.82–0.92) for high drinking (>3 cups/day), suggesting a dose–risk relation. The pooled RR for coffee consumption of ≥4 cups/day was 0.87 (95 % CI 0.83–0.91) based on 14 studies.

After the publication of the meta-analysis, an American cohort study found a slightly increased risk of total mortality in subjects younger than 55 years drinking >4 cups/day, with no linear trend in risk [6, 7].

The effects of decaffeinated coffee have been less studied. The NIH-AARP Diet and Health Study reported that decaffeinated coffee had the same inverse relation with total mortality as did regular coffee [4]. An inverse association for decaffeinated coffee was also found in the two meta-analyses, although it was based on only a few studies, including persons who often drunk both decaffeinated and regular coffee [5, 7]. These findings suggest that substances other than caffeine may be responsible for the beneficial effect of coffee on total mortality.

The issue of the causality of the inverse association is still open. It cannot be excluded that people with chronic diseases associated with higher mortality rates chose to consume less coffee than healthier people, thereby leading to a spurious protective association. However, the prospective cohort studies collected information many years before death, and in most studies subjects with cancer or cardiovascular disease (CVD) at baseline were excluded. This indicates that reverse causation cannot totally explain the favorable effect. Moreover, a real favorable effect of coffee on total mortality is supported by the dose–risk relation; the consistency of results across strata of several covariates, including sex and geographic regions with different amounts of coffee intake; and biological plausibility. Thus, although the causality of the inverse association of coffee drinking with total mortality is still debated, overall, coffee consumption up to 3 cups/day does not seem to be a risk factor for health and might even have a somewhat favorable effect.

Cardiovascular Disease

The effect of coffee on CVD risk factors and CVD incidence and mortality has long been debated [8]. Coffee consumption and its association with blood pressure, serum lipid profile, diabetes, and stroke have been studied intensively.

Coffee and Main CVD Risk Factors

Blood Pressure

Hypertension is a strong risk factor for both stroke and coronary heart disease (CHD), and caffeine intake has been related with increased blood pressure in the short term after consumption [9]. A meta-analysis of clinical trials found a cumulative mean increase of 2.0–2.4 mmHg of systolic blood pressure and of 0.8–1.2 mmHg of diastolic blood pressure after 4 cups/day of coffee [10]. The authors concluded that these increases do not necessarily imply an increased CVD risk; they suggested that the caffeine-dependent increased risk could be counterbalanced by the favorable effects on the CV system of other coffee components (such as antioxidants). Moreover, caffeine effects on blood pressure are short lasting and are lowered by chronic administration, as tolerance to caffeine rapidly develops in habitual coffee consumers. A meta-analysis of six prospective cohort studies showed a slightly increased blood pressure in drinkers of 1–3 cups/day of coffee, but no risk of hypertension in consumers of 3 or more cups/day [11]. Another more recent meta-analysis of ten clinical trials and five cohort studies showed no clinically relevant effects of coffee intake on blood pressure or risk of hypertension [12].

In hypertensive patients drinking coffee, a slight blood pressure increase followed the intake of 2–3 cups of coffee in the first 3 h, with no long-term effects and no evidence of increased CVD risk [13].

Serum Lipids

Coffee beans contain diterpenes, such as kahweol and cafestol, which have been reported to increase cholesterol levels and whose concentration in the final beverage depends mainly on the methods of preparation [8]. A meta-analysis of 14 clinical trials found increased serum levels of cholesterol and low-density lipoproteins (LDL) only in drinkers of boiled/nonfiltered coffee [14], as diterpenes are mostly retained by filters. These results were confirmed in another meta-analysis of five studies showing that total cholesterol, triglycerides, and high-density lipoproteins (HDL) and LDL were not increased in drinkers of filtered coffee [15].

Diabetes

Coffee increases adiponectin levels, has favorable effects on inflammation, and decreases insulin resistance [8]. Chlorogenic acid and other antioxidants have been shown to improve glucose metabolism, and caffeine activates insulin-independent transport of glucose in muscles [8].

A meta-analysis, based on 28 cohort studies, showed RRs for an increment of 1 cup/day of 0.91 (95 % CI 0.89–0.94) for regular coffee and 0.94 (95 % CI 0.91–0.98) for decaffeinated coffee, suggesting that coffee drinking may have a real favorable effect on the incidence of type 2 diabetes [16]. Moreover, the NIH-AARP Diet and Health Study found an inverse relationship between coffee drinking and diabetes mortality [4]. In diabetic subjects drinking coffee, two cohort studies, one in men and one in women, showed no increased risk of total mortality and CVD incidence and mortality [17, 18].

Coffee and Overall CVD

Older studies suggested that coffee intake could increase the risk of CHD and stroke. However, most recent studies did not confirm those observations, possibly because they adjusted for smoking and other potential confounders [8].

The NIH-AARP Diet and Health Study found no relation between coffee drinking and mortality from CVD, heart disease, and stroke in men and stroke in women. However, it did observe a dose-related inverse association for coffee drinking with mortality from heart disease in women, with a 28 % reduced risk in drinkers of 6 or more cups/day [4]. A meta-analysis that pooled 17 smoking-adjusting cohort studies reported an inverse association of borderline significance between CVD mortality and coffee intake [5]. The pooled RRs for the increment of 1 cup/day of coffee were 0.98 (95 % CI 0.95–1.00; RR 0.99 in men and RR 0.95 in women; 16 studies) for CVD, 1.00 (95 % CI 0.97–1.04; 12 studies) for CHD, and 0.97 (95 % CI 0.94–1.01; 7 studies) for stroke. A more recent meta-analysis that included 13 prospective cohort studies found RRs of 0.89 for 1 cup/day, 0.81 for 2 cups/day, 0.79 for 3 cups/day, 0.80 for 4 cups/day, and 0.85 for 6 cups/day, all statistically significant, but with no linear dose relation [19]. However, in occasional drinkers, some short-term harmful effect after ingestion of coffee cannot be excluded. A study on 503 cases of CVD mentioned coffee among triggers for acute myocardial infarction (AMI), sudden death, or ischemic stroke in the first hour after ingestion in nondrinkers or occasional drinkers, with no effect in regular drinkers [20].

A meta-analysis pooled 36 studies of CVD and included both incidence and mortality [21]. It observed a nonlinear relationship between coffee and CVD risk. The inverse association was significant for moderate intake (i.e., 3–5 cups/day), with no relationship for higher intake (>6 cups/day).

Taking the evidence as a whole, it seems that a moderate intake of coffee is associated with a modest reduction in risk of CVD. However, the causality of this association is uncertain as reverse causation cannot be excluded.

As for secondary prevention, a large Italian randomized clinical trial found that coffee intake up to 4 cups/day did not increase risk of new CV events (AMI, stroke, sudden death) in more than 11,000 post-AMI patients [22], although after CV events medical advice is necessary.

Coffee and Heart Disease

The association between coffee and CHD/AMI is inconsistent. At least 20–25 prospective cohort studies suggested no association between moderate coffee consumption and CHD, while at least 15 case–control studies suggested that consumption higher than 3–4 cups/day might slightly increase the risk. Two meta-analyses published in 1994 and 2007 found no relationship between coffee drinking and heart disease in cohort studies and a slight increased risk in case–control studies [23, 24]. A meta-analysis published in 2009, based on 21 cohort studies, reported no association with coffee drinking [25], while a meta-analysis published in 2014, based on 30 studies, found a nonlinear inverse relationship with the strongest association for moderate consumption [21]. Thus, in healthy subjects a moderate coffee intake (up to 3 cups/day) is unlikely to increase risk of CHD.

A meta-analysis that included >6500 subjects with heart failure showed a J-shaped curve in relation to coffee intake, with the strongest inverse association for 4 cups/day and an increased risk for higher doses [26]. This association was consistent in strata of sex and history of diabetes and previous AMI.

A moderate intake of coffee does not increase risk of cardiac arrhythmias in healthy subjects. In five controlled trials, the amount of caffeine contained in approximately 4–5 cups of coffee did not increase the severity or frequency of ventricular arrhythmias [27], and there is evidence that drinkers of small amounts of coffee could have fewer episodes of atrial fibrillation [28]. The mechanisms for the eventual protective effects of coffee on arrhythmias are largely unknown, but they could include the competitive action of caffeine against endogenous adenosine on the adenosine receptor [8].

Stroke

The relationship between coffee intake and risk of stroke has been widely analyzed, and a meta-analysis of 11 cohort studies (with about 10,000 cases) found a nonlinear relation with a weak inverse association for an intake of 2–4 cups/day [29]. The relationship was similar in both sexes and for both ischemic and hemorrhagic stroke, although for the latter it was not statistically significant, probably because of the smaller number of subjects. The inverse relationship was confirmed in a more recent large Japanese cohort study [30]. A recent meta-analysis, based on 22 studies, found a nonlinear relationship, with the strongest inverse relationship seen for moderate coffee intake [21]. However, in non- and occasional drinkers coffee may slightly increase the risk of stroke in the first hour after ingestion [24].

Cancer

Mortality for All Cancers

A meta-analysis summarized the evidence concerning the association between coffee consumption and mortality from all cancers based on 13 cohort studies [5]. The pooled RR for ten smoking-adjusted studies for the highest versus lowest (≤1 cup/day) categories of coffee drinking was 1.03 (95 % CI 0.97–1.10; 1.07 in men and 0.98 in women), and the combined RR for an increment of 1 cup/day of coffee was 1.00 (95 % CI 0.99–1.01; similar in men and women). Overall, therefore, coffee appears to pose no risk of causing death from cancer.

Cancers of the Oral Cavity and Pharynx

The many antioxidants contained in coffee may prevent the oxidative damage induced on the oral and pharyngeal mucosa by tobacco smoking and alcohol drinking, which are the main risk factors for the disease.

A meta-analysis, based on a total of 2633 cases from eight case–control studies and one cohort study, found a pooled RR of 0.64 (95 % CI 0.51–0.80) for the highest versus the lowest category of coffee drinking. The pooled RRs were consistent for case–control (odds ratios, OR 0.67) and cohort studies (RR 0.35) and for various geographic regions with different coffee intakes and dietary correlates [31]. A pooled analysis including nearly 4000 cases from nine case–control studies (three of which were also included in the meta-analysis) found a cumulative OR for drinkers of >4 cups/day compared with nondrinkers of 0.61 for cancer of the oral cavity and pharynx combined, 0.46 for oral cavity, 0.58 for oropharynx/hypopharynx, and 0.61 for nonspecified or overlapping sites, with significant trends in risk [32]. Another case–control study on the risk of cancer of the mouth and oropharynx published after the meta-analysis found a reduced risk of about 60 % for the highest versus the lowest quartile of lifelong consumption of coffee [33]. Of the three cohort studies published after the meta-analysis, two found a decreased risk of about 40 % for the highest intake compared with the lowest one, with an inverse trend in risk with exposure [34, 35], and the third found no relation with either oral or pharyngeal cancer risk [36]. An update of the meta-analysis of papers adjusting for tobacco smoking and alcohol drinking published up to March 2013 found a cumulative RR for the highest intake of coffee drinking compared with the lowest one of 0.72 (95 % CI 0.59–0.87), based on about 7000 cases [37]. The inverse association was apparently consistent in strata of tobacco and alcohol users, although difficult to study given the small number of subjects with oral and pharyngeal cancer among nonsmokers and nondrinkers of alcohol [32]. The inverse association was also consistent in men and women and in strata of vegetable and fruit intake [32].

Thus, overall, epidemiological evidence suggests a real protective role of coffee in the etiology of oral and pharyngeal cancer, supported by the dose relationship, a biological plausibility, and the consistency in different settings, populations, and strata of major covariates.

Cancer of the Colorectum

Besides the possible protective benefit of antioxidant and antimutagenic compounds with potential anticarcinogenic effects, there are other actions of coffee drinking in the colon that might reduce the risk of colorectal cancer. These include a reduction in bile acid secretion and an increase in colonic motility.

A pooled analysis of 13 cohort studies, including about 5600 incident colon cancer cases, found an overall RR of 1.07 (95 % CI 0.89–1.30) for coffee consumption of >6 cups/day versus nondrinkers. The RR did not differ by sex, smoking status, alcohol consumption, body mass index, physical activity, or tumor site [38]. Of the two cohort studies published after the pooled analysis, the NIH-AARP Diet and Health Study found a moderate inverse association [39], while the National Cancer Institute's Prostate, Lung, Colorectal, and Ovarian Cancer Screening Trial found no relationship [40]. A meta-analysis of case–control studies on coffee consumption and colorectal cancer risk, including 24 studies for a total of 14,846 cases of colorectal, colon, or rectal cancer, suggests an overall moderately favorable effect of coffee consumption [41]. The OR for an increment of 1 cup/day of coffee was 0.94 (95 % CI 0.91–0.98). Compared with non-/low drinkers, the highest coffee drinkers had ORs of 0.70 (95 % CI 0.60–0.81) for colorectal cancer, 0.75 (95 % CI 0.64–0.88) for colon, and 0.87 (95 % CI 0.75–1.00) for rectal cancer. The reduced risk was consistent across study design (hospital versus population based), geographic area, and various confounding factors [41]. The inverse relationship found in case–control studies might reflect a real association, or reverse causation, i.e., decreased coffee consumption among cases following the onset of intestinal symptoms.

In summary, cohort studies indicate no consistent association, whereas case–control studies suggest that coffee has some favorable effect. These discrepant results leave the issue still open to discussion.

Cancer of the Liver

It has been suggested that chlorogenic acid and other antioxidants from coffee beans inhibit liver carcinogenesis. Studies in cell cultures and animal models have pointed to potential anticarcinogenic effects of cafestol and kahweol against aflatoxin B1-induced genotoxicity, although it is not clear if these compounds reach sufficient levels for such action after coffee intake. Coffee may help to prevent type 2 diabetes, a known risk factor for liver cancer, and coffee drinking has been inversely related to the activity of glutamyl transferase and alanine transferase, indicators of liver status, and also with the risk for developing cirrhosis [42].

A meta-analysis of eight cohort and eight case–control studies, including a total of 3153 cases of liver cancer, found a summary RR of 0.60 (95 % CI 0.50–0.71) for coffee drinkers versus nondrinkers (0.64 from cohort and 0.56 from case–control studies) [43]. The inverse relationship persisted after adjusting for major risk factors for liver cancer (such as hepatitis B and C, liver cirrhosis, other liver diseases, alcohol drinking, and tobacco smoking) and was consistent across various subjects at increased risk of liver cancer (such as history of hepatitis infection, other liver diseases, and alcohol drinking). The RR for an increment of 1 cup/day of coffee was 0.80 (95 % CI 0.77–0.84) [43]. A recent publication on a cohort of Finnish male smokers with a low prevalence of HBV and HCV confirmed the results of the meta-analysis [44]. Compared with men drinking <1 cup/day of coffee, drinkers of >2 cups/day had a 50 % reduction in risk of liver cancer. Moreover, men drinking >4 cups/day had a 90 % reduction of mortality for chronic liver diseases. The inverse associations were consistent during the follow-up period and across strata of history of diabetes, age, body mass index, serum cholesterol levels, the amount of alcohol consumed, and cigarette smoking [44].

Thus, several lines of evidence suggest that coffee drinking really does reduce liver cancer incidence. The key evidence is as follows: the dose relationship, the biological plausibility, and the consistency of clinical and epidemiological evidence from liver enzymes to cirrhosis to liver cancer [45]. However, reverse causation (i.e., decreased coffee consumption among cases following the onset of liver symptoms) cannot be excluded. It is important to emphasize, however, that about 90 % of cases of primary liver cancer worldwide can be avoided through alcohol drinking reduction, hepatitis B vaccination, and control of hepatitis C transmission.

Cancer of the Pancreas

In the early 1980s, a case–control study found that consumption of 3 or more cups/day of coffee increased the risk of pancreatic cancer about threefold, independently of cigarette smoking [46]. However, findings in more recent studies have failed to confirm this. A meta-analysis, based on 37 case–control and 17 cohort studies and including a total of 10,594 pancreatic cancer cases, found an overall RR of 1.13 (95 % CI 0.99–1.29) for the highest versus lowest coffee intake [47]. The pooled RRs were 1.25 (95 % CI 0.96–1.63) in the 17 studies that did not adjust for tobacco smoking and 1.08 (95 % CI 0.94–1.25) for the 37 studies that did adjust for it. These findings were consistent across strata of sex, geographic region, type of controls, and other covariates. The pooled RRs for an increment of 1 cup/day of coffee was 1.03 (95 % CI 0.99–1.06), based on the smoking-adjusting studies [47]. A pooled analysis, published after the meta-analysis and including data from 14 cohort studies and 2185 incident pancreatic cancer cases, found a multivariate overall RR of 1.10 (95 % CI 0.81–1.48) in drinkers of ≥900 g/day of coffee beverage compared with nondrinkers [48]. The lack of an association was consistent across levels of sex, smoking status, and body mass index. Thus, the evidence as a whole suggests a lack of any clear relationship between coffee drinking and pancreatic cancer risk.

Cancer of the Endometrium

Caffeine intake has been directly associated with sex hormone-binding globulin levels and inversely to bioavailable testosterone. These changes may be protective against endometrial cancer. Coffee drinking has been inversely related to the risk of type 2 diabetes, a risk factor for endometrial cancer; this association is independent of measures of overweight and obesity.

A meta-analysis, including two cohort (201 cases) and seven case–control studies (2409 cases), found an overall RR of 0.80 (95 % CI 0.68–0.94) for coffee drinkers versus nondrinkers [49]. The summary RR was 0.87 (95 % CI 0.78–0.97) for low-to-moderate drinking and 0.64 (95 % CI 0.48–0.86) for heavy drinking, and the RR for an increase of 1 cup/day was 0.93 (95 % CI 0.89–0.97). This indicates a dose-dependent inverse relationship between coffee intake and endometrial cancer risk. A recent meta-analysis, which included ten case–control and six cohort studies and 6628 endometrial cancer cases, found a pooled RR for the highest versus the lowest categories of coffee drinking of 0.71 (95 % CI 0.62–0.81; 0.69 for case–control studies and 0.70 for cohort studies) [50]. The pooled RR for an increment of 1 cup/day of coffee was 0.92 (95 % CI 0.90–0.95).

The results of cohort and case–control studies, together with the potential biological mechanisms, therefore, suggest that coffee is protective against endometrial cancer. However, it cannot be excluded that the inverse association between coffee and risk of the cancer may in part be due to residual confounding from diabetes.

Cancer of the Bladder

Caffeine and other substances contained in coffee have a wide spectrum of direct and indirect metabolic activities. This might induce changes in the levels of carcinogens or anticarcinogens in the bladder epithelium, since most substances or metabolites are secreted through the urinary tract and are consequently in direct contact with the bladder mucosa.

A monograph of the International Agency for Research on Cancer (IARC) summarized the results of 22 studies published before 1990 [51]. A moderately increased risk of bladder cancer in coffee drinkers compared to nondrinkers was reported in 16 studies; the direct relationship was significant in seven of these and showed a dose–risk relation in three studies. No association was observed in the other six studies. As smoking is an important risk factor for bladder cancer, lifelong non-smokers were also considered separately to obtain information on the potential distorting effect of tobacco. The relationship with coffee was still observed, although it was less clear, in part because of the smaller numbers.

After the publication of this report, many other studies provided information on the relationship between coffee and bladder cancer. In a pooled analysis of ten European studies, including 564 cases, there was no excess risk in ever drinkers of coffee (RR 1.0); a significant excess risk was seen in subjects drinking ≥10 cups/day (RR 1.8, 95 % CI 1.0–3.3), with no linear relationship with dose or duration, and a small excess risk in nonsmokers who were also heavy drinkers of coffee [52]. A meta-analysis, which included 3 cohort and 34 case–control studies, found an overall RR for drinkers versus nondrinkers of 1.18 (95 % CI 1.03–1.36) for coffee and 1.18 (95 % CI 0.99–1.40) for decaffeinated coffee [53]. The RR was 1.26 (95 % CI 1.09–1.46) for studies considering only men and 1.08 (nonsignificant) for those considering only women. A later review included 4 cohort and 17 case–control studies published between 1991 and 2007 [54]. Three cohort studies found a nonsignificant increased risk, and one study found a significant decreased risk only in women. Among the 17 case–control studies, 8 found a moderate statistically significant increased risk, with a dose–risk relation in three studies.

Thus, the overall data on the relationship between coffee and risk of bladder cancer excludes a strong association. It is not clear whether the weak direct association reported in many studies is causal. Possible sources of residual confounding, partly responsible for the direct relationship, might include smoking, exposure to chemicals at work, and diet. However, residual confounding is unlikely to completely explain the association, leaving the issue still open.

Other Cancers

The evidence on the relationship of coffee drinking with cancer at other anatomical sites is reassuring. A modest inverse association has been reported for coffee intake with advanced or fatal cases of prostate cancer [55, 56]. No association has been reported with cancer of the esophagus [31], stomach [57], larynx [31, 32, 41], lung in nonsmokers [58], breast [59], ovary [60], kidney [61], brain [62], and thyroid [63]. The information is scanty but reassuring for gallbladder and biliary tract cancers, melanoma, cervical cancer, lymphomas, and sarcomas.

Conclusions for Cancer

Coffee drinking does not increase cancer risk, except for a possible weak increase of bladder cancer, whose causality is uncertain. No association was found with the most frequent cancers, such as cancers of the breast, lung, colorectum, and prostate, while coffee may have favorable effects on the risk of cancer of the oral cavity and pharynx, liver, and endometrium.

Neurologic Diseases

A few studies have shown a weak inverse association between moderate coffee intake and cognitive impairment. A meta-analysis of nine cohort and two case–control studies reported a RR of 0.84 (95 % CI 0.72–0.99) for the highest versus lowest coffee consumption; the RR was 0.93 (95 % CI 0.83–1.04) in cohort and 0.49 (95 % CI 0.31–0.79) in case–control studies [64]. The RR was 0.62 (95 % CI 0.45–0.87) for Alzheimer's disease (based on two cohort and two case–control studies), while there was no relationship for other types of cognitive impairment. However, a cohort study found a favorable effect of coffee only in the 0–4 years of follow-up and no relation in the long term [65]. Thus, although overall evidence suggests a weak protection, data are still inconclusive. Moreover, causality is still uncertain because of the inconsistency of results in the two study designs and because healthier subjects, living longer, usually drink more coffee.

A weak protection of coffee intake on the risk of Parkinson's disease has been observed in a meta-analysis summarizing the results of 7 cohort studies, 16 case–control studies, 2 case–control studies nested in a cohort, and one cross-sectional study [66]. The RR was 0.75 (95 % CI 0.68–0.82) for the highest intake compared with the lowest one, with a dose–exposure relationship. Conceivably, withdrawal from coffee might be an early indicator of the disease. If true, that would argue against the hypothesis of a causal relationship. However, the favorable effect has only been seen in cohort studies (RR 0.80, 95 % CI 0.71–0.90), where exposure has been recorded a long time before the onset of the disease.

Osteoporosis

Elevated caffeine levels increase the release of calcium from bones to balance circulating calcium levels. However, with a moderate coffee intake, calcium balance is relatively stable. A meta-analysis summarizing the results of 14 epidemiological studies found no association between coffee intake and risk of osteoporosis or fractures [67].

Pregnancy and Breastfeeding

During the last trimester of pregnancy, caffeine metabolism and elimination are slowed by about 15-fold. Caffeine passes freely across the placental barrier; the fetus does not express the main enzymes to inactivate it, and caffeine metabolites may accumulate in the fetal brain.

The issue of the safety of coffee consumption during pregnancy has been considered in many papers. The risks considered are miscarriage, stillbirth, preterm delivery, low birth weight, and giving birth to a small-for-gestational-age baby. However, the interpretation of data is limited by measurement errors and by the confounding by pregnancy symptoms (such as nausea and vomiting), which limits coffee drinking, and environmental factors (such as smoking which is often associated with coffee drinking) [68]. A recent large prospective investigation concluded that coffee intake was not related to spontaneous preterm delivery, while it was associated with marginally increased gestational length, decreased birth weight, and increased risk of giving birth to a small-for-gestational-age baby [68]. A recent meta-analysis found that, for an increment of caffeine intake of 100 mg/day, the RRs were 1.14 (95 % CI 1.10–1.19) for miscarriage (based on 14 prospective and 12 case–control studies), 1.19 (95 % CI 1.05–1.35) for stillbirth (based on 3 prospective and 2 case–control studies),

1.07 (95 % CI 1.01–1.12) for low birth weight (based on 6 prospective and 5 case–control studies), and 1.10 (95 % CI 1.06–1.14) for small-for-gestational-age birth (based on 10 prospective and 5 case–control studies) [69]. No relation was found with preterm delivery (RR 1.02, 95 % CI 0.98–1.06). A Cochrane evaluation of clinical trials found one study only [70] and reported that no conclusions can be reached as there is insufficient evidence of the effect of caffeine on birth weight or other pregnancy outcomes [71]. Thus, the evidence suggests a potentially harmful effect of coffee during pregnancy. Consequently, in the absence of solid evidence, coffee drinking should be kept to a low level. The American College of Obstetricians and Gynecologists, the Nordic Nutrition Recommendations, and the Norwegian Food Safety Authority recommend a caffeine intake below 200 mg/day (less than 2 cups of coffee) for pregnant women [68].

Caffeine is found in breast milk after ingestion of coffee. There is no clear information on the effect of caffeine in the breastfed baby, except for irritability. However, caffeine is metabolized very slowly by young children; thus, an accumulation is possible after high maternal ingestion. Maternal drinking over 3 cups/day may reduce the absorption of iron and other minerals in the newborn. A low consumption of coffee during breastfeeding is therefore recommended.

Conclusion

How can we answer the question "is coffee healthy"? The main points of this question are summarized in Table 3.3.

Table 3.3 Impact of coffee intake on human health

Favorable effects on	• Total mortality
	• Oral and pharyngeal cancer incidence
	• Endometrial cancer incidence
	• Liver cancer incidence
	• Liver cirrhosis incidence
	• Type 2 diabetes incidence and mortality
	• Stroke incidence
	• Alzheimer's disease
	• Parkinson's disease
Unfavorable effects on	• Short-term increase in blood pressure
	• Moderate if any increase in bladder cancer incidence
Coffee intake should be avoided/limited in	• Children
	• Pregnant and lactating women
	• Patients with liver cirrhosis
	• Patients with gastritis and ulcer
	• People who metabolize caffeine slowly

Is Coffee Dangerous for Health?

As far as we know, the only coffee component having a potential unfavorable effect on health is caffeine. The chemical can weakly increase blood pressure in the short term, but it has no long-term effect on risk of CVD. Caffeine intake (and consequently caffeinated coffee intake) should be minimized in children and in pregnant and lactating women, and it should be limited by those who metabolize it slowly, that is all those who empirically "feel that caffeine has strong effects." Caffeine intake should also be reduced in patients with specific diseases, such as gastritis and peptic ulcers. The only potentially dangerous effect of coffee not dependent on caffeine is the weak, if any, increase of bladder cancer risk; however, the causality of this association is still uncertain.

Does Coffee Consumption Improve Our Health?

Caffeine reduces tiredness and reaction time and increases alertness, digestion, and gastrointestinal motility; it has ergogenic and anti-inflammatory effects and potentiates analgesic effects of salicylates and nonsteroidal anti-inflammatory drugs. Coffee is a major contributor of dietary antioxidants, even in populations with high intakes of fruit and vegetables. Coffee components other than caffeine are probably responsible for the potentially favorable effect of coffee on total mortality, the incidence of stroke, type 2 diabetes, liver cirrhosis, and Alzheimer's and Parkinson's diseases and of cancers of the oral cavity and pharynx, liver, and endometrium. The causality of these associations is still uncertain as reverse causation may be responsible, at least to some degree.

Summarizing the above, a moderate intake of coffee up to 3 cups/day in healthy people is not dangerous, while it can even have some favorable effects on health.

References

1. Viani R. The composition of coffee. In: Garattini S, editor. Caffeine, coffee, and health. New York: Raven; 1993. p. 17–41.
2. Sharwood LN, Elkington J, Meuleners L, Ivers R, Boufous S, Stevenson M. Use of caffeinated substances and risk of crashes in long distance drivers of commercial vehicles: case–control study. BMJ. 2013;346:f1140.
3. Arria AM, O'Brien MC. The "high" risk of energy drinks. JAMA. 2011;305:600–1.
4. Freedman ND, Park Y, Abnet CC, Hollenbeck AR, Sinha R. Association of coffee drinking with total and cause-specific mortality. N Engl J Med. 2012;366:1891–904.
5. Malerba S, Turati F, Galeone C, et al. A meta-analysis of prospective studies of coffee consumption and mortality for all causes, cancers and cardiovascular diseases. Eur J Epidemiol. 2013;28:527–39.
6. Liu J, Lavie CJ, Hebert JR, Earnest CP, Blair SN. Association of coffee consumption with all-cause and cardiovascular disease mortality. Mayo Clin Proc. 2013;88:1066–74.

7. Je Y, Giovannucci E. Coffee consumption and total mortality: a meta-analysis of twenty prospective cohort studies. Br J Nutr. 2014;111:1162–73.
8. O'Keefe JH, Bhatti SK, Patil HR, DiNicolantonio JJ, Lucan SC, Lavie CJ. Effects of habitual coffee consumption on cardiometabolic disease, cardiovascular health, and all-cause mortality. J Am Coll Cardiol. 2013;62:1043–51.
9. James JE. Is habitual caffeine use a preventable cardiovascular risk factor? Lancet. 1997;349:279–81.
10. Noordzij M, Uiterwaal CS, Arends LR, Kok FJ, Grobbee DE, Geleijnse JM. Blood pressure response to chronic intake of coffee and caffeine: a meta-analysis of randomized controlled trials. J Hypertens. 2005;23:921–8.
11. Zhang Z, Hu G, Caballero B, Appel L, Chen L. Habitual coffee consumption and risk of hypertension: a systematic review and meta-analysis of prospective observational studies. Am J Clin Nutr. 2011;93:1212–9.
12. Winkelmayer WC, Stampfer MJ, Willett WC, Curhan GC. Habitual caffeine intake and the risk of hypertension in women. JAMA. 2005;294:2330–5.
13. Mesas AE, Leon-Munoz LM, Rodriguez-Artalejo F, Lopez-Garcia E. The effect of coffee on blood pressure and cardiovascular disease in hypertensive individuals: a systematic review and meta-analysis. Am J Clin Nutr. 2011;94:1113–26.
14. Jee SH, He J, Appel LJ, Whelton PK, Suh I, Klag MJ. Coffee consumption and serum lipids: a meta-analysis of randomized controlled clinical trials. Am J Epidemiol. 2001;153:353–62.
15. Cai L, Ma D, Zhang Y, Liu Z, Wang P. The effect of coffee consumption on serum lipids: a meta-analysis of randomized controlled trials. Eur J Clin Nutr. 2012;66:872–7.
16. Ding M, Bhupathiraju SN, Chen M, van Dam RM, Hu FB. Caffeinated and decaffeinated coffee consumption and risk of type 2 diabetes: a systematic review and a dose–response meta-analysis. Diabetes Care. 2014;37:569–86.
17. Zhang W, Lopez-Garcia E, Li TY, Hu FB, van Dam RM. Coffee consumption and risk of cardiovascular diseases and all-cause mortality among men with type 2 diabetes. Diabetes Care. 2009;32:1043–5.
18. Zhang WL, Lopez-Garcia E, Li TY, Hu FB, van Dam RM. Coffee consumption and risk of cardiovascular events and all-cause mortality among women with type 2 diabetes. Diabetologia. 2009;52:810–7.
19. Crippa A, Discacciati A, Larsson SC, Wolk A, Orsini N. Coffee consumption and mortality from all causes, cardiovascular disease, and cancer: a dose–response meta-analysis. Am J Epidemiol. 2014;180:763–75.
20. Nawrot TS, Perez L, Kunzli N, Munters E, Nemery B. Public health importance of triggers of myocardial infarction: a comparative risk assessment. Lancet. 2011;377:732–40.
21. Ding M, Bhupathiraju SN, Satija A, van Dam RM, Hu FB. Long-term coffee consumption and risk of cardiovascular disease: a systematic review and a dose–response meta-analysis of prospective cohort studies. Circulation. 2014;129:643–59.
22. Silletta MG, Marfisi R, Levantesi G, et al. Coffee consumption and risk of cardiovascular events after acute myocardial infarction: results from the GISSI (Gruppo Italiano per lo Studio della Sopravvivenza nell'Infarto miocardico)-Prevenzione trial. Circulation. 2007;116:2944–51.
23. Kawachi I, Colditz GA, Stone CB. Does coffee drinking increase the risk of coronary heart disease? Results from a meta-analysis. Br Heart J. 1994;72:269–75.
24. Sofi F, Conti AA, Gori AM, et al. Coffee consumption and risk of coronary heart disease: a meta-analysis. Nutr Metab Cardiovasc Dis. 2007;17:209–23.
25. Wu JN, Ho SC, Zhou C, et al. Coffee consumption and risk of coronary heart diseases: a meta-analysis of 21 prospective cohort studies. Int J Cardiol. 2009;137:216–25.
26. Mostofsky E, Rice MS, Levitan EB, Mittleman MA. Habitual coffee consumption and risk of heart failure: a dose–response meta-analysis. Circ Heart Fail. 2012;5:401–5.
27. Myers MG. Caffeine and cardiac arrhythmias. Ann Intern Med. 1991;114:147–50.
28. Caldeira D, Martins C, Alves LB, Pereira H, Ferreira JJ, Costa J. Caffeine does not increase the risk of atrial fibrillation: a systematic review and meta-analysis of observational studies. Heart. 2013;99:1383–9.

29. Larsson SC, Orsini N. Coffee consumption and risk of stroke: a dose–response meta-analysis of prospective studies. Am J Epidemiol. 2011;174:993–1001.
30. Kokubo Y, Iso H, Saito I, et al. The impact of green tea and coffee consumption on the reduced risk of stroke incidence in Japanese population: the Japan public health center-based study cohort. Stroke. 2013;44:1369–74.
31. Turati F, Galeone C, La Vecchia C, Garavello W, Tavani A. Coffee and cancers of the upper digestive and respiratory tracts: meta-analyses of observational studies. Ann Oncol. 2011;22:536–44.
32. Galeone C, Tavani A, Pelucchi C, et al. Coffee and tea intake and risk of head and neck cancer: pooled analysis in the international head and neck cancer epidemiology consortium. Cancer Epidemiol Biomarkers Prev. 2010;19:1723–36.
33. Biazevic MG, Toporcov TN, Antunes JL, et al. Cumulative coffee consumption and reduced risk of oral and oropharyngeal cancer. Nutr Cancer. 2011;63:350–6.
34. Hildebrand JS, Patel AV, McCullough ML, et al. Coffee, tea, and fatal oral/pharyngeal cancer in a large prospective US cohort. Am J Epidemiol. 2013;177:50–8.
35. Radoi L, Paget-Bailly S, Menvielle G, et al. Tea and coffee consumption and risk of oral cavity cancer: results of a large population-based case–control study, the ICARE study. Cancer Epidemiol. 2013;37:284–9.
36. Ren JS, Freedman ND, Kamangar F, et al. Tea, coffee, carbonated soft drinks and upper gastrointestinal tract cancer risk in a large United States prospective cohort study. Eur J Cancer. 2010;46:1873–81.
37. Tavani A, Galeone C, Turati F, Cavalli L, Vecchia CL. Epidemiological evidence on the relation between coffee intake and the risk of head and neck cancer. In: Preedy VR, editor. Coffee in health and disease prevention. New York: Elsevier; 2014. p. 349–58.
38. Zhang X, Albanes D, Beeson WL, et al. Risk of colon cancer and coffee, tea, and sugar-sweetened soft drink intake: pooled analysis of prospective cohort studies. J Natl Cancer Inst. 2010;102:771–83.
39. Sinha R, Cross AJ, Daniel CR, et al. Caffeinated and decaffeinated coffee and tea intakes and risk of colorectal cancer in a large prospective study. Am J Clin Nutr. 2012;96:374–81.
40. Dominianni C, Huang WY, Berndt S, Hayes RB, Ahn J. Prospective study of the relationship between coffee and tea with colorectal cancer risk: the PLCO Cancer Screening Trial. Br J Cancer. 2013;109:1352–9.
41. Galeone C, Turati F, La Vecchia C, Tavani A. Coffee consumption and risk of colorectal cancer: a meta-analysis of case–control studies. Cancer Causes Control. 2010;21:1949–59.
42. Klatsky AL, Morton C, Udaltsova N, Friedman GD. Coffee, cirrhosis, and transaminase enzymes. Arch Intern Med. 2006;166:1190–5.
43. Bravi E, Bosetti C, Tavani A, Gallus S, La Vecchia C. Coffee reduces risk for hepatocellular carcinoma: an updated meta-analysis. Clin Gastroenterol Hepatol. 2013;11:1413–21.
44. Lai GY, Weinstein SJ, Albanes D, et al. The association of coffee intake with liver cancer incidence and chronic liver disease mortality in male smokers. Br J Cancer. 2013;109:1344–51.
45. Hu G, Tuomilehto J, Pukkala E, et al. Joint effects of coffee consumption and serum gamma-glutamyltransferase on the risk of liver cancer. Hepatology. 2008;48:129–36.
46. MacMahon B, Yen S, Trichopoulos D, Warren K, Nardi G. Coffee and cancer of the pancreas. N Engl J Med. 1981;304:630–3.
47. Turati F, Galeone C, Edefonti V, et al. A meta-analysis of coffee consumption and pancreatic cancer. Ann Oncol. 2012;23:311–8.
48. Genkinger JM, Li R, Spiegelman D, et al. Coffee, tea, and sugar-sweetened carbonated soft drink intake and pancreatic cancer risk: a pooled analysis of 14 cohort studies. Cancer Epidemiol Biomarkers Prev. 2012;21:305–18.
49. Bravi F, Scotti L, Bosetti C, et al. Coffee drinking and endometrial cancer risk: a metaanalysis of observational studies. Am J Obstet Gynecol. 2009;200:130–5.
50. Je Y, Giovannucci E. Coffee consumption and risk of endometrial cancer: findings from a large up-to-date meta-analysis. Int J Cancer. 2012;131:1700–10.

51. IARC. Coffee, tea, mate, methylxanthines and methylglyoxal, IARC monographs on the evaluation of carcinogenic risks to humans. Lyon: IARC; 1991.

52. Sala M, Cordier S, Chang-Claude J, et al. Coffee consumption and bladder cancer in nonsmokers: a pooled analysis of case–control studies in European countries. Cancer Causes Control. 2000;11:925–31.

53. Zeegers MP, Tan FE, Goldbohm RA, van den Brandt PA. Are coffee and tea consumption associated with urinary tract cancer risk? A systematic review and meta-analysis. Int J Epidemiol. 2001;30:353–62.

54. Pelucchi C, La Vecchia C. Alcohol, coffee, and bladder cancer risk: a review of epidemiological studies. Eur J Cancer Prev. 2009;18:62–8.

55. Discacciati A, Orsini N, Andersson SO, et al. Coffee consumption and risk of localized, advanced and fatal prostate cancer: a population-based prospective study. Ann Oncol. 2013;24:1912–8.

56. Bosire C, Stampfer MJ, Subar AF, Wilson KM, Park Y, Sinha R. Coffee consumption and the risk of overall and fatal prostate cancer in the NIH-AARP Diet and Health Study. Cancer Causes Control. 2013;24:1527–34.

57. Botelho F, Lunet N, Barros H. Coffee and gastric cancer: systematic review and meta-analysis. Cad Saude Publica. 2006;22:889–900.

58. Tang N, Wu Y, Ma J, Wang B, Yu R. Coffee consumption and risk of lung cancer: a meta-analysis. Lung Cancer. 2010;67:17–22.

59. Gierach GL, Freedman ND, Andaya A, et al. Coffee intake and breast cancer risk in the NIH-AARP diet and health study cohort. Int J Cancer. 2012;131:452–60.

60. Steevens J, Schouten LJ, Verhage BA, Goldbohm RA, van den Brandt PA. Tea and coffee drinking and ovarian cancer risk: results from the Netherlands Cohort Study and a meta-analysis. Br J Cancer. 2007;97:1291–4.

61. Lee JE, Hunter DJ, Spiegelman D, et al. Intakes of coffee, tea, milk, soda and juice and renal cell cancer in a pooled analysis of 13 prospective studies. Int J Cancer. 2007;121:2246–53.

62. Malerba S, Galeone C, Pelucchi C, et al. A meta-analysis of coffee and tea consumption and the risk of glioma in adults. Cancer Causes Control. 2013;24:267–76.

63. Mack WJ, Preston-Martin S, Dal Maso L, et al. A pooled analysis of case–control studies of thyroid cancer: cigarette smoking and consumption of alcohol, coffee, and tea. Cancer Causes Control. 2003;14:773–85.

64. Santos C, Costa J, Santos J, Vaz-Carneiro A, Lunet N. Caffeine intake and dementia: systematic review and meta-analysis. J Alzheimers Dis. 2010;20 Suppl 1:S187–204.

65. Mirza SS, Tiemeier H, de Bruijn RF, et al. Coffee consumption and incident dementia. Eur J Epidemiol. 2014;29:735–41.

66. Costa J, Lunet N, Santos C, Santos J, Vaz-Carneiro A. Caffeine exposure and the risk of Parkinson's disease: a systematic review and meta-analysis of observational studies. J Alzheimers Dis. 2010;20 Suppl 1:S221–38.

67. Sheng J, Qu X, Zhang X, et al. Coffee, tea, and the risk of hip fracture: a meta-analysis. Osteoporos Int. 2014;25:141–50.

68. Sengpiel V, Elind E, Bacelis J, et al. Maternal caffeine intake during pregnancy is associated with birth weight but not with gestational length: results from a large prospective observational cohort study. BMC Med. 2013;11:42.

69. Greenwood DC, Thatcher NJ, Ye J, et al. Caffeine intake during pregnancy and adverse birth outcomes: a systematic review and dose–response meta-analysis. Eur J Epidemiol. 2014;29:725–34.

70. Bech BH, Obel C, Henriksen TB, Olsen J. Effect of reducing caffeine intake on birth weight and length of gestation: randomised controlled trial. BMJ. 2007;334:409.

71. Jahanfar S, Jaafar SH. Effects of restricted caffeine intake by mother on fetal, neonatal and pregnancy outcome. Cochrane Database Syst Rev. 2013;2:CD006965.

Chapter 4
Health Benefits of Tea Consumption

Takuji Suzuki, Noriyuki Miyoshi, Sumio Hayakawa, Shinjiro Imai, Mamoru Isemura, and Yoriyuki Nakamura

Keywords Tea • Green tea • Black tea • Polyphenol • (−)-Epigallocatechin gallate • Catechin • Cancer • Obesity

Key Points

1. Tea is manufactured from the leaves of the *Camellia sinensis* Theaceae plant.
2. Tea exhibits anticancer, antiobesity, antiatherosclerotic, antidiabetic, antibacterial, and antiviral effects.
3. Various types of brewed tea are consumed worldwide and may have an impact on human health.
4. Many of the biological effects of tea have been attributed to the activities of (−)-epigallocatechin gallate (EGCG), a major component of tea catechins.
5. The beneficial health effects of tea and EGCG have also been demonstrated in cellular and animal experiments.

T. Suzuki
Faculty of Education, Art and Science, Yamagata University, Yamagata 990-8560, Japan

N. Miyoshi • S. Imai • M. Isemura (⊠) • Y. Nakamura
Graduate School of Nutritional and Environmental Sciences, University of Shizuoka, Shizuoka 422-8526, Japan
e-mail: isemura@u-shizuoka-ken.ac.jp

S. Hayakawa
Department of Cellular and Molecular Medicine, Medical Research Institute, Tokyo Medical and Dental University, Tokyo 113-8510, Japan

© Springer International Publishing Switzerland 2016
T. Wilson, N.J. Temple (eds.), *Beverage Impacts on Health and Nutrition*, Nutrition and Health, DOI 10.1007/978-3-319-23672-8_4

Introduction

Tea, a product of the leaves and buds of the *Camellia sinensis* (Theaceae) plant, is one of the world's most popular beverages. Tea can be broadly classified according to the production method as unfermented (green tea), half-fermented (oolong tea), fully fermented (black tea), or post-fermented (pu-erh tea). Green tea is mainly consumed in Japan and China, whereas black tea is primarily consumed in Western countries, India, and other parts of the world. The global production of green tea accounts for only 20 % of the total amount of tea produced, which is approximately one fourth of that of black tea [1]. However, green tea has been the primary target for investigations on health and nutrition among the various teas as indicated by a search conducted in the PubMed database in January 2015, which showed approximately 6020, 3340, 330, and 100 publications for the keywords "green tea," "black tea," "oolong tea," and "pu-erh tea," respectively. When combined with cancer, for example, the corresponding numbers of publications were approximately 2000, 670, 40, and 10, respectively.

Tea contains various components with potential health-promoting effects. Green tea polyphenols and catechins (Fig. 4.1) are considered to have protective effects against diseases such as cancer, obesity, type 2 diabetes mellitus (T2D), cardiovascular disease (CVD), and atherosclerosis [2–5]. They may also have antibacterial, antiviral, hepatoprotective, and neuroprotective effects. Of these catechins, (−)-epigallocatechin gallate (EGCG) displays the strongest bioactivity. In addition to these

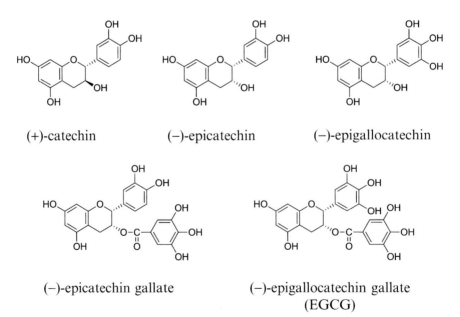

Fig. 4.1 Chemical structure of catechins. (−)-Epicatechin, (−)-epigallocatechin, (−)-epicatechin gallate, and EGCG are major green tea catechins

catechins, black tea and oolong tea contain various bioactive catechin derivatives that are generated during the production process.

Caffeine, another component of tea, induces wakefulness, decreases the sensation of fatigue, and has a diuretic effect. Theanine and γ-aminobutyric acid contained in green tea lower blood pressure and regulate brain function. Vitamin C has antiscorbutic activity and is believed to prevent cataracts and strengthen the immune system [6, 7].

Many studies have investigated the effects of tea on human health. The majority of evidence from cellular and animal experiments indicates that tea has positive effects for human health; however, clinical evidence relating to its effects in humans remains inconclusive. This chapter describes recent advances in studies on the health-promoting effects of drinking tea, especially green tea, with some mechanistic considerations.

Tea Components

Green tea leaves are produced by steaming fresh tea leaves at elevated temperatures to inactivate the enzymes that oxidize polyphenols. Green tea is made by brewing and contains various water-soluble polyphenols such as catechins. The major catechins are (–)-epicatechin, (–)-epicatechin gallate, (–)-epigallocatechin, and EGCG (Fig. 4.1). A single 200 mL cup of green tea supplies 17, 28, 65, and 140 mg of these catechins, respectively [8]. Various other compounds are also present in green tea, including caffeine, theanine, γ-aminobutyric acid, vitamins, theobromine, theophylline, and gallic acids (Table 4.1) [9, 10].

Black tea is made by promoting the enzymatic oxidation of fresh leaves. The total level of the catechins is reduced by this process from 40 % in green tea to 10 % in black tea (Table 4.1). Catechins, theaflavins, and thearubigins may account for 3–10 %, 2–6 %, and greater than 20 % of the dry weight in brewed black tea, respectively [5]. The caffeine content in black tea is similar to that in green tea.

Oolong tea contains monomeric catechins, theaflavins, and thearubigins, and brewed tea may have catechin levels of 8–20 % of the total dry matter [9]. Several polyphenolic derivatives such as theasinensins and chaflosides are also present [5, 11].

Table 4.2 shows the total polyphenol content (the sum of the five catechins listed in Fig. 4.1), ascorbic acid, and caffeine in some of the tea beverages marketed in Japan [12]. A representative Japanese brand of green tea beverage with a high content of catechins contains 154 mg catechins and 23 mg of caffeine per 100 mL. An epidemiological study in Japan revealed that many people drink more than 10 cups per day [13]. Their catechin intake is estimated to be >800 mg/day.

According to data obtained from diet history interviews of 15,371 people across Germany, aged 14–80 years, the mean intakes of total flavanols, flavan-3-ol monomers, proanthocyanidins, and theaflavins were 386, 120, 196, and 70 mg/day, respectively [14]. The major contributor of total flavanols in all subjects was pome fruits (27 %), followed by black tea (25 %).

Table 4.1 Principal components of green and black tea beverage (measured in wt.% of extract solids)

Components	Green tea	Black tea
Catechins	30–42	3–10
Flavanols	5–10	6–8
Other flavonoids	2–4	–
Theogallin	2–3	–
Ascorbic acid	1–2	–
Gallic acid	0.5	–
Quinic acid	2	–
Other organic acids	4–5	–
Theanine	4–6	–
Other amino acids	4–6	13–15
Methylxanthines	7–9	8–11
Carbohydrates	10–15	15
Minerals	6–8	10
Volatiles	0.02	<0.1
Theaflavins	–	3–6
Thearubigins	–	12–18
Caffeine	3–4	3–4

Modified from Shukla [9]

Table 4.2 Contents of tea components in three types of commercial tea beverages (mg/100 mL)

| Component (analytical method) | Tea type | | |
	Green ($n=20$)	Black ($n=3$)	Oolong ($n=8$)
Total polyphenols (Folin–Ciocalteu)	41–83	67–70	39–61
Sum of five catechins listed in Fig. 4.1 (HPLC)	5.2–39.2	4.6–9.2	4.2–14.4
Ascorbic acid (HPLC)	12–68	<0.5–21	<0.5–17
Caffeine (HPLC)	7.2–15.9	12.8–17.4	12.6–18.2

Modified from Shohin Test Hokoku [12]

Health Benefits

Cancer

Epidemiology

The use of epidemiological studies to demonstrate the relationship between consumption of tea and risk of cancer has proven to be challenging. In 1989, Oguni and his colleagues observed that the rate of death from stomach cancer in males in the town of Nakakawane in Japan was approximately one fifth of the average for all Japanese men and suggested that this low rate may have been associated with the consumption of green tea [15]. On the other hand, Tewes et al. [16] carried out a case–control study and reported an increased risk of lung cancer among Chinese

Table 4.3 Studies on tea consumption and the risk of cancer in humans

Site	Type of tea	Cohort studies		Case–control studies	
		Risk reduction	No risk reduction	Risk reduction	No risk reduction
Breast	Green	3	4	3	0
	Black	1	8	1	9
Colon	Green	2	5	4	3
	Black	2	8	4	12
Kidney and bladder	Green	0	1	0	4
	Black	1	4	2	5
Lung	Green	0	3	2	3
	Black	0	8	6	4
Esophagus	Green	0	2	3	4
	Black	0	1	2	1
Ovary	Green	1	0	1	0
	Black	2	3	0	6
Pancreas	Green	0	2	1	1
	Black	0	4	1	3
Prostate	Green	2	0	2	0
	Black	1	2	1	3
Stomach	Green	2	6	8	8
	Black	0	6	4	5
Other	Green	0	2	5	1
	Black	2	3	1	3

The number of studies showing risk reduction or no risk reduction is shown.
Modified from Yang and Hong [5]

women in Hong Kong who drank green tea. Recent large-scale prospective cohort studies reported that tea consumption did not correlate with the risk of stomach cancer [4]. However, a more recent study revealed an inverse association between green tea consumption and distal gastric cancer among Japanese women [17].

Yang et al. [3] summarized the findings that had been reported by 2008 (Table 4.3). These findings suggested that green tea and tea catechins have a preventive action against some types of cancer. Further support has come from more recent results. However, the evidence lacks consistency. More studies are needed, therefore, before we can firmly conclude that green tea is indeed preventive against some types of cancer. It should be noted that the inconsistent findings may be due to several different factors, including the methods of quantifying tea consumption, tea temperature, cigarette smoking, alcohol consumption, and genetic polymorphisms [2–5].

Several human studies reported an inverse relationship between consumption of black tea and the risk of cancer. For example, McCann et al. observed a significant inverse association between the consumption of >2 cups/day black tea and the risk of endometrial cancer [18]. Regular drinking of green tea, black tea, and/or oolong tea was associated with a lower risk of ovarian cancer, with the adjusted odds ratio being

0.29, in a case–control study conducted in southern China [19]. Dietary flavonoid intake and black tea consumption were associated with a decreased risk of advanced prostate cancer in the Netherlands Cohort Study involving 58,000 men [20].

However, many studies have reported no or positive associations between drinking black tea and risk of cancer [21–24]. For example, a meta-analysis based on 24 case–control and cohort studies showed no significant association against esophageal cancer risk for the highest versus non-/lowest intake of black tea [22]. In a cohort study among Chinese men in Singapore, a statistically significant positive association of black tea intake with prostate cancer risk was observed when comparing those with daily intake versus no intake [23]. Similarly, in a case–control study conducted in Taiwan, the odds ratio of bladder cancer for drinkers of oolong tea was 3.0 and was 14.9 for drinkers of black and/or green tea, relative to nondrinkers of tea [25]. Whether the apparently harmful effects of drinking black tea are limited to cancer at a few specific sites needs to be clarified in future studies.

There have been few studies regarding the effects of oolong tea on risk of cancer or other diseases, perhaps owing to low global consumption.

Intervention Studies

Intervention studies may also provide useful information for the chemopreventive effects of tea or tea components. Yamane [26] reported that the administration of green tea powder capsules was effective in reducing the number of recurrent polyps in patients with adenomatous polyps following colectomy. Shimizu and colleagues [27] also demonstrated that green tea extract was an effective supplement for the chemoprevention of metachronous colorectal adenomas.

In a study in Italy, 30 men with high-grade prostate intraepithelial neoplasias were given 600 mg of green tea catechins daily for 12 months. While only one patient in the treated group developed prostate cancer, nine of the 30 patients in the placebo group developed the disease [28]. This chemopreventive effect was also observed 2 years later in a follow-up study in which 13 subjects in the treated group and 9 in the placebo groups agreed to continue the study [29]. There were one and two newly diagnosed cases of prostate cancer in the treated and placebo groups, respectively. The statistical analysis indicated that the catechin treatment led to an overall 80 % reduction in prostate cancer diagnosis.

The standardized green tea polyphenol preparation Polyphenon® E has been examined in many clinical trials and approved for the treatment of genital warts by the US Food and Drug Administration [4]. More than 30 human trials with Polyphenon or sinecatechins are in progress [30]. Many findings are encouraging, and this is leading to further clinical studies on the chemopreventive effects of tea catechins and their derivatives.

Animal Studies

Carcinogen-induced carcinogenesis is markedly reduced in animal models following the intake of green tea or catechins. In addition, the growth and metastasis of inoculated cancer cells were inhibited by the consumption of tea and tea catechins [2–5]. However, several other animal experiments have failed to show anticancer activity of green tea or catechins [5].

Mechanisms of Anticancer Activity

(a) Apoptosis induction by EGCG

The major compound contributing to the anticancer activity of green tea was shown to be EGCG in most cases [2–5]. One of the leading candidates for the mechanism of action involves apoptosis, i.e., programmed cell death. Apoptosis is physiological cell death by which unnecessary cells are eliminated. The induction of apoptosis in cancer cells leads to the prevention of cancer development, and many anticancer drugs are known to induce apoptosis in cancer cells [4].

A study tested the effect of the peroral administration of EGCG in rats after they were treated with azoxymethane, a chemical that causes colon cancer in these animals. EGCG was apparently protective in two ways: it significantly reduced the number of colonic aberrant crypt foci (a precancerous lesion) and also increased apoptosis [4]. Gupta and colleagues [31] demonstrated that green tea catechins significantly inhibited cancer development, increased survival rates, and induced apoptosis in prostate cancer cells in an experimental animal model that spontaneously develops metastatic prostate cancer [31].

EGCG has been shown to induce apoptosis by binding to a cell surface protein called Fas in cultured human leukemia cells [4]. This binding causes the activation of protease caspase-8, which activates a caspase-dependent deoxyribonuclease that degrades DNA leading to cell death. Tachibana [32] also reported that a cell surface protein called 67 kDa laminin receptor was involved in EGCG-induced apoptosis. EGCG has a stronger apoptosis-inducing effect on cancer cells than on normal cells [2, 4], which is desirable for anticancer drugs.

Another mechanism for EGCG-induced apoptosis has recently been proposed. MicroRNA, referred to as miRNA, is a single strand RNA that contains 20–25 nucleotides. EGCG was found to induce apoptosis in hepatoma cells by upregulating the miRNA named miR-16, which led to the downregulation of the antiapoptotic protein Bcl-2 [33]. The involvement of miRNA in EGCG-induced apoptosis has also been reported in other tumor cells [34]. These and other effects of EGCG epigenetic regulation may be involved in various mechanisms including the induction of apoptosis; this has been comprehensively reviewed by Pan et al. [35].

Theaflavin and theaflavin digallate were shown to induce apoptosis in certain tumor cells, and this may be related to the anticancer action of black tea [36]. These mechanisms include cell-cycle inhibition [37] and the involvement of Fas/caspase-8 and Akt/pBad pathways [38].

Pan et al. [39] demonstrated the induction of apoptosis by the oolong tea polyphenol theasinensin A through the release of cytochrome c and activation of caspases 9 and 3.

(b) Other anticancer mechanisms

Several lines of evidence have indicated that EGCG elicits anticancer activity by mechanisms other than the induction of apoptosis. These include antioxidative actions, the inhibition of cell-cycle progression, inhibition of nuclear factor κB, activation of the mitogen-activated protein kinase cascade, and epigenetic modifications [3–5].

The antibacterial action of EGCG against *Helicobacter pylori* may also contribute to the preventive effect of green tea against gastric cancer [2]. Many of these events may be related to the induction of apoptosis.

Chiang et al. [40] demonstrated that supplementation with pu-erh tea suppressed fatty acid synthase (Fasn) expression in the rat liver by downregulating Akt and JNK signaling, as demonstrated in human hepatoma HepG2 cells. Fasn is a key enzyme in lipogenesis and may be a target for anticancer drugs [41]. Pu-erh tea may therefore have both antiobesity and anticancer actions.

(c) Activity of other tea components

Other tea components may also have anticancer activities. Aqueous nondialyzable high molecular weight components derived from green tea, black tea, oolong tea, and pu-erh tea have been shown to induce apoptosis [4]. These components may inhibit tumorigenesis at the initiation stage because they inhibit the AP-1 transcription activity of tumor cells.

The risk of sunlight-induced nonmelanoma skin cancer may be reduced by caffeine through a mechanism that includes the inhibition of thymine dimer formation and induction of apoptosis [42]. Caffeine may exhibit anticancer properties by inducing apoptosis [43].

Antimetastatic Effect

Green tea and tea catechins have been shown to inhibit tumor metastasis in animal experiments [3, 4]. The mechanisms responsible for this effect may include antioxidative activity, the inhibition of matrix metalloproteinase (MMP) activity, and induction of apoptosis [3, 4]. Membrane-type 1 MMP (MT1-MMP), which hydrolyzes type I collagen and activates MMP-2, is deeply involved in angiogenesis as well as in tumor cell invasion and metastasis. Previous studies demonstrated that EGCG inhibited the enzymatic activity and gene expression of MT1-MMP and angiogenesis [3, 4].

EGCG was shown to inhibit the adhesion of tumor cells to fibronectin and laminin [4]. EGCG also inhibited the spreading of tumor cells on the fibrinogen substratum [44]. These activities may contribute to the antimetastatic action of EGCG [4].

The Metabolic Syndrome (MetS)

The MetS is a cluster of associated variables including body mass index (BMI), body fat, waist circumference, blood pressure, triglycerides, HDL cholesterol, blood glucose concentration, and hemoglobin A1c. The presence of MetS indicates an elevated risk of CVD and T2D. MetS is discussed in more detail in Chap. 13.

Brown et al. [45] reported a reduction in diastolic blood pressure in obese men, aged 40–65 years, who ingested a capsule containing 400 mg of EGCG twice a day for 8 weeks; however, no other significant effects were observed on MetS-related indices such as the insulin resistance index [5]. Epidemiological studies have found no correlation between intake of green tea and MetS [46, 47]. However, in a study examining the association between tea consumption (evaluating hot and iced tea independently) and markers for MetS in a sample of 6472 adults, an inverse association between hot tea intake with MetS markers was observed, which continues to support the protective effects suggested by cell culture and animal studies [48]. It is noteworthy that this association was reversed for iced tea consumption [48]. Thus, the efficacy of tea as a preventive agent for MetS lacks solid supporting evidence.

Obesity

Several lines of research have confirmed the fat-suppressing effects of green tea and tea catechins [4, 5].

Epidemiological and Intervention Studies

An epidemiological study showed that consumption of hot tea was inversely associated with obesity [48]. Tea consumers had significantly lower mean waist circumference and lower BMI than nonconsumers (25 vs. 28 kg/m^2 in men; 26 vs. 29 kg/m^2 in women).

Basu et al. [49] reported that body weight and the blood lipid oxidation index were decreased in patients with the MetS in the USA when they consumed green tea and green tea catechins for 8 weeks. Similarly, in a study on 45 elderly patients with MetS, the green tea group ($n=24$) consumed 3 cups of green tea brewed from 1 g tea bags per day for 60 days. The results showed that the green tea was effective in reducing BMI and waist circumference [50]. Nagao et al. [51] demonstrated that the continuous ingestion of green tea rich in catechins led to a reduction in body fat, systolic blood pressure, and LDL cholesterol. The ingestion of pu-erh tea had significant effects on 36 preobese Japanese adults by reducing the mean waist circumference, BMI, and visceral fat values [52].

In Vitro and Animal Experiments

Findings from several studies suggest that the inhibition of pancreatic lipase may be involved in the antiobesity actions of tea components [53]. EGCG inhibited pancreatic lipase ($IC_{50} = 7.5$ μmol/L) in a noncompetitive manner with respect to substrate concentration; (−)-epicatechin gallate exhibited similar inhibitory activity [54].

The results of animal experiments revealed that a diet with tea catechin enhanced the hepatic gene expression of enzymes involved in β-oxidation [55]. This indicates that tea catechins may reduce body fat by preferentially enhancing the utilization of fat as an energy source.

Tea catechins may inhibit cell growth by suppressing lipogenesis in human MCF-7 breast cancer cells through the downregulation of Fasn gene expression in the nucleus and stimulation of cell energy expenditure in mitochondria [56]. Experimental findings indicated that the molecular mechanism underlying Fasn gene suppression by tea polyphenols (EGCG and theaflavins) may be the downregulation of EGFR/PI3K/Akt/Sp-1 signal transduction pathways. Supplementation with green, black, and pu-erh tea leaves significantly decreased hepatic Fasn mRNA and protein levels in an animal study [57].

A catechin-free fraction of green tea was also shown to reduce the hepatic gene expression in mice of lipogenic enzymes including Fasn [4]. This fraction reduced the gene expression of sterol regulatory element-binding transcription factor (Srebf)1 and/or Srebf2, which suggests that the reduction in Srebfs contributes to the downregulation of lipogenic enzymes. These findings suggest that, in addition to EGCG, green tea contains some component(s) that may help prevent obesity and arteriosclerosis.

Cardiovascular and Related Diseases

In a study to examine the relationship between the consumption of tea beverages and risk of mortality from CVD, the results of one million person-years of follow-up showed that the consumption of coffee, green, and oolong tea and total caffeine intake are associated with a reduced risk of mortality from CVD [4]. When databases were searched for relevant epidemiological and clinical studies published between 1990 and 2004, strong evidence was obtained showing risk reductions in coronary heart disease by intakes of three or more cups per day of black tea and for improved antioxidant status at intakes of one to six cups per day [58].

A recent review described that tea consumption may reduce the risk of stroke [59]. For example, a cohort study examining 75,000 Swedish women and men suggested that the daily consumption of four or more cups of black tea may be inversely associated with the risk of stroke [60]. Pu-erh tea may also be used to reduce the risk of cardiovascular disorders [61]. A comprehensive review has been published that examines the mechanistic aspects responsible [5].

Elevated blood pressure is a major risk factor in the development of cerebrovascular disease. The findings from a recent meta-analysis of randomized controlled studies revealed that consumption of both green tea and black tea significantly reduce blood pressure [62]. Systolic and diastolic blood pressures were lowered by 2.1 and 1.7 mmHg, respectively, by green tea and by 1.4 and 1.1 mmHg, respectively, by black tea. A similar study also showed that regular consumption of black tea reduces blood pressure [63].

Type 2 Diabetes

Epidemiological and Intervention Studies

Several epidemiological studies have described the antidiabetic effects of green tea [4, 5]. Iso and colleagues [64] carried out a large cohort study and found that consumption of green tea, coffee, and total caffeine was associated with a reduced risk of T2D. However, no association was found between consumption of black or oolong teas and risk of T2D. A cohort study conducted in 26 centers in eight European countries, with a total of 340,000 participants and four million person-years of follow-up, revealed that tea consumption was inversely associated with the incidence of T2D; the hazard ratio was 0.84 when participants who drank ≥4 cups of tea per day were compared with nondrinkers [65].

The results of a case–control study conducted in China with 4800 subjects indicated that the consumption of green or rock tea (a kind of oolong tea) may protect against the development of T2D, particularly in those who drink 16–30 cups per week [66]. The results of a study on the relationship between consumption of black tea and a selection of key health indicators in 50 countries showed a significant inverse association between the intake of black tea and prevalence of T2D [67].

The results of an intervention study on 60 residents in Shizuoka Prefecture, Japan, with mild hyperglycemia revealed that the ingestion of green tea extracts decreased the blood levels of hemoglobin A1c, an indicator of glucose control and a marker used to diagnose T2D [68]. Nagao et al. [69] suggested that a catechin-rich beverage may have several therapeutic uses: the prevention of obesity, the recovery of insulin-secretory ability, and maintaining low hemoglobin A1c levels in certain patients with T2D.

Thus, the results of the studies looked at above indicate that tea has beneficial effects on T2D. However, several studies have failed to show such results [70–72]. For example, the results of a cohort study that followed 47,000 participants aged 30–69 years suggested that African American women who drank moderate amounts of caffeinated coffee or alcohol have a reduced risk of T2D, while the intake of decaffeinated coffee and tea was not associated with the risk of T2D [70]. Similarly, an epidemiological study was conducted in Japan with 5897 male and 7643 female subjects [73]. The study showed that green tea, black tea, and oolong tea each had no clear association with T2D in either men or women. Associations were erratic (negative or positive) but with no trends.

In light of these conflicting studies, the possible antidiabetic benefit of tea therefore needs to be clarified. Future studies must pay careful attention to the various confounding factors that may be a source of error.

Cellular and Animal Experiments

T2D is a disease in which there are high blood glucose levels over a prolonged period. Any intervention that reduces aberrantly high levels of glucose may contribute to the disease control. Several mechanisms of action are involved in the effects of tea and catechins, including (1) inhibition of α-amylase activity and glucose absorption [74], which is involved in the production of sugar from starch in digestive secretions, resulting in a reduction in glucose production and uptake in the digestive tract; (2) promotion of glucose intake into skeletal muscle and adipose tissue [75]; (3) enhancement of insulin sensitivity and the protection of pancreatic β-cells [76]; and (4) suppression of hepatic gluconeogenesis (in vivo glucose production from noncarbohydrates) to prevent an increase in postprandial blood glucose levels [4].

It is believed that the increase in endogenous glucose production (i.e., gluconeogenesis in the liver) contributes to the development of hyperglycemia [4]. The rate-controlling gluconeogenic enzymes are phosphoenolpyruvate carboxykinase (PEPCK) and glucose-6-phosphatase (G6Pase). The failure of insulin to regulate the transcription of these enzymes may contribute to T2D [4]. EGCG was shown to mimic the cellular effects of insulin, including its reductive effect on the gene expression of these gluconeogenic enzymes in experiments using rat hepatoma H4IIE cells [4]. In a later animal study, the administration of green tea caused a reduction in the level of mRNA of these enzymes in the liver of normal mice [4]. Wolfram and colleagues [77] demonstrated that EGCG downregulated the gene expression of these enzymes in normal and db/db mice.

One possible mechanism is that tea catechins, including EGCG, suppress the expression of the transcription factors HNF4 and HNF1, which control the expression of gluconeogenic enzymes, leading to their reduced activities and diminished glucose synthesis [4] (Fig. 4.2).

Hepatoprotective Effects

In a study on the galactosamine-induced hepatitis rat model, the oral administration of green tea rich in catechins restored the levels of inflammatory cytokines in the treated group to near control values, suggesting that EGCG may contribute to the

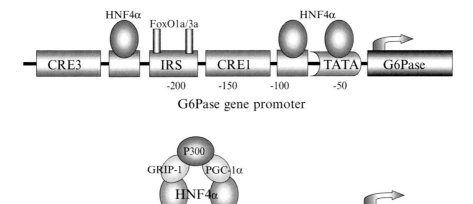

Fig. 4.2 HNF4α-mediated gene expression of gluconeogenic enzymes. *CRE* cyclic AMP responsive element, *DR* direct repeat spaced by one nucleotide, *FoxO* forkhead/winged helix box gene group O, *GRIP* glucocorticoid receptor-interacting protein, *IRS* insulin response sequence, *PGC* peroxisome proliferator-activated receptor-γ coactivator

reduction of inflammation [78]. EGCG was also shown to prevent alcohol-induced liver injury in rats [79]. Tumor necrosis factor-α (TNF-α) protein levels were shown to be increased by alcohol, and this increase was attenuated by the green tea extract. Another study also demonstrated the reducing effect of green tea on TNF-α [80]. In this study the increase in TNF-α protein levels in the mesenteric adipose pad of mice given a high-fat diet was attenuated by daily supplementation with 400 mg green tea extract per kg body weight. These studies suggest that the modulation of TNF-α appears to be the key action of tea and/or EGCG.

Abe and colleagues [81] showed that green tea effectively prevented the progression of hepatitis to liver fibrosis in an experiment examining its semi-chronic effects. The ingestion of green tea reduced the gene expression of collagen and transforming growth factor-β. These proteins are fibrosis-promoting factors; it is likely that the decrease in their production contributes to the antifibrotic action of green tea.

Using obese and hypertensive nonalcoholic steatohepatitis model rats, Kochi et al. demonstrated that the administration of 0.1 % EGCG inhibited the development of hepatic premalignant lesions [82]. The mechanism of this was by improving liver fibrosis, inhibiting activation of the renin–angiotensin system, and attenuating inflammation and oxidative stress. This suggests that EGCG may prevent nonalcoholic steatohepatitis-related liver fibrosis and tumorigenesis.

An informative clinical trial was performed on nine cases of intractable chronic hepatitis C with a very high viral load of >850 kIU/mL. The patients received a combination therapy regimen of 6 g of green tea powder per day and interferon/

ribavirin. The therapy with green tea was 3.5 times more effective than treatment without green tea [83]. The results also indicated the absence of serious side effects.

Other Health Effects

There are many possible beneficial health effects of tea besides those described here, including effects on brain function, bone health, dental health, allergies, the common cold, and influenza [4, 5, 84]. Future studies should provide more detailed information on these issues.

Possible Deleterious Effects and a Safe Level

Mazzanti and colleagues [85] reported that the intake of a green tea supplement was associated with liver damage. Therefore, the ingestion of green tea containing extremely high concentrations of catechins and supplements with a high catechin content should be avoided or done with caution.

A study by Tsubono and colleagues [86] stated that the intake of green tea in men may be associated with a higher risk of stomach cancer. The intake of green, black, and oolong teas may also increase the risk of bladder cancer [25]. Shirai et al. [87] reported 21 cases of asthma that were attributable to green tea. In addition, hypersensitivity pneumonitis was seen in a 51-year-old man who underwent tea catechin inhalation therapy for 1 month and tuberculosis treatment for 3.5 months [88].

Overall, however, tea is generally considered to be safe and few reports of toxicity from tea consumption have been reported [2, 5]. Phase I trials performed among healthy volunteers have defined the basic biodistribution patterns, pharmacokinetic parameters, and preliminary safety profiles for short-term oral administration of various green tea preparations [2]. Pisters et al. [89] determined that even in persons with solid tumors, participants could safely consume up to 1 g of green tea solids three times daily, which is the equivalent of approximately 900 mL of green tea.

Conclusion

Evidence has steadily accumulated showing the generally beneficial effects of tea drinking on human health. However, conflicting results have also been reported, which indicate that future studies are warranted to better understand the health effects of different types of tea. Further research is also needed to reveal the underlying biological mechanisms for the action of teas. Nevertheless, the results of recent human studies, which have demonstrated the inverse association between tea consumption and mortality, suggest that we may be able to enjoy healthy longevity by drinking tea [90–92].

References

1. Thakur VS, Gupta K, Gupta S. The chemopreventive and chemotherapeutic potentials of tea polyphenols. Curr Pharm Biotechnol. 2012;13:191–9.
2. Carlson JR, Bauer BA, Vincent A, Limburg PJ, Wilson T. Reading the tea leaves: anticarcinogenic properties of (−)-epigallocatechin-3-gallate. Mayo Clin Proc. 2007;82:725–32.
3. Yang CS, Wang X, Lu G, Picinich SC. Cancer prevention by tea: animal studies, molecular mechanisms and human relevance. Nat Rev Cancer. 2009;9:429–39.
4. Suzuki Y, Miyoshi N, Isemura M. Health-promoting effects of green tea. Proc Jpn Acad Ser B Phys Biol Sci. 2012;88:88–101.
5. Yang CS, Hong J. Prevention of chronic diseases by tea: possible mechanisms and human relevance. Annu Rev Nutr. 2013;33:161–81.
6. Weikel KA, Garber C, Baburins A, Taylor A. Nutritional modulation of cataract. Nutr Rev. 2014;72:30–47.
7. Sorice A, Guerriero E, Capone F, Colonna G, Castello G, Costantini S. Ascorbic acid: its role in immune system and chronic inflammation diseases. Mini Rev Med Chem. 2014;14:444–52.
8. Smith TJ. Green tea polyphenols in drug discovery – a success or failure? Expert Opin Drug Discov. 2011;6:589–95.
9. Shukla Y. Tea and cancer chemoprevention: a comprehensive review. Asian Pac J Cancer Prev. 2007;8:155–66.
10. Chow HH, Hakim IA. Pharmacokinetic and chemoprevention studies on tea in humans. Pharmacol Res. 2011;64:105–12.
11. Ishida H, Wakimoto T, Kitao Y, Tanaka S, Miyase T, Nukaya H. Quantitation of chafurosides A and B in tea leaves and isolation of prechafurosides A and B from oolong tea leaves. J Agric Food Chem. 2009;57:6779–86.
12. Shohin Test Hokoku (Commercial products test reports). Kochi Prefecture Consumer Center. 2000;35:1–17 (in Japanese)
13. Imai K, Suga K, Nakachi K. Cancer-preventive effects of drinking green tea among a Japanese population. Prev Med. 1997;26:769–75.
14. Vogiatzoglou A, Heuer T, Mulligan AA, Lentjes MA, Luben RN, Kuhnle GG. Estimated dietary intakes and sources of flavanols in the German population (German National Nutrition Survey II). Eur J Nutr. 2014;53:635–43.
15. Oguni I, Nasu K, Kanaya S, Ota Y, Yamamoto S, Komura T. Epidemiological and experimental studies on the antitumor activity by green tea extracts. Jpn J Nutr. 1989;47:93–102.
16. Tewes FJ, Koo LC, Meisgen TJ, Rylander R. Lung cancer risk and mutagenicity of tea. Environ Res. 1990;52:23–33.
17. Sasazuki S, Tamakoshi A, Matsuo K, et al. Research Group for the Development and Evaluation of Cancer Prevention Strategies in Japan. Green tea consumption and gastric cancer risk: an evaluation based on a systematic review of epidemiologic evidence among the Japanese population. Jpn J Clin Oncol. 2012;42:335–46.
18. McCann SE, Yeh M, Rodabaugh K, Moysich KB. Higher regular coffee and tea consumption is associated with reduced endometrial cancer risk. Int J Cancer. 2009;124:1650–3.
19. Lee AH, Su D, Pasalich M, Binns CW. Tea consumption reduces ovarian cancer risk. Cancer Epidemiol. 2013;37:54–9.
20. Geybels MS, Verhage BA, Arts IC, van Schooten FJ, Goldbohm RA, van den Brandt PA. Dietary flavonoid intake, black tea consumption, and risk of overall and advanced stage prostate cancer. Am J Epidemiol. 2013;177:1388–98.

21. Yuan JM, Sun C, Butler LM. Tea and cancer prevention: epidemiological studies. Pharmacol Res. 2011;64:123–35.
22. Zheng JS, Yang J, Fu YQ, Huang T, Huang YJ, Li D. Effects of green tea, black tea, and coffee consumption on the risk of esophageal cancer: a systematic review and meta-analysis of observational studies. Nutr Cancer. 2013;65:1–16.
23. Montague JA, Butler LM, Wu AH, et al. Green and black tea intake in relation to prostate cancer risk among Singapore Chinese. Cancer Causes Control. 2012;23:1635–41.
24. Shafique K, McLoone P, Qureshi K, Leung H, Hart C, Morrison DS. Tea consumption and the risk of overall and grade specific prostate cancer: a large prospective cohort study of Scottish men. Nutr Cancer. 2012;64:790–7.
25. Lu CM, Lan SJ, Lee YH, Huang JK, Huang CH, Hsieh CC. Tea consumption: fluid intake and bladder cancer risk in Southern Taiwan. Urology. 1999;54:823–8.
26. Yamane T. Clinical trial involving 8 patients with familial adenomatous polyposis. In: Isemura M, editor. Beneficial health effect of green tea. Kerala: Research Signpost; 2008. p. 105–12.
27. Shimizu M, Fukutomi Y, Ninomiya M, et al. Green tea extracts for the prevention of metachronous colorectal adenomas: a pilot study. Cancer Epidemiol Biomarkers Prev. 2008;17:3020–5.
28. Bettuzzi S, Brausi M, Rizzi F, Castagnetti G, Peracchia G, Corti A. Chemoprevention of human prostate cancer by oral administration of green tea catechins in volunteers with high-grade prostate intraepithelial neoplasia: a preliminary report from a one-year proof-of-principle study. Cancer Res. 2006;66:1234–40.
29. Brausi M, Rizzi F, Bettuzzi S. Chemoprevention of human prostate cancer by green tea catechins: two years later. A follow-up update. Eur Urol. 2008;54:472–3.
30. Hara Y. Tea catechins and their applications as supplements and pharmaceutics. Pharmacol Res. 2011;64:100–4.
31. Gupta S, Hastak K, Ahmad N, Lewin JS, Mukhtar H. Inhibition of prostate carcinogenesis in TRAMP mice by oral infusion of green tea polyphenols. Proc Natl Acad Sci U S A. 2001;98:10350–5.
32. Tachibana H. Green tea polyphenol sensing. Proc Jpn Acad Ser B Phys Biol Sci. 2011;87:66–80.
33. Tsang WP, Kwok TT. Epigallocatechin gallate up-regulation of miR-16 and induction of apoptosis in human cancer cells. J Nutr Biochem. 2010;21:140–6.
34. Chakrabarti M, Ai W, Banik NL, Ray SK. Overexpression of miR-7-1 increases efficacy of green tea polyphenols for induction of apoptosis in human malignant neuroblastoma SH-SY5Y and SK-N-DZ cells. Neurochem Res. 2013;38:420–32.
35. Pan MH, Lai CS, Wu JC, Ho CT. Epigenetic and disease targets by polyphenols. Curr Pharm Des. 2013;19:6156–85.
36. Hibasami H, Komiya T, Achiwa Y, et al. Black tea theaflavins induce programmed cell death in cultured human stomach cancer cells. Int J Mol Med. 1998;1:725–7.
37. Halder B, Das Gupta S, Gomes A. Black tea polyphenols induce human leukemic cell cycle arrest by inhibiting Akt signaling: possible involvement of Hsp90, Wnt/beta-catenin signaling and FOXO1. FEBS J. 2012;279:2876–91.
38. Lahiry L, Saha B, Chakraborty J, et al. Theaflavins target Fas/caspase-8 and Akt/pBad pathways to induce apoptosis in p53-mutated human breast cancer cells. Carcinogenesis. 2010;31:259–68.
39. Pan MH, Liang YC, Lin-Shiau SY, Zhu NQ, Ho CT, Lin JK. Induction of apoptosis by the oolong tea polyphenol theasinensin A through cytochrome c release and activation of caspase-9 and caspase-3 in human U937 cells. J Agric Food Chem. 2000;48:6337–46.
40. Chiang CT, Weng MS, Lin-Shiau SY, Kuo KL, Tsai YJ, Lin JK. Pu-erh tea supplementation suppresses fatty acid synthase expression in the rat liver through downregulating Akt and JNK signalings as demonstrated in human hepatoma HepG2 cells. Oncol Res. 2005;16:119–28.
41. Wang J, Hudson R, Sintim HO. Inhibitors of fatty acid synthesis in prokaryotes and eukaryotes as anti-infective, anticancer and anti-obesity drugs. Future Med Chem. 2012;4:1113–51.
42. Conney AH, Lu YP, Lou YR, Kawasumi M, Nghiem P. Mechanisms of caffeine-induced inhibition of UVB carcinogenesis. Front Oncol. 2013;3:144.

43. Miwa S, Sugimoto N, Yamamoto N, et al. Caffeine induces apoptosis of osteosarcoma cells by inhibiting AKT/mTOR/S6K, NF-kappaB and MAPK pathways. Anticancer Res. 2012;32:3643–9.

44. Suzuki Y, Isemura M. Binding interaction between (−)-epigallocatechin gallate causes impaired spreading of cancer cells on fibrinogen. Biomed Res. 2013;34:301–8.

45. Brown AL, Lane J, Coverly J, et al. Effects of dietary supplementation with the green tea polyphenol epigallocatechin-3-gallate on insulin resistance and associated metabolic risk factors: randomized controlled trial. Br J Nutr. 2009;101:886–94.

46. Hino A, Adachi H, Enomoto M, et al. Habitual coffee but not green tea consumption is inversely associated with metabolic syndrome: an epidemiological study in a general Japanese population. Diabetes Res Clin Pract. 2007;76:383–9.

47. Takami H, Nakamoto M, Uemura H, et al. Inverse correlation between coffee consumption and prevalence of metabolic syndrome: baseline survey of the Japan Multi-Institutional Collaborative Cohort (J-MICC) Study in Tokushima. Jpn J Epidemiol. 2013;23:12–20.

48. Vernarelli JA, Lambert JD. Tea consumption is inversely associated with weight status and other markers for metabolic syndrome in US adults. Eur J Nutr. 2013;52:1039–48.

49. Basu A, Sanchez K, Leyva MJ, et al. Green tea supplementation affects body weight, lipids, and lipid peroxidation in obese subjects with metabolic syndrome. J Am Coll Nutr. 2010;29:31–40.

50. Vieira Senger AE, Schwanke CH, Gomes I, Valle Gottlieb MG. Effect of green tea (*Camellia sinensis*) consumption on the components of metabolic syndrome in elderly. J Nutr Health Aging. 2012;16:738–42.

51. Nagao T, Hase T, Tokimitsu I. A green tea extract high in catechins reduces body fat and cardiovascular risks in humans. Obesity. 2007;15:1473–83.

52. Kubota K, Sumi S, Tojo H, et al. Improvements of mean body mass index and body weight in preobese and overweight Japanese adults with black Chinese tea (Pu-Erh) water extract. Nutr Res. 2011;31:421–8.

53. Yuda N, Tanaka M, Suzuki M, Asano Y, Ochi H, Iwatsuki K. Polyphenols extracted from black tea (*Camellia sinensis*) residue by hot-compressed water and their inhibitory effect on pancreatic lipase in vitro. J Food Sci. 2012;77:H254–61.

54. Grove KA, Sae-tan S, Kennett MJ, Lambert JD. (−)-Epigallocatechin-3-gallate inhibits pancreatic lipase and reduces body weight gain in high fat-fed obese mice. Obesity. 2012;20:2311–3.

55. Murase T, Nagasawa A, Suzuki J, Hase T, Tokimitsu I. Beneficial effects of tea catechins on diet-induced obesity: stimulation of lipid catabolism in the liver. Int J Obes Relat Metab Disord. 2002;26:1459–64.

56. Yeh CW, Chen WJ, Chiang CT, Lin-Shiau SY, Lin JK. Suppression of fatty acid synthase in MCF-7 breast cancer cells by tea and tea polyphenols: a possible mechanism for their hypolipidemic effects. Pharmacogenomics J. 2003;3:267–76.

57. Huang HC, Lin JK. Pu-erh tea, green tea, and black tea suppresses hyperlipidemia, hyperleptinemia and fatty acid synthase through activating AMPK in rats fed a high-fructose diet. Food Funct. 2012;3:170–7.

58. Gardner EJ, Ruxton CH, Leeds AR. Black tea--helpful or harmful? A review of the evidence. Eur J Clin Nutr. 2007;61:3–18.

59. Larsson SC. Coffee, tea, and cocoa and risk of stroke. Stroke. 2014;45:309–14.

60. Larsson SC, Virtamo J, Wolk A. Black tea consumption and risk of stroke in women and men. Ann Epidemiol. 2013;23:157–60.

61. Hou Y, Shao W, Xiao R, et al. Pu-erh tea aqueous extracts lower atherosclerotic risk factors in a rat hyperlipidemia model. Exp Gerontol. 2009;44:434–9.

62. Liu G, Mi XN, Zheng XX, Xu YL, Lu J, Huang XH. Effects of tea intake on blood pressure: a meta-analysis of randomised controlled trials. Br J Nutr. 2014;112:1043–54.

63. Greyling A, Ras RT, Zock PL, et al. The effect of black tea on blood pressure: a systematic review with meta-analysis of randomized controlled trials. PLoS One. 2014;9:e103247.

64. Iso H, Date C, Wakai K, Fukui M, Tamakoshi A, JACC Study Group. The relationship between green tea and total caffeine intake and risk for self-reported type 2 diabetes among Japanese adults. Ann Intern Med. 2006;144:554–62.

65. van Woudenbergh GJ, Kuijsten A, Drogan D, et al. Tea consumption and incidence of type 2 diabetes in Europe: the EPIC-InterAct case-cohort study. PLoS One. 2012;7:e36910.

66. Huang H, Guo Q, Qiu C, et al. Associations of green tea and rock tea consumption with risk of impaired fasting glucose and impaired glucose tolerance in Chinese men and women. PLoS One. 2013;8:e79214.

67. Beresniak A, Duru G, Berger G, Bremond-Gignac D. Relationships between black tea consumption and key health indicators in the world: an ecological study. BMJ Open. 2012;2:e000648.

68. Maruyama K, Iso H, Sasaki S, Fukino Y. The association between concentrations of green tea and blood glucose levels. J Clin Biochem Nutr. 2009;44:41–5.

69. Nagao T, Meguro S, Hase T, et al. A catechin-rich beverage improves obesity and blood glucose control in patients with type 2 diabetes. Obesity. 2009;17:310–7.

70. Boggs DA, Rosenberg L, Ruiz-Narvaez EA, Palmer JR. Coffee, tea, and alcohol intake in relation to risk of type 2 diabetes in African American women. Am J Clin Nutr. 2010;92:960–6.

71. Hayashino Y, Fukuhara S, Okamura T, Tanaka T, Ueshima H. High oolong tea consumption predicts future risk of diabetes among Japanese male workers: a prospective cohort study. Diabet Med. 2011;28:805–10.

72. Pham NM, Nanri A, Kochi T, et al. Coffee and green tea consumption is associated with insulin resistance in Japanese adults. Metabolism. 2014;63:400–8.

73. Oba S, Nagata C, Nakamura K, et al. Consumption of coffee, green tea, oolong tea, black tea, chocolate snacks and the caffeine content in relation to risk of diabetes in Japanese men and women. Br J Nutr. 2010;103:453–9.

74. Williamson G. Possible effects of dietary polyphenols on sugar absorption and digestion. Mol Nutr Food Res. 2013;57:48–57.

75. Anderson RA, Polansky MM. Tea enhances insulin activity. J Agric Food Chem. 2002;50:7182–6.

76. Han MK. Epigallocatechin gallate, a constituent of green tea, suppresses cytokine-induced pancreatic beta-cell damage. Exp Mol Med. 2003;35:136–9.

77. Wolfram S, Raederstorff D, Preller M, et al. Epigallocatechin gallate supplementation alleviates diabetes in rodents. J Nutr. 2006;136:2512–8.

78. Abe K, Ijiri M, Suzuki T, Taguchi K, Koyama Y, Isemura M. Green tea with a high catechin content suppresses inflammatory cytokine expression in the galactosamine-injured rat liver. Biomed Res. 2005;26:187–92.

79. Bharrhan S, Koul A, Chopra K, Rishi P. Catechin suppresses an array of signalling molecules and modulates alcohol-induced endotoxin mediated liver injury in a rat model. PLoS One. 2011;6:e20635.

80. Cunha CA, Lira FS, Rosa Neto JC, et al. Green tea extract supplementation induces the lipolytic pathway, attenuates obesity, and reduces low-grade inflammation in mice fed a high-fat diet. Mediators Inflamm. 2013;2013:635470.

81. Abe K, Suzuki T, Ijiri M, Koyama Y, Isemura M, Kinae N. The anti-fibrotic effect of green tea with a high catechin content in the galactosamine-injured rat liver. Biomed Res. 2007;28:43–8.

82. Kochi T, Shimizu M, Terakura D, et al. Non-alcoholic steatohepatitis and preneoplastic lesions develop in the liver of obese and hypertensive rats: suppressing effects of EGCG on the development of liver lesions. Cancer Lett. 2014;342:60–9.

83. Sameshima Y, Ishida Y, Ono Y, Hujita M, Kuriki Y. Green tea powder enhances the safety and efficacy of interferon α-2b plus ribavirin combination therapy in chronic hepatitis C patients with a very high genotype 1 HCV load. In: Isemura M, editor. Beneficial health effect of green tea. Kerala: Research Signpost; 2008. p. 113–9.

84. Mandel SA, Youdim MB. In the rush for green gold: can green tea delay age-progressive brain neurodegeneration? Recent Pat CNS Drug Discov. 2012;7:205–17.

85. Mazzanti G, Menniti-Ippolito F, Moro PA, et al. Hepatotoxicity from green tea: a review of the literature and two unpublished cases. Eur J Clin Pharmacol. 2009;65:331–41.

86. Tsubono Y, Nishino Y, Komatsu S, et al. Green tea and the risk of gastric cancer in Japan. N Engl J Med. 2001;344:632–6.
87. Shirai T, Sato A, Chida K, et al. Epigallocatechin gallate-induced histamine release in patients with green tea-induced asthma. Ann Allergy Asthma Immunol. 1997;79:65–9.
88. Otera H, Tada K, Sakurai T, Hashimoto K, Ikeda A. Hypersensitivity pneumonitis associated with inhalation of catechin-rich green tea extracts. Respiration. 2011;82:388–92.
89. Pisters KM, Newman RA, Coldman B, et al. Phase I trial of oral green tea extract in adult patients with solid tumor. J Clin Oncol. 2001;19:1830–8.
90. Kuriyama S, Shimazu T, Ohmori K, et al. Green tea consumption and mortality due to cardiovascular disease, cancer, and all causes in Japan: the Ohsaki study. JAMA. 2006;296:1255–65.
91. Qiu L, Sautter J, Gu D. Associations between frequency of tea consumption and health and mortality: evidence from old Chinese. Br J Nutr. 2012;108:1686–97.
92. Gardener H, Rundek T, Wright CB, Elkind MS, Sacco RL. Coffee and tea consumption are inversely associated with mortality in a multiethnic urban population. J Nutr. 2013;143:1299–308.

Chapter 5
What Are the Health Implications of Alcohol Consumption?

Norman J. Temple

Keywords Alcohol • Fetal alcohol syndrome • Cancer • Obesity • Coronary heart disease • Blood pressure • Stroke • Pattern of drinking

Key Points

1. Consumption of alcohol is associated with many effects harmful to health, including accidents, violence, suicide, fetal alcohol syndrome, and cancer.
2. There is little evidence linking alcohol with weight gain.
3. Strong evidence indicates that moderate consumption of alcohol is protective against coronary heart disease.
4. There is also evidence suggesting that alcohol in moderation may be protective against several other conditions including elevated blood pressure, gallstones, loss of bone mineral density, hearing loss, dementia, benign prostatic hyperplasia, type 2 diabetes, and lung disease.
5. For many conditions, the relationship is J-shaped: the lowest risk is associated with consumption of alcohol in moderation whereas risk climbs with higher levels of alcohol consumption.
6. For people aged 50–80 years, the lowest risk of death is seen at an alcohol intake of around 1.0–1.5 drinks/day in men and 0.5–1.0 drinks/day in women. However, for people below age 40 years, alcohol consumption does not reduce mortality.
7. Alcohol is most protective when consumed in small regular amounts rather than binge drinking.

N.J. Temple (✉)
Centre for Science, Athabasca University, Athabasca, AB, Canada, T9S 3A3
e-mail: normant@athabascau.ca

© Springer International Publishing Switzerland 2016
T. Wilson, N.J. Temple (eds.), *Beverage Impacts on Health and Nutrition*,
Nutrition and Health, DOI 10.1007/978-3-319-23672-8_5

Introduction

The harmful effects of alcohol are far better known than the beneficial effects. This is scarcely surprising: it requires no training in epidemiology to recognize the devastating harm that often comes with both drunkenness and chronic alcohol abuse. However, findings that have emerged in recent years have uncovered several surprising associations between moderate intake of alcohol and enhanced health and well-being.

In this chapter, we use the American definition of a drink, namely, 12.5–13.0 g of alcohol. This quantity of alcohol is approximately the amount contained in 12 oz (356 g) of regular beer, 4–5 oz (118–148 g) of wine, or 1.5 oz (42 g) of spirits. We also use the USDA dietary guidelines' definition of moderate alcohol consumption as up to two drinks a day for men and one drink a day for women.

Harmful Effects of Alcohol

Accidents, Violence, and Suicide

It is well established that abuse of alcohol is associated with accidents, violence, and suicide. The most dramatic evidence of this has come from Russia. Following the collapse of the Soviet Union in 1989, Russia experienced serious economic decline and much political turmoil. During the early 1990s, life expectancy fell by 4 years in men and by 2 years in women. A major factor in this was apparently widespread alcohol abuse, particularly binge drinking, which led to large increases in deaths from accidents, homicide, and suicide, as well as cardiovascular disease [1, 2]. This severe health crisis continued for a long period. In 2006, in comparison with Western Europe, the mortality rate for Russians aged 15–54 years was five times higher for men and three times higher for women. Alcohol is apparently the dominant factor that explains this [3].

Approximately 10,200 people were killed in the USA in 2010 in alcohol-impaired driving crashes. This represents nearly one-third of all traffic-related deaths [4]. This figure includes alcohol intake by persons other than the driver, such as a pedestrian. This was the highest level since 1992, suggesting that the trend toward lower levels of alcohol-related car crashes has gone into reverse.

Chronic Alcohol Abuse

For many persons, years of alcohol abuse eventually leads to chronic health and nutritional problems. Alcohol is rich in calories and typically devoid in nutrients, especially alcohol- and sugar-rich hard liquors. The body often compensates for the high caloric intake by decreasing the stimulus to eat regular nutrient-rich foods. As a result, there is a high probability of malnutrition, especially of folate and thiamin. The thiamin deficiency associated with alcohol abuse is known as Wernicke–Korsakoff syndrome. Liver disease is also a likely result with a downward spiral from fatty liver, to alcoholic hepatitis, and, eventually, to cirrhosis.

Fetal Alcohol Syndrome

Pregnancy is another situation where alcohol misuse can have tragic consequences. This induces fetal alcohol syndrome (FAS). FAS encompasses a variety of symptoms including prenatal and postnatal growth retardation, abnormal facial features, and an increased frequency of major birth defects. Children born with FAS never recover.

A subclinical form of FAS is known as fetal alcohol effects (FAE). Children with FAE may be short or have only minor facial abnormalities or develop learning disabilities, behavioral problems, or motor impairments.

FAS occurs at a level of alcohol intake that is well below the amount that would be considered alcohol abuse in a nonpregnant woman. Four drinks per day poses a real threat of FAS, although 1 or 2 drinks/day may still retard growth; the epidemiological data are weaker and somewhat inconsistent at these lower levels of consumption. Although women who have an occasional drink during pregnancy should not fear they are doing irreparable harm to their fetus, it is now generally accepted that any woman who is or may become pregnant should abstain from alcohol.

Cancer

Alcohol greatly increases the risk of several types of cancer. An alcohol intake at the high end of moderation (two drinks per day in women, four in men) is associated with relative risks (RRs) for different types of cancer as follows: 1.16 for colorectal cancer, 1.8 for mouth and pharynx, 2.4 for esophagus, and 3.0 for liver [5]. Our best evidence is that lower intakes of alcohol produce proportionately smaller RRs. For all cancer combined, a significant risk is seen starting at an alcohol intake of 2 drinks/day, with a RR of 1.22 at 4 drinks/day [6].

Many studies have investigated the mechanisms by which alcohol may enhance risk of cancer. It is likely that metabolites of alcohol, such as acetaldehyde, are carcinogenic. Alcohol can act as a solvent enhancing the penetration of carcinogens into cells. For breast cancer, it is less likely that ethanol is directly toxic since the increase has been seen at relatively low levels. It is more likely that alcohol influences circulating estrogen levels which may impact on disease occurrence [7, 8].

Obesity

Alcohol, of course, is a source of calories (7 kcal/g). Its final metabolite acetate can be either oxidized to ATP or utilized for fatty acid synthesis (weight gain). It is important to remember that most types of wine and beer also contain carbohydrates that add additional calories. A half liter of wine contains about 350 kcal, while three cans of beer supply about 250–450 kcal, clearly enough to tip the energy balance well into positive territory. These numbers explain the popularity of low-calorie "light beers." It is predictable, therefore, that alcohol consumption should be associated with excess weight gain. But, is this actually the case in the real world?

Intervention studies are inconclusive. Alcohol consumption causes an increase in energy intake [9]. However, Cordain et al. [10] reported that when men consumed 35 g/day of alcohol (a little less than three glasses of wine) for a period of 6 weeks, this did not affect body weight. Similar results were seen this when overweight women consumed 25 g/day of alcohol, 5 days/week, for 10 weeks [11].

Several long-term cohort studies have been carried out. In a cohort study of 16,600 men aged 40–75, change in alcohol intake was not associated with change in waist circumference over 9 years of follow-up [12]. In a cohort study of 19,200 women of normal BMI at baseline, alcohol intake displayed a clear negative association with risk of becoming overweight or obese over the following 13 years [13]. In sharp contrast, other cohort studies have reported a positive association between alcohol consumption and weight gain [14]. At present, therefore, it is far from clear whether alcohol intake is a risk factor for weight gain.

Protective Effects of Alcohol

Coronary Heart Disease

A convincing body of evidence suggests that the risk of coronary heart disease (CHD) is reduced by 20–40 % in persons who consume alcohol in moderation [5]. In some populations, this association can be skewed if individuals at higher risk for CHD reduce or eliminate alcohol consumption due to a diagnosis of a related chronic disease (e.g., hypertension or diabetes). This is frequently described as the "sick quitter" syndrome and can much exaggerate the strength of the inverse association between alcohol and CHD [15]. Because conditions such as hypertension and diabetes increase the risk of CHD by two- to threefold, a study which does not take these conditions into account may find that moderate drinkers have as much as 50–70 % less heart disease. However, even in large cohort studies where "sick quitters" are removed or moderate drinkers are compared to lifelong abstainers, alcohol has been found to have a strong and clear cardiovascular benefit [16, 17].

There has been much speculation that wine, particularly red wine, may be more potent than beer or spirits in preventing CHD. This is largely based on findings from ecological studies (i.e., countries with a high intake of wine tend to have relatively low rates of CHD) [18]. As France is the country most closely associated with this observation, it has often been referred to as the "French paradox." But it has been repeatedly shown that such associations can easily be spurious. This is indicated by the findings from case–control and cohort studies: these show no clear trend for one type of alcohol to be more consistently associated with protection from CHD [16, 18]. Where one type of alcohol does manifest a stronger association than other types, this is likely due to confounding by such factors as smoking and drinking pattern or to differences in other lifestyle factors such as eating patterns or physical activity.

Findings from major cohort studies indicate that HDL-C explains much of the association between alcohol and CHD [16] (i.e., alcohol consumption helps prevent CHD by increasing the blood level of HDL-C). HbA_{1c} may also be an important factor, as is, to a lesser extent, fibrinogen. HbA_{1c} is a measure of blood glucose levels over the long term. A raised level is an indicator of poor glucose tolerance; this is linked to risk of CHD. Fibrinogen is part of the blood clotting mechanism and is also a risk factor for CHD.

Blood Pressure and Stroke

A relatively high alcohol intake (>4 drinks/day) has been shown to be associated with elevated blood pressure [19, 20] and an increased risk of stroke [5]. However, evidence from cohort studies suggest that the association between alcohol and hypertension may be J-shaped such that light and moderate drinkers have a modestly reduced risk of developing the condition [21]. Although the results of large epidemiological studies have not been consistent, the data as a whole indicate that there is also a J-shaped relationship between alcohol intake and risk of stroke [5]. The protective effect of moderate consumption of alcohol is seen only for ischemic stroke (the more common type), not for hemorrhagic stroke [5].

More work is needed to determine if drinking patterns influence risk of stroke (i.e., frequent consumption of small amounts of alcohol versus binge drinking). Binge drinking is typically defined as consuming five or more drinks on a single occasion, for a man, or four or more for a woman.

Impotence

The relationship between excessive alcohol intake and poor erectile function is well known. As Shakespeare put it: "It provokes the desire, but takes away from the performance" (Macbeth). But, as in the case of alcohol and blood pressure, recent findings have revealed an apparently beneficial effect, or at least no ill effects, of moderate alcohol consumption [22].

Although erectile dysfunction was originally thought to be purely psychogenic in nature, 80–90 % is likely due to biological factors that may share a similar profile to atherosclerosis.

Gallstones

The balance of evidence points to a protective association between alcohol and risk of gallstones. For instance, Leitzmann et al. [23] observed that men who consume alcohol frequently (5–7 days/week) have a reduced risk of gallstones but not those who consume alcohol less frequently (1–2 days/week). These findings suggest that frequency of alcohol consumption rather than quantity is the critical factor.

Bone Health

While findings are not consistent, several studies have reported that compared to nondrinking, moderate alcohol intake is associated with higher bone mineral density, especially in postmenopausal women [24–26]. This indicates that alcohol may help prevent osteoporosis. However, as osteoporosis is so dependent on lifetime diet, physical activity, obesity, and other factors, it is probable that alcohol does not play an important role. In contrast to the situation with osteoporosis, high levels of drinking cause loss of balance and falls leading to an increased risk of hip or wrist fracture.

Hearing Loss

A cross-sectional study of subjects aged 50–91 years reported that moderate alcohol intake was associated with better hearing [27]. Again, like bone health, many other environmental and genetic effects play a more important role in the etiology of hearing loss.

Cognitive Function and Dementia

It is well known that heavy drinking has a damaging effect on brain function. Nevertheless, alcohol manifests a J-shaped relationship with the decline in brain function with aging. In several studies, mostly carried out on older adults, moderate consumption of alcohol was associated with enhanced cognitive ability or a slower rate of decline with aging. This effect is generally more pronounced in women [28–32].

While results have not been entirely consistent, several cohort studies have reported a protective association between moderate alcohol consumption and the development of dementia (mainly Alzheimer's disease) [32–35].

Benign Prostatic Hyperplasia

A cohort study reported that moderate alcohol intake (2.5–4 drinks/day) was associated with a reduced risk of benign prostatic hyperplasia (RR of 0.59) [36]. The mechanisms for this action are speculative but may include the effects of alcohol on steroid hormone levels.

Diabetes

Cohort studies have suggested that alcohol may be protective against type 2 diabetes. Moderate consumers have a 33–56 % reduced risk of developing the condition [37]. Interestingly, several studies have suggested that moderate consumption of alcohol among men and women with type 2 diabetes is also associated with a much reduced risk of subsequent CHD [38–41], the number one killer of diabetics.

Lung Disease

Alcohol may also be protective against chronic obstructive pulmonary disease (COPD). A cohort study of middle-aged men in Finland, Netherlands, and Italy revealed a protective association between alcohol intake and risk of death from COPD [42]. The lowest risk was seen at an intake of up to about 3 drinks/day. Alcohol intake has also been observed to manifest a protective association with emphysema in smokers [43].

Effect of Alcohol on Total Mortality

The effects of alcohol consumption represent a complex mixture of harm and benefit. Overall, alcohol certainly causes more deaths than it prevents. In an estimate by Danaei and colleagues [5], alcohol causes 90,000 deaths per year in the USA. These are due to a variety of causes, the main ones being traffic accidents and other injuries, violence, chronic liver disease, cancer, alcohol use disorders, and hemorrhagic stroke. At the same time, alcohol prevents 26,000 deaths from CHD, ischemic stroke, and diabetes. Alcohol therefore causes 64,000 more deaths than it prevents.

When intake is moderate and binge drinking is avoided, the beneficial health effects of alcohol on the cardiovascular system outweigh most detrimental effects. As a result, the net effect of alcohol on total mortality is a J-shaped curve with minimum mortality associated with a moderate intake of alcohol but with a rising curve as consumption increases, especially when there is binge drinking. As an example, a major study by the American Cancer Society on subjects with a mean age of 56 years reported that in each sex, persons consuming one drink daily had a risk of death from all causes about 20 % below those of nondrinkers [44]. To put this in perspective, among American men and women aged 35–69 years, a moderate consumption of alcohol prevents approximately one death for every six deaths caused by smoking [44].

The benefits of alcohol are most apparent in the middle-aged and elderly. This is because alcohol reduces risk of CHD and stroke, the first and third leading cause of death, respectively, in those age groups. By contrast, the leading cause of death in Americans under age 40 years is accidents, with homicide and suicide being other major causes, especially in males. These are all associated with alcohol. This age effect is illustrated by a report from the Nurses' Health Study. A moderate intake of alcohol has a protective relationship with total mortality in women aged over 50 years (RR is 0.80–0.88) but is associated with a doubling of the risk of death in those aged 34–39 years [45]. Similar findings were reported from England and Wales: a net favorable mortality outcome was seen only in men over age 55 and women over 65 years [46].

The alcohol intake corresponding to the nadir for mortality is still unclear but in people aged 50–80 years is around 1.0–1.5 drinks/day in men and 0.5–1.0 drinks/day in women [47, 48]. However, as this is based on self-reported intake, which represents a substantial underestimation, the true nadir is almost certainly higher [47].

Drinking Patterns

Research in recent years has focused on the importance of pattern of drinking on health outcomes. Not surprisingly, alcohol is most protective when consumed in small regular amounts rather than episodic heavy drinking (binge drinking). This was demonstrated in cohort studies in the USA [49] and Finland [50]. People who engaged in occasional heavy drinking had a higher risk of death than persons with the same alcohol intake but who did not engage in binge drinking. Similar observations were made on cardiovascular disease in Canada. The data from that study revealed that while alcohol consumption has a protective association with both CHD and hypertension, binge drinking increases the risk of both, especially in men [51]. In a study of US male health professionals, frequency of consumption (days/week) was more important than quantity consumed. Men who consumed alcohol at least 5 days/week had the lowest risk of both type 2 diabetes [52] and myocardial infarction [16], regardless of the total amount consumed. These findings are hardly surprising: many dietary components cause no harm in small, frequent doses but are toxic when a large dose is taken.

Recent Controversy

A note of caution must at this point be injected into the discussion. Reference was made earlier to the "sick quitter" syndrome and how this can increase the magnitude of the inverse association between alcohol and CHD. Most of the evidence referred to in this chapter has come from cohort studies. It has been argued that such evidence may have serious flaws and as a result the protective benefit of moderate consumption of alcohol has been much exaggerated. This may apply not only to CHD but also to the other conditions mentioned earlier [53, 54]. The source of this problem is not only the "sick quitter" syndrome but also that lifelong abstainers are at raised risk of various diseases as a result of having important differences from people who drink in moderation.

Supporting evidence for this viewpoint came from a recent investigation that combined the results from 56 studies involving a total of 262,000 people of European origin [55]. For every subject, the investigators determined if he/she had a particular allele for the gene that codes for alcohol dehydrogenase. Persons with this allele consume, on average, 17 % less alcohol than the rest of the subjects. The presence of this variant is independent of all other aspects of lifestyle and health. The results revealed that persons with the allele had a lower risk of CHD than the rest of the subjects. This indicates that alcohol does not lower the risk of CHD.

A contrary interpretation was made by Roerecke and Rehm [56]. They made a detailed analysis of the evidence and argued that the negative association seen between moderate intake of alcohol and CHD is real and cannot be dismissed.

Clearly, the extent to which alcohol is protective against CHD and other conditions is still open to debate.

Conclusion

It is important to bear in mind that the harmful effects of alcohol frequently occur at a much younger age than the apparent benefits. Consequently, if the effects of alcohol are measured in terms of quality years of life (lost or gained), then the harm done to one (usually younger) person by alcohol is likely to be far greater than the benefit gained by another (usually older) person.

The large majority of the harmful effects of alcohol can be avoided by sensible drinking, by drinking in moderation, and by the avoidance of alcohol when driving. For the person who can drink sensibly and can avoid alcohol's negative side, alcohol may be of considerable benefit. Like so much else in life, it's a matter of balance. While alcohol should perhaps not be prescribed [57], neither should it be proscribed.

Researchers in Australia estimated that for people aged over 60 years, the cost per life year gained by moderate consumption of alcohol was A$5700 in men and A$19,000 in women [58]. This estimate was published in 2000; the numbers translate to about \$8000 in men and \$26,000 in women in 2014 US dollars. On this basis, alcohol can be considered a cost-effective medication. This conclusion rests, of course, on the assumption that alcohol consumption in moderation does indeed have a protective benefit.

The findings discussed in this chapter have implications for public health policy. But what are those implications? One possible policy is the following: all adults aged over 40 years should be encouraged to consume moderate amounts of alcohol daily, unless there is a specific reason to the contrary, such as religion, medication use, or a history of alcohol abuse. There are two potential problems with such a policy. First, the evidence referred to above suggests that the belief that alcohol helps prevent CHD and other diseases may be false. Second, there is a risk that encouraging more alcohol consumption may lead to a rise in the prevalence of alcohol abuse. Typically, about 5–10 % of people in any society where alcohol is available become abusers of the beverage. The actual proportion is related to the mean alcohol intake: the higher the mean alcohol intake, the higher is the proportion of alcohol abusers [59]. Thus, a policy that encourages greater use of alcohol will likely also lead to more problems associated with abuse.

Arguably, the most prudent policy is one that explains that alcohol in moderation may possibly have several health benefits for people in middle age and above, while also stressing the hazards of abuse.

References

1. Leon DA, Chenet L, Shkolnikov VM, et al. Huge variation in Russian mortality rates 1984–94: artefact, alcohol, or what? Lancet. 1997;350:383–8.
2. Walberg P, McKee M, Shkolnikov V, Chenet L, Leon DA. Economic change, crime, and mortality crisis in Russia: regional analysis. BMJ. 1998;317:312–8.
3. Zaridze D, Brennan P, Boreham J, et al. Alcohol and cause-specific mortality in Russia: a retrospective case–control study of 48,557 adult deaths. Lancet. 2009;373:2201–14.
4. Centers for Disease Control and Prevention. Injury prevention & control: motor vehicle safety. 2013. http://www.cdc.gov/motorvehiclesafety/impaired_driving/impaired-drv_factsheet.html. Accessed 8 Apr 2014.
5. Danaei G, Ding EL, Mozaffarian D, et al. The preventable causes of death in the United States: comparative risk assessment of dietary, lifestyle, and metabolic risk factors. PLoS Med. 2009;6:e1000058.
6. Bagnardi V, Blangiardo M, Vecchia CL, Corrao G. A meta-analysis of alcohol drinking and cancer risk. Br J Cancer. 2001;85:1700–5.
7. Hankinson SE, Willett WC, Manson JE, et al. Alcohol, height, and adiposity in relation to estrogen and prolactin levels in postmenopausal women. J Natl Cancer Inst. 1995;87:1297–302.
8. Dorgan JF, Baer DJ, Albert PS, et al. Serum hormones and the alcohol-breast cancer association in postmenopausal women. J Natl Cancer Inst. 2001;93:710–5.
9. Yeomans MR. Alcohol, appetite and energy balance: is alcohol intake a risk factor for obesity? Physiol Behav. 2010;100:82–9.
10. Cordain L, Bryan ED, Melby CL, Smith MJ. Influence of moderate daily wine consumption on body weight regulation and metabolism in healthy free-living males. J Am Coll Nutr. 1997;16:134–9.

11. Cordain L, Melby CL, Hamamoto AE, et al. Influence of moderate chronic wine consumption on insulin sensitivity and other correlates of syndrome X in moderately obese women. Metabolism. 2000;49:1473–8.
12. Koh-Banerjee P, Chu NF, Spiegelman D, Rosner B, Colditz G, Willett W, Rimm E. Prospective study of the association of changes in dietary intake, physical activity, alcohol consumption, and smoking with 9-y gain in waist circumference among 16 587 US men. Am J Clin Nutr. 2003;78:719–27.
13. Wang L, Lee IM, Manson JE, Buring JE, Sesso HD. Alcohol consumption, weight gain, and risk of becoming overweight in middle-aged and older women. Arch Intern Med. 2010;170:453–61.
14. Mozaffarian D, Hao T, Rimm EB, Willett WC, Hu FB. Changes in diet and lifestyle and long-term weight gain in women and men. N Engl J Med. 2011;364:2392–404.
15. Shaper AG, Wannamethee G, Walker M. Alcohol and mortality in British men: explaining the U-shaped curve. Lancet. 1988;2:1267–73.
16. Mukamal KJ, Jensen MK, Grønbaek M, Stampfer MJ, Manson JE, Pischon T, Rimm EB. Drinking frequency, mediating biomarkers, and risk of myocardial infarction in women and men. Circulation. 2005;112:1406–13.
17. Rimm E. Alcohol and cardiovascular disease. Curr Atheroscler Rep. 2000;2:529–35.
18. Rimm EB, Klatsky A, Grobbee D, Stampfer MJ. Review of moderate alcohol consumption and reduced risk of coronary heart disease: is the effect due to beer, wine, or spirits? BMJ. 1996;312:731–6.
19. Corrao G, Bagnardi V, Zambon A, La Vecchia C. A meta-analysis of alcohol consumption and the risk of 15 diseases. Prev Med. 2004;38:613–9.
20. Puddey IB, Beilin LJ, Vandongen R, Rouse IL, Rogers P. Evidence for a direct effect of alcohol consumption on blood pressure in normotensive men. A randomized controlled trial. Hypertension. 1985;7:707–13.
21. Thadhani R, Camargo Jr CA, Stampfer MJ, Curhan GC, Willett WC, Rimm EB. Prospective study of moderate alcohol consumption and risk of hypertension in young women. Arch Intern Med. 2002;162:569–74.
22. Bacon CG, Mittleman MA, Kawachi I, Giovannucci E, Glasser DB, Rimm EB. Sexual function in men older than 50 years of age: results from the health professionals follow-up study. Ann Intern Med. 2003;139:161–8.
23. Leitzmann MF, Giovannucci EL, Stampfer MJ, et al. Prospective study of alcohol consumption patterns in relation to symptomatic gallstone disease in men. Alcohol Clin Exp Res. 1999;23:835–41.
24. Rapuri PB, Gallagher JC, Balhorn KE, Ryschon KL. Alcohol intake and bone metabolism in elderly women. Am J Clin Nutr. 2000;72:1206–13.
25. Feskanich D, Korrick SA, Greenspan SL, Rosen HN, Colditz GA. Moderate alcohol consumption and bone density among postmenopausal women. J Womens Health. 1999;8:65–73.
26. Macdonald HM, New SA, Golden MH, Campbell MK, Reid DM. Nutritional associations with bone loss during the menopausal transition: evidence of a beneficial effect of calcium, alcohol, and fruit and vegetable nutrients and of a detrimental effect of fatty acids. Am J Clin Nutr. 2004;79:155–65.
27. Popelka MM, Cruikshanks KJ, Wiley TL, et al. Moderate alcohol consumption and hearing loss: a protective effect. J Am Geriatr Soc. 2000;48:1273–8.
28. Britton A, Singh-Manoux A, Marmot M. Alcohol consumption and cognitive function in the Whitehall II Study. Am J Epidemiol. 2004;160:240–7.
29. Leroi I, Sheppard JM, Lyketsos CG. Cognitive function after 11.5 years of alcohol use: relation to alcohol use. Am J Epidemiol. 2002;156:747–52.
30. Kalmijn S, van Boxtel MP, Verschuren MW, Jolles J, Launer LJ. Cigarette smoking and alcohol consumption in relation to cognitive performance in middle age. Am J Epidemiol. 2002;156:936–44.
31. Stampfer MJ, Kang JH, Chen J, Cherry R, Grodstein F. Effects of moderate alcohol consumption on cognitive function in women. N Engl J Med. 2005;352:245–53.

32. Espeland MA, Gu L, Masaki KH, et al. Association between reported alcohol intake and cognition: results from the Women's Health Initiative Memory Study. Am J Epidemiol. 2005;161:228–38.
33. Ruitenberg A, van Swieten JC, Witteman JC, et al. Alcohol consumption and risk of dementia: the Rotterdam Study. Lancet. 2002;359:281–6.
34. Huang W, Qiu C, Winblad B, Fratiglioni L. Alcohol consumption and incidence of dementia in a community sample aged 75 years and older. J Clin Epidemiol. 2002;55:959–64.
35. Mukamal KJ, Kuller LH, Fitzpatrick AL, Longstreth Jr WT, Mittleman MA, Siscovick DS. Prospective study of alcohol consumption and risk of dementia in older adults. JAMA. 2003;289:1405–13.
36. Platz EA, Rimm EB, Kawachi I, et al. Alcohol consumption, cigarette smoking, and risk of benign prostatic hyperplasia. Am J Epidemiol. 1999;149:106–15.
37. Howard AA, Arnsten JH, Gourevitch MN. Effect of alcohol consumption on diabetes mellitus: a systematic review. Ann Intern Med. 2004;140:211–9.
38. Tanasescu M, Hu FB, Willett WC, Stampfer MJ, Rimm EB. Alcohol consumption and risk of coronary heart disease among men with type 2 diabetes mellitus. J Am Coll Cardiol. 2001;38:1836–42.
39. Ajani UA, Gaziano JM, Lotufo PA, et al. Alcohol consumption and risk of coronary heart disease by diabetes status. Circulation. 2000;102:500–5.
40. Solomon CG, Hu FB, Stampfer MJ, et al. Moderate alcohol consumption and risk of coronary heart disease among women with type 2 diabetes mellitus. Circulation. 2000;102:494–9.
41. Valmadrid CT, Klein R, Moss SE, Klein BE, Cruickshanks KJ. Alcohol intake and the risk of coronary heart disease mortality in persons with older-onset diabetes mellitus. JAMA. 1999;282:239–46.
42. Tabak C, Smit HA, Rasanen L, et al. Alcohol consumption in relation to 20-year COPD mortality and pulmonary function in middle-aged men from three European countries. Epidemiology. 2001;12:239–45.
43. Pratt PC, Vollmer RT. The beneficial effect of alcohol consumption on the prevalence and extent of centrilobular emphysema. Chest. 1984;85:372–7.
44. Thun MJ, Peto R, Lopez AD, Monaco JH, Henley SJ, Heath Jr CW, Doll R. Alcohol consumption and mortality among middle-aged and elderly U.S. adults. N Engl J Med. 1997;337:1705–14.
45. Fuchs CS, Stampfer MJ, Colditz GA, et al. Alcohol consumption and mortality among women. N Engl J Med. 1995;332:1245–50.
46. Britton A, McPherson K. Mortality in England and Wales attributable to current alcohol consumption. J Epidemiol Community Health. 2001;55:383–8.
47. White IR. The level of alcohol consumption at which all-cause mortality is least. J Clin Epidemiol. 1999;52:967–75.
48. Lee SJ, Sudore RL, Williams BA, Lindquist K, Chen HL, Covinsky KE. Functional limitations, socioeconomic status, and all-cause mortality in moderate alcohol drinkers. J Am Geriatr Soc. 2009;57:955–62.
49. Rehm J, Greenfield TK, Rogers JD. Average volume of alcohol consumption, patterns of drinking, and all-cause mortality: results from the US National Alcohol Survey. Am J Epidemiol. 2001;153:64–71.
50. Laatikainen T, Manninen L, Poikolainen K, Vartiainen E. Increased mortality related to heavy alcohol intake pattern. J Epidemiol Community Health. 2003;57:379–84.
51. Murray RP, Connett JE, Tyas SL, et al. Alcohol volume, drinking pattern, and cardiovascular disease morbidity and mortality: is there a U-shaped function? Am J Epidemiol. 2002;155:242–8.
52. Conigrave KM, Hu BF, Camargo Jr CA, Stampfer MJ, Willett WC, Rimm EB. A prospective study of drinking patterns in relation to risk of type 2 diabetes among men. Diabetes. 2001;50:2390–5.
53. Fekjaer HO. Alcohol-a universal preventive agent? A critical analysis. Addiction. 2013;108:2051–7.

54. Stockwell T, Chikritzhs T. Commentary: another serious challenge to the hypothesis that moderate drinking is good for health? Int J Epidemiol. 2013;42:1792–4.
55. Holmes MV, Caroline E, Dale CE, Zuccolo L. Association between alcohol and cardiovascular disease: Mendelian randomisation analysis based on individual participant data. BMJ. 2014;349:g4164.
56. Roerecke M, Rehm J. Alcohol consumption, drinking patterns, and ischemic heart disease: a narrative review of meta-analyses and a systematic review and meta-analysis of the impact of heavy drinking occasions on risk for moderate drinkers. BMC Med. 2014;12:182.
57. Wannamethee SG, Shaper AG. Taking up regular drinking in middle age: effect on major coronary heart disease events and mortality. Heart. 2002;87:32–6.
58. Simons LA, McCallum J, Friedlander Y, Ortiz M, Simons J. Moderate alcohol intake is associated with survival in the elderly: the Dubbo Study. Med J Aust. 2000;173:121–4.
59. Colhoun H, Ben-Shlomo Y, Dong W, Bost L, Marmot M. Ecological analysis of collectivity of alcohol consumption in England: importance of average drinker. BMJ. 1997;314:1164–8.

Chapter 6
Nonalcoholic Components of Wine and Atherosclerotic Cardiovascular Disease

Abigail J. O'Connor, Georges M. Halpern, and Rosemary L. Walzem

Keywords Atherosclerotic cardiovascular disease • Atherogenesis • Inflammation • Microbiota • Wine

Key Points

1. Wine is believed to be protective against atherosclerotic cardiovascular disease.
2. Wine phenolics are generally poorly absorbed and rapidly metabolized.
3. Direct antioxidant actions appear biologically implausible as the primary mechanism of the health benefit of wine phenolics.
4. Biologically plausible mechanisms for the nonalcoholic components of wine now include beneficial modulation of microbiota composition and function perhaps through generation of beneficial or suppression of deleterious microbial metabolites, or both.
5. New lower-cost methods to characterize microbiota, gene expression, and metabolomics, coupled with increasingly powerful computational strategies, are allowing interrogation of the host/microbiota/diet relationships to assess whether biological plausibility can be verified as actual health mechanisms through which the nonalcoholic components of wine can act.

Wine is the most healthful and most hygienic of beverages.—*Louis Pasteur*

A.J. O'Connor
Nutrition Graduate Program, Department of Nutrition and Food Science, Texas A&M University, College Station, TX 77843, USA

G.M. Halpern, M.D., Ph.D.
Department of Biomedical Sciences, City University of Hong Kong, Kowloon, Hong Kong, China

R.L. Walzem, R.D., Ph.D. (✉)
Nutrition Graduate Program, Department of Poultry Science, Texas A&M University, College Station, TX 77843, USA
e-mail: rwalzem@poultry.tamu.edu

© Springer International Publishing Switzerland 2016
T. Wilson, N.J. Temple (eds.), *Beverage Impacts on Health and Nutrition*, Nutrition and Health, DOI 10.1007/978-3-319-23672-8_6

Introduction

Cardiovascular disease (CVD) represents a collection of diseases and symptoms that affect the heart and blood vessels. A plethora of terms are used to specify particular forms of CVD, for example, coronary heart disease to identify dysfunction in the entire heart and coronary artery disease to identify disease within the arteries of the heart itself, while peripheral artery disease refers to disease in the arms and legs [1]. Despite the abundance of names, coronary and peripheral artery diseases arise from a process termed atherosclerosis and are combined by health professionals under the term atherosclerotic cardiovascular disease (ASCVD). This is the disease process for which data are most available in relation to the effects of the nonalcoholic components (NAC) of wine. ASCVD develops due to chronic inflammation of the vascular wall in association with low-density lipoprotein (LDL) oxidation, platelet aggregation, and reduced availability of nitric oxide [2–5]. Failed processes of vascular wall health produce characteristic "hardening" of arteries typified by monocyte/macrophage infiltration of the vascular wall, accumulation of cholesteryl esters in the subendothelium (aka plaque), thickening of the artery wall, and loss of vascular compliance [6]. ASCVD drives the majority of CVD including angina (chronic chest pain), arrhythmias, as well as heart attacks and strokes. In 2010, CVD accounted for 31.9 % of deaths in the United States [7]. ASCVD was reported to cause over half of the CVD and cost $109 billion per year [1].

The multifactorial nature of ASCVD pathology includes lifestyle, and, historically, consumption of a "Western diet" has been viewed as a key risk factor. The Western diet is most often consumed by northern Europeans and Americans and is enriched in saturated fats and cholesterol. Consumption of this is often associated with high blood lipids, particularly cholesterol carried in LDL [4]. Regular moderate wine consumption was linked to a reduced risk for ASCVD mortality by Renaud and de Lorgeril in the early 1990s and was the key factor in what they dubbed "the French paradox" [4]. The paradox is that the French population, in comparison with the United States and northern European countries, had a similarly unhealthy lifestyle but exhibited a lower total ASCVD mortality rate. Indeed, France had high rates of smoking and consumed a diet high in fat and saturated fats. For example, using a diet quality index, Gerber found that only 10 of 146 subjects studied in the Languedoc area of southern France had a healthful diet [8]. The typical French diet more closely resembles the American and north European diets than a "Mediterranean diet" [2]. The Mediterranean diet differed from typical diets consumed in France in that it was rather richer in vegetables and fruits, with olive oil rather than butter as the primary dietary fat. In this dietary pattern less meat and more fish or other n-3 fatty acid sources were consumed along with more pulses and nuts [2]. Thus, the distinctive difference of the French as opposed to other Europeans as well as Americans consuming a Western-type diet was the common practice of regular moderate wine consumption by the French [4]. The initial proposal was that regular moderate ethanol intake via consumption of wine with meals inhibits platelet aggregation and so counteracts the pro-aggregatory effects of consuming a diet rich in saturated fats [4, 9] or the hyperaggregability associated with weekend "binge"-type drinking [10]. The concept that regular, moderate ethanol consumption during meals in the form of wine could reduce the risk of ASCVD was shortly followed by the proposal that a closer association between risk reduction and red wine consumption was possible [11] due to the ability of NAC to act as antioxidants able to protect LDL from in vitro oxidative damage [12]. This latter proposal provided impetus for a vast amount of research seeking to link wine consumption to improved cardiovascular health. Indeed increased phytochemical intakes afforded by the Mediterranean diet, for which regular moderate wine consumption is also a feature, seems to have strengthened the perception of health benefit being provided by the NAC of wine.

The alcohol component of wine has several effects on health as discussed in Chap. 5 where the role of ethanol and the definition of optimal alcohol intake are explored. However, as noted above, wine can be rich in phenolic compounds including anthocyanins, flavanols, flavonols, resveratrol, and a variety of phenolic acids [13, 14] (Table 6.1 and Fig. 6.1). These compounds have all shown activity in cardioprotective mechanisms, and their concentrations in wine vary based on the type of wine, environmental factors during grape growth and development, as well as vintification and preparation techniques [5, 9]. An online database (www.phenol-explorer.eu) is a useful tool as it presents published information on the phenolic content of beverages and foods and allows for the estimation of metabolite production and processing effects [15]. Red wine, which is fermented with the skin and stems of grapes, has a phenolic content 6–12 times greater than white wines which are removed from their skins during fermentation [16]. As a result red wines were expected to provide greater cardiovascular protection than what is seen with white wines or other alcoholic beverages. This has not yet been shown in prospective epidemiological studies; in some studies red wine consumption was not distinguished from total wine or alcohol consumption [17, 18], and in one study that sought to distinguish red wine consumption from alcohol consumption [19], no difference in magnitude of effect was observed due to the high correlation between total alcohol intake and red wine consumption ($r^2 = 0.92$). Two recent crossover-type studies of 20-day [20] and 28-day [21] duration for each intervention period compared the effects of red wine, dealcoholized red wine, and gin on inflammatory cytokines, leukocyte adhesion molecules, circulating concentrations of the microbially produced inflammogen lipopolysaccharide, LPS, and microbiota composition. Intake of NAC derived from red wine, as opposed to intake of alcohol, was associated with favorable changes in adhesion molecules and correlated with increases in *Bifidobacterium* and *Prevotella* which correlated negatively with LPS. Both ethanol and NAC were associated with reductions in inflammatory cytokines.

Holahan et al. [22] reconfirmed the association of moderate ethanol intake and reduced all-cause mortality compared to abstainers. However, the interesting aspect of this study was that the initial advantage of moderate ethanol consumption, which was predominantly in the form of wine, could be explained by lifestyle factors; low wine drinkers were more likely to be male, smokers, less physically active, lower socioeconomic level, and have more self-reported health problems. The authors noted a number of limitations of this study including self-reporting of ethanol. This

Table 6.1 Nonalcoholic wine components[a,i]

Component	Red wine (mg/100 g)	Nonphytochemical (g/L)	White wine (mg/100 g)
Total phenols and phenolic acids	1200 (900–2500)		200 (190–290)
Nonflavonoid[b]	240–500		160–260
• Hydroxybenzoic acids	0–260		0–100
• Hydroxycinnamic acids	162 (62–334)		130–154
• Stilbenes	12.3 (4–19)		1.8 (0.04–3.5)
(*trans*-Resveratrol)	1.0 (0.1–2.3)		0.22 (0.003–2.0)
Flavonoids[c]	750–1060		25–30
• Flavonols	98 (10–203)		Trace
• Flavanols	168 (48–440)		15–30
• Anthocyanins[d]	281 (20–500)		0
Water		800–900	
Carbohydrate[e]		<1–200	
Glycerol[f]		3–14	
Betaine		0.010–0.011	
Nitrogenous compounds		0.1–0.9	
Minerals		1.5–4.0	
Oligosaccharides[g]		0.102–0.127	
Organic acids: tartaric, lactic, succinic, acetic, *p*-hydroxyglutaric, galacturonic, amino, malic, citric, fumaric, oxalic, α-ketoglutaric, aconic, citramalic, malonic, pyrorocemic, and pantothenic		3–11	

[a]Tabular values, except oligosaccharides, summarized from [1]. Mean values were calculated from literature reports; the range of values contributing to the mean is in parentheses
[b]Hydroxybenzoic acids, hydroxycinnamic acids, and stilbenes
[c]Flavonols, flavanols, and anthocyanins
[d]Anthocyanins impart a red color to wine, which includes 3-monoglucosides of delphinidin, cyanidin, petunidin, peonidin, and malvidin
[e]Concentration varies with style of wine—dry (low carbohydrate) or sweet (high carbohydrate). Dessert wines are the sweetest and contain 140–240 g sugar/L. In contrast, a dry red might contain 2.5 g sugar/L. Residual sugar may appear on the label
[f]Glycerol imparts mouthfeel to a wine. A dry white wine contains about 5 g glycerol/L
[g]Values shown are the determinations of a single laboratory [63]
[h]Includes in decreasing concentration, tartaric, lactic, succinic, acetic, *p*-hydroxyglutaric, galacturonic, amino, malic, citric, fumaric, oxalic, α-ketoglutaric, aconic, citramalic, malonic, pyrorocemic, and pantothenic
[i]Varies with location of vineyard and equipment used in wine making

study did not measure markers of polyphenol intake which may be important as the putative phytochemicals that may mitigate ASCVD have expanded to include those in fruits, vegetables, and even phytochemical supplements. Additionally, changes over time in the intakes from these phytochemical sources are often not measured in observational studies. In a separate strategy, Mangoni et al. [23] sought to evaluate

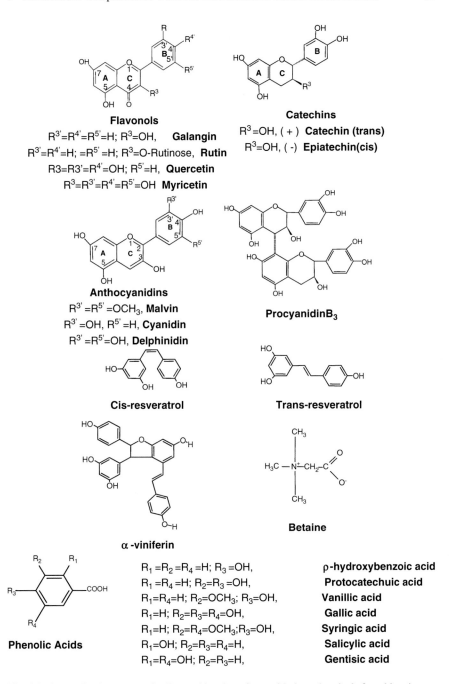

Flavonols

R$^{3'}$=R$^{4'}$=R$^{5'}$=H; R^3=OH,   **Galangin**

R$^{3'}$=R$^{4'}$=H; =R$^{5'}$=H; R^3=O-Rutinose, **Rutin**

R3=R3'=R$^{4'}$=OH; R$^{5'}$=H, **Quercetin**

R^3=R$^{3'}$=R$^{4'}$=R$^{5'}$=OH **Myricetin**

Catechins

R^3=OH, (+) **Catechin (trans)**

R^3=OH, (-) **Epiatechin(cis)**

Anthocyanidins

R$^{3'}$ =R$^{5'}$ =OCH$_3$, **Malvin**

R$^{3'}$ =OH, R$^{5'}$ =H, **Cyanidin**

R$^{3'}$ =R$^{5'}$=OH, **Delphinidin**

ProcyanidinB$_3$

Cis-resveratrol

Trans-resveratrol

α -viniferin

Betaine

Phenolic Acids

R$_1$ =R$_2$ =R$_4$ =H; R$_3$ =OH,   **p-hydroxybenzoic acid**

R$_1$ =R$_4$ =H; R$_2$=R$_3$ =OH,   **Protocatechuic acid**

R$_1$=R$_4$=H; R$_2$=OCH$_3$; R$_3$=OH,   **Vanillic acid**

R$_1$=H; R$_2$=R$_3$=R$_4$=OH,   **Gallic acid**

R$_1$=H; R$_2$=R$_4$=OCH$_3$;R$_3$=OH,   **Syringic acid**

R$_1$=OH; R$_2$=R$_3$=R$_4$=H,   **Salicylic acid**

R$_1$=R$_4$=OH; R$_2$=R$_3$=H,   **Gentisic acid**

Fig. 6.1 Generalized structures for flavonoid and nonflavonoid phytochemicals found in wine

published evidence relating red wine NAC to established markers of arterial structure and function in healthy subjects and ASCVD patients. The review provides clear explanations of methodologies used to evaluate arterial health but found that outcomes from the 26 studies evaluated were inconclusive, largely due to underpowered statistical designs, inadequate documentation of background polyphenolic intake, and relatively short intervention duration. While the present chapter focuses on the NAC of wine and their possible cardioprotective effects, we cannot lose sight of the benefits of wine, the beverage, as a whole, and its usual role in the diet. Thus, while research into the mechanisms of individual compounds is critical, wine is a beverage that delivers many compounds that may affect multiple targets by a variety of mechanisms simultaneously. This realization is particularly important in the context of newer aspects of the French paradox.

French Paradox: Old Paradigm

Following establishment of the concept of the French paradox, there was a dramatic increase in Europe and the United States in research investigations into the cardioprotective effects of wine and of the observed inverse relationship between CVD incidence and regular moderate wine consumption. Originally, the proposed mechanisms for the beneficial effects of wine included the consideration of the direct antioxidant capabilities of some of the polyphenolic compounds in wine within the vasculature itself in connection with LDL oxidation [3, 12, 13]. Hypothesized mechanisms grew to include reduction in platelet aggregation, increased NO production, inhibition of superoxide production, as well as some indications of a lowering blood pressure [3, 5, 13, 24, 25]. The proposed effects that dominated the early explanations of the French paradox linked wine consumption to the reduction in the risk of suffering from ASCVD and are well covered in reviews of the time [3, 5, 13, 25, 26]. However, continued research innovations are improving our understanding of both the causes of ASCVD and possible cardioprotective mechanisms of the NAC in wine; both are moving away from the original hypothesis of direct antioxidant actions.

Polyphenol Bioavailability Is Limited

The absorbability of wine NAC was recognized early on as an essential part of the hypothesis of systemic direct antioxidant activity as a mechanism to the French paradox [27]. Ultimately, demonstration of the poor bioavailability of wine phenolics led investigators away from red wine antioxidant capacity in the vascular wall as a major explanation for the French paradox [28–31]. It has long been pointed out that much of what has been reported about the actions of polyphenols, especially the proposed antioxidant effects, is based on in vitro rather than in vivo experimentation

[9, 13, 24]. Such studies are often not readily translated to in vivo situations due to the utilization of concentrations far greater than what can be expected in the body and because in vitro experiments often do not take into consideration the extensive metabolism and chemical alterations that occur through phase II metabolic processes once phenolics enter the body [28, 29, 32]. When modifications such as methylation of the hydroxyl rings are considered [32], antioxidant activity is greatly diminished and compound polarity altered. D'Archivio [24] recently summarized a number of factors and considerations relevant to food producers that impact polyphenolic availability. A recent in-depth review and evaluation by the Functional Foods Task Force of the European Union in connection with proposed health claims could not establish biological relevance for direct antioxidant actions of polyphenolics in ASCVD [33].

Newly Recognized Sources of Inflammation That Provoke ASCVD

A second step away from direct antioxidant actions has been the appreciation of ASCVD as an outcome of chronic systemic inflammation—an inflammation that can be driven by factors other than elevated LDL concentration per se, including altered immune responsiveness. The original French paradox noted that despite high intakes of saturated fat, ASCVD mortality in France was relatively low [4]. Interestingly it has been concluded that the cholesterol and saturated fat content of red meat may not be high enough to account for the observed increased risk for ASCVD in populations where red meat is a major component of the diet [34, 35]. However, other food components provide new sources of concern, albeit through different mechanisms [7, 34, 36, 37].

French Paradox: New Paradigm

Recent technological breakthroughs in sequencing, metabolomics, and computational biology are rapidly improving our ability to assess the impact of the complex materials we call food on our physiology, health, and well-being. Importantly, these new capacities have allowed characterization of what has come to be thought of as our newest and largest "organ," our microbiome [38]. The microbiome refers to the total number of microorganisms and their genetic material, while microbiota refers to a consortium of microbes present at various sites on the body. Microbiota composition varies by location, but the total number of cells comprising the microbiota outnumbers our own by 10 to 1. Within the gut particularly, the microbiota vary by region, are responsive to diet [39], and influence incidence of various intestinal disorders, obesity, allergic disease, and neuropsychiatric illnesses [38]. The poor absorbability of wine polyphenols becomes extremely relevant in this context as these substances may influence either the composition or function of microbiota. Recent studies have shown that wine NAC are metabolized by the microbiota to new molecules [40, 41] whose specific actions are the topic of ongoing investigation. As we learn more about microbially produced compounds, our understanding of potential mechanisms responsible for the French paradox is expanded.

New Mechanisms of ASCVD: Influence of the Gut Microbiota

New mechanisms of ASCVD causation have surfaced, and as they do, so do newly proposed mechanisms of the French paradox. The gut microbiome is the primary component of newly focused studies into overall human health [42]. The bacteria in our gut can metabolize, or further metabolize, nutrients in our food resulting in the formation of new compounds that affect our health [43, 44]; the best understood compounds at present are short-chain fatty acids and metabolites of tryptophan, carnitine, and choline metabolites [45, 46]. In addition, the types of bacteria living in the gut can be affected by diet; diet can also affect the metabolic processes active within the microbiome [43, 47–49]. In relation to ASCVD risk, microbiota-derived factors may alter gut function or otherwise result in increased systemic inflammation that ultimately compromises function of the vascular endothelium [38]. Factors that increase gut permeability, including obesity and diet components, may allow the microbial LPS to enter the systemic circulation and damage the vascular endothelium and initiate ASCVD [50–52]. Both microbial nitrogen and sulfur metabolism are considered critically relevant to gut health as they form bioactive compounds at several levels of oxidation that can affect both local intestinal processes and systemic processes following absorption into the body [53, 54]. Dysregulated cross talk between the gut immune system and the brain may be an important contributor to several neuropsychiatric illnesses, perhaps through microbiota-produced chemicals that cause changes in blood-brain barrier integrity [38] or perhaps due to microbiota-mediated immune tolerance, e.g., the "Old Friends" theory of stress resilience [55, 56].

Saturated Fat, Red Meat, and ASCVD Redux

L-Carnitine and choline are nitrogenous conditionally essential nutrients. They are novel ASCVD risk factors that may help explain the protective effects of red wine phenolics [7, 36, 37, 57]. They can be metabolized by gut bacteria into trimethylamine (TMA), a gas that can be absorbed into the circulation. In the liver, the enzyme flavin monooxygenase-3 quickly oxidizes this gas to form TMA oxide (TMAO). It appears that TMAO is directly inflammatory to vascular endothelium, thereby increasing ASCVD risk [7, 34, 37, 57] (Fig. 6.2). Notably, this process does not require any increase in gut permeability to allow TMA transfer to the systemic

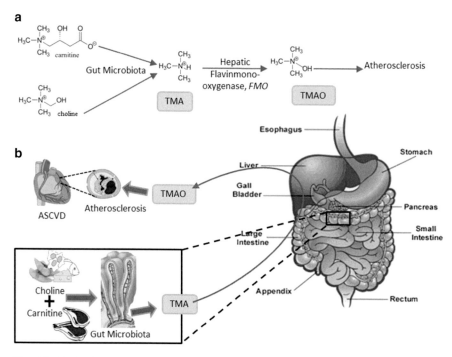

Fig. 6.2 Mechanism and illustration of the metabolism of carnitine and choline into trimethylamine and trimethylamine oxide. Adapted from [34, 57]. (**a**) Microbial conversion of diet components to trimethylamine (TMA) that is converted in liver to atherogenic trimethylamine oxide (TMAO). (**b**) Multi-organ transport and genesis of atherogenic TMAO

circulation. While red meat and eggs are often cited as the source of dietary L-carnitine and choline, and thus the main source of TMA, both are readily available in other foods. Fish is a rich source of preformed TMAO [58] (Table 6.2), but fish consumption is not associated with increased ASCVD risk. Clearly, many questions remain to be answered regarding diet and TMA/TMAO metabolism in humans as well as the ability of wine NAC to mitigate any untoward health effects that they create. It has been shown, however, that transplantation of cecal microbiota from ASCVD-susceptible inbred mouse strains to ASCVD-resistant inbred mouse strains increases susceptibility of resistant mice to choline-provoked ASCVD and increased TMAO concentrations [60].

With the gut microbiome increasingly implicated in ASCVD, a clear understanding of the metabolism of poorly available wine NAC becomes more important. In fact, this shift in attention to the gut microbiome has sparked interest in previously unstudied wine NAC, namely oligosaccharides. Breast milk oligosaccharides are often linked to the increased health benefits seen in breast-fed infants compared to formula fed [61, 62]. The link between oligosaccharides and improved health outcomes prompted characterization of oligosaccharides present in wine [63]. Breast milk oligosaccharides are typically oligolactates and are observed in concentrations

Table 6.2 Carnitine and choline concentrations in various food products[a]

	Carnitine (mg/100 g)		Choline[b] (mg/100 g)	
Meat products				
Beef	75.98	(64.6–87.5)	164.51	(78.15–418.22)
Poultry	31.05	(1.5–94.0)	144.87	(65.83–290.03)
Lamb and pork	28.63	(13.0–53.5)	113.83	(102.76–124.89)
Veal	72.50	(6.5–132.8)		
Processed meat	21.28	(2.9–66.3)	62.22	(51.36–73.07)
Fish and seafood[c]	2.13	(0.7–5.8)	62.00	(28.32–83.63)
Milk and dairy products				
Milk and butter	3.06	(1.3–10.0)	5.08	(0.65–16.40)
Cheese	7.99	(0.0–19.8)	16.50	9
Yogurt	6.95	(1.3–12.5)	14.62	(14.04–15.20)
Egg[d]	0.55	(0.3–0.8)	147.00	
Fruits	0.34	(0.0–0.8)	5.06	(1.94–9.76)
Vegetables	1.28	(0.0–8.1)	14.58	(5.96–27.51)
Nut and seeds	0.87	(0.0–2.2)	31.81	(11.14–52.47)
Cereal grains and pasta	0.00	not detected	4.37	(2.08–6.66)

[a]The range of values contributing to the mean is in parenthesis
[b]Total choline = sum of choline, phosphatidylcholine, glycerophosphocholine, and phosphocholine [39, 59]
[c]The median TMAO content of 226 samples from 86 fresh and saltwater fish species was 97 mg/100 g (range = 0.5–380 mg/100 g) [58]
[d]Value for one large egg, 50 g, as consumed. http://ndb.nal.usda.gov/ndb/foods. Accessed on June 17, 2014

of 7–12 g/L of milk [61]. Wines, by contrast, possess oligosaccharide concentrations of 102–127 mg/L and do not typically include oligolactates [63]. However, Cani and colleagues reported that the non-oligolactate prebiotic oligofructose reversed metabolic endotoxemia by reducing gut permeability, circulating LPS concentrations, and vascular inflammation [49, 50]. Moreover, the polyphenolic NAC in wine have also shown prebiotic effects [64] and so may act through mechanisms more often associated with oligosaccharides.

Diet and the Microbiome

The importance of the relationships between microbiota, immune function, and vascular health seems obvious as immune dysfunction leads to chronic inflammation which contributes to the development of a number of diseases including ASCVD. Relationships between the microbiome and our health are an area of intensive research [65]. It is now well documented that diet can impact the microbiota [39], and rapid progress is being made in understanding how metabolites produced by the microbiota affect immune function [45, 65]. There is a need for more research so that we learn how to maximize the health-promoting potential of the gut microbiota. Each individual's microbiome is shaped by genetics and environmental exposures, such as diet, hygiene, and social behavior, as well as the physical environment they inhabit [38, 39, 49, 66, 67]. Improved culture-independent methods to determine the structure of the microbiota community are being coupled with microbial transcriptomics to document global microbial gene expression, termed metagenomes, that determine microbial metabolite production as measurable by metabolomic techniques [39, 68, 69].

Studies using beverage and food challenges demonstrate that overall microbial gene expression is strongly linked to the host diet and that change in diet can quickly modulate the bacteria present in an individual's gut [39]. Metabolite profiles demonstrate that the metagenome activity is driven by substrate availability and that the metagenome changes in order to process those substrates rather than to maintain a fixed community structure for the microbiome [66]. Of particular note, while individuals are highly consistent in their microbiome-mediated metabolic responses to diet (reflecting a relatively constant microbiota), there is significant interindividual difference in microbial metabolism (reflecting significant interindividual variation in microbiota community structure) [41, 66, 70]. This implies that differing consortia of microbes contain core metabolic capacities but differ in final metabolite end products from core pathways. Feasibility studies that employ biomarker measurements within time-defined windows to identify the effects of diet components on measurable metabolomes of both of the host and microbiome show that such a strategy may be the next critical step toward personalizing nutrition recommendations for optimal health outcomes.

Wine and the Gut Microbiota

The previous discussion may be of much relevance to the specific question of how wine affects the gut microbiota and thence health. Red wine consumption has been shown to have a significant influence on the growth of select gut microbiota in humans, suggestive of prebiotic effects of red wine polyphenols [64]. Phytochemicals, specifically tannins and polyphenolics found in wine, are known to decrease the production of short-chain fatty acids at the level of the microbiota; additional effects may be caused by metabolites generated by microbial actions on nonabsorbed wine NAC. Recent studies have begun to use metabolomic analysis to characterize wine components or polyphenols and their microbially produced metabolites in plasma and urine following consumption [41, 66, 69, 71, 72]. At least one group has performed metabolite measurements of microbiota composition [64]. The number of hosts and microbiota that produce metabolites of wine NAC is large; studies have found that of the some 75 phenolics found in wines [68], the host generates at least 97 metabolites of parent compounds through phase II enzyme activities, mostly sulfated, glucuronidated, and methylated derivatives [68]. Further, the microbiota gives rise to additional metabolites of phenolic acids via hydrolysis, ring cleavage,

Table 6.3 Microbial metabolites showing the greatest increase in urinary concentration after 4 weeks of consumption of 272 mL of dealcoholized red wine (DRW) per day, $n = 36$ men [73]

Metabolite	Baseline (μmol/24 h)	Post-DRW (μmol/24 h)	Fold change	Likely precursors [73]
Syringic acid	0.73 ± 0.15	2.03 ± 032	2.78	Malvidin
Gallic acid	0.85 ± 0.18	4.76 ± 0.53	5.60	Tannins/anthocyanins
Ethyl gallate	1.06 ± 0.37	4.97 ± 0.73	4.69	Fermentation by-product
3-Hydroxyphenyl acetic acid	24.72 ± 3.50	56.57 ± 6.90	2.29	Proanthocyanidins
p-Coumaric acid	0.64 ± 0.07	1.48 ± 0.15	2.31	Cinnamic acid, anthocyanins, proanthocyanidins
Dihydroxyphenyl-valerolactone 1	6.73 ± 1.21	13.61 ± 2.68	2.02	Procyanidin components such as epicatechin, its gallates, or epigallocatechins
Dihydroxyphenyl-valerolactone 2	18.50 ± 3.67	37.04 ± 4.31	2.00	
Pyrogallol	1.96 ± 0.43	8.08 ± 1.78	4.12	Gallic acid, tannis
Ethyl glucuronide [74]	ND	ND	–	Ethanol
Tartaric acid [75]	ND	ND	–	Wine—red or white

decarboxylation, demethylation, reduction, and dehydroxylation. Boto-Ordóñez et al. [56] identified and quantified 24 host-derived phase II metabolites and 33 microbiome-derived phenolic acid metabolites in the urine of 36 men at high risk for ASCVD after 4 weeks of drinking dealcoholized red wine (Table 6.3). Others have identified markers for ethanol and phenolic intake [66, 72] (Table 6.3); Loke et al. [69] identified 11 metabolites arising from quercetin alone. New research strategies that address the expected large and divergent pattern of metabolites produced by individuals possessing different microbiota and phase II enzyme activities are the subject of critical discussion in the recent literature [45, 76, 77]. New experimental approaches include creation of animal models harboring "humanized" microbiota [41] in order to understand key variables within simplified environmental settings.

One of the most intriguing possibilities for the health-promoting potential of wine is of a chemical link between microbial metabolites of wine NAC and neurobiology. Good evidence is now available to support a microbiome-gut-brain axis [78]. Germ-free mice have exaggerated stress responses, and there appears to be a critical window for microbiota exposure to correct this behavior [79]. Wine is a complex beverage, and a contentious aspect of the French paradox has been whether the traditional consumption pattern for wine, namely, the positive effects of a shared meal and enjoyment of beverage and food, plays a role beyond avoidance of binge drinking. What we eat and drink is absorbed, thanks to our genes and microbiota, but in general, we only eat and drink what we like [80–82], and what we enjoy depends greatly on social memory [83–85]. Wine is not a simple food; it is bitter and acidic and complex in aroma and flavors and can be sweet or dry. It is a beverage whose nuances must be learned and whose "appreciation" often occurs in a rich social context with rituals that may include specialized utensils for its consumption [86]. There is reward in persevering, sharing, and learning in a positive setting how to appreciate wine as the circuitry around the *nucleus accumbens* [87] enables the identification of pleasurable vintages. We are only at the threshold of understanding the complex interplay between the brain, ingestive behaviors, microbiota, and health [88].

Learning how to enjoy meals, friends, and life may be the most complex task set before any individual. It is known that host physiology can alter our perception of food flavors. For example, Piombino et al. found that the saliva of obese individuals possessed a different microbiota than that of normal weight individuals and that it suppressed the release of wine aroma volatiles [89]. Really tasting wine adds an extra dimension to the basic daily routines of eating and drinking. It turns obligation into pleasure, a daily necessity into a celebration of life [9]. Conversely, reducing NAC to their medicinal role to create "wine pills" circumvents the pleasurable aspects of wine drinking, and such strategies, which have been tried with resveratrol [90], use pharmacologic doses that are impossible to achieve through moderate wine consumption and have not proved successful.

Conclusion

Our understanding of the mechanisms behind the cardioprotective nature of wine is far from complete. However, new technologies are allowing breakthroughs that further our understanding of how wine, as well as other beverages, influences our overall health including ASCVD risk. We are moving away from simplistic hypotheses of direct antioxidant actions and toward integrated hypotheses based on the recognition that our microbiota plays a crucial role and modulates the healthfulness of beverages. The concepts underlying the new lines of investigation into the French paradox reveal the complexity of the interactions between the practice of regular moderate wine consumption and cardiovascular health. With the multitude of proposed mechanisms, there seems to be nothing left but to sit and ponder the possibilities, perhaps over a glass of wine?

References

1. Centers for Disease Control. Heart disease. www.cdc.gov/heartdisease. Accessed 10 Jan 2015.
2. de Lorgeril M, Salen P, Paillard F, Laporte F, Boucher F, de Leiris J. Mediterranean diet and the French paradox: two distinct biogeographic concepts for one consolidated scientific theory on the role of nutrition in coronary heart disease. Cardiovasc Res. 2002;54:503–15.
3. Folts J. Potential health benefits from the flavonoids in grape products on vascular disease. In: Buslig B, Manthey J, editors. Flavonoids in cell function. New York: Springer; 2002. p. 95–111.
4. Renaud S, de Lorgeril M. Wine, alcohol, platelets, and the French paradox for coronary heart disease. Lancet. 1992;339:1523–6.

5. Walzem RL, German JB. The French Paradox: mechanisms of action of nonalcoholic wine components on cardiovascular disease. In: Wilson T, Temple N, editors. Nutrition and health. Totowa: Humana; 2004. p. 31–48.

6. Ross R. The pathogenesis of atherosclerosis: a perspective for the 1990s. Nature. 1993;362:801–9.

7. Bennett BJ, de Aguiar Vallim TQ, Wang Z, et al. Trimethylamine-n-oxide, a metabolite associated with atherosclerosis, exhibits complex genetic and dietary regulation. Cell Metab. 2013;17:49–60.

8. Gerber MJ, Scali JD, Michaud A, et al. Profiles of a healthful diet and its relationship to biomarkers in a population sample from Mediterranean southern France. J Am Diet Assoc. 2000;100:1164–71.

9. Walzem RL. Wine and health: state of proofs and research needs. Inflammopharmacology. 2008;16:265–71.

10. Ruf JC, Berger JL, Renaud S. Platelet rebound effect of alcohol withdrawal and wine drinking in rats. Relation to tannins and lipid peroxidation. Arterioscler Thromb Vasc Biol. 1995;15:140–4.

11. St Leger AS, Cochrane AL, Moore F. Factors associated with cardiac mortality in developed countries with particular reference to the consumption of wine. Lancet. 1979;1:1017–20.

12. Frankel EN, Kanner J, German JB, Parks E, Kinsella JE. Inhibition of oxidation of human low-density lipoprotein by phenolic substances in red wine. Lancet. 1993;341:454–7.

13. German JB, Walzem RL. The health benefits of wine. Annu Rev Nutr. 2000;20:561–93.

14. Xia EQ, Deng GF, Guo YJ, Li HB. Biological activities of polyphenols from grapes. Int J Mol Sci. 2010;11:622–46.

15. Rothwell JA, Perez-Jimenez J, Neveu V, et al. Phenol-Explorer 3.0: a major update of the Phenol-Explorer database to incorporate data on the effects of food processing on polyphenol content. Database (Oxford). 2013;2013:bat070.

16. Lippi G, Franchini M, Favaloro EJ, Targher G. Moderate red wine consumption and cardiovascular disease risk: beyond the "French Paradox". Semin Thromb Hemost. 2010;36:59–70.

17. Levantesi G, Marfisi R, Mozaffarian D, et al. Wine consumption and risk of cardiovascular events after myocardial infarction: results from the gissi-prevenzione trial. Int J Cardiol. 2013;163:282–7.

18. Pai JK, Mukamal KJ, Rimm EB. Long-term alcohol consumption in relation to all-cause and cardiovascular mortality among survivors of myocardial infarction: the health professionals follow-up study. Eur Heart J. 2012;33:1598–605.

19. Beulens JW, Algra A, Soedamah-Muthu SS, et al. Alcohol consumption and risk of recurrent cardiovascular events and mortality in patients with clinically manifest vascular disease and diabetes mellitus: the second manifestations of arterial (smart) disease study. Atherosclerosis. 2010;212:281–6.

20. Chiva-Blanch G, Urpi-Sarda M, Llorach R, et al. Differential effects of polyphenols and alcohol of red wine on the expression of adhesion molecules and inflammatory cytokines related to atherosclerosis: a randomized clinical trial. Am J Clin Nutr. 2012;95:326–34.

21. Clemente-Postigo M, Queipo-Ortuno MI, Boto-Ordonez M, et al. Effect of acute and chronic red wine consumption on lipopolysaccharide concentrations. Am J Clin Nutr. 2013;97:1053–61.

22. Holahan CJ, Schutte KK, Brennan PL, et al. Wine consumption and 20-year mortality among late-life moderate drinkers. J Stud Alcohol Drugs. 2012;73:80–8.

23. Mangoni AA, Stockley CS, Woodman RJ. Effects of red wine on established markers of arterial structure and function in human studies: current knowledge and future research directions. Expert Rev Clin Pharmacol. 2013;6:613–25.

24. D'Archivio M, Filesi C, Vari R, Scazzocchio B, Masella R. Bioavailability of the polyphenols: status and controversies. Int J Mol Sci. 2010;11:1321–42.

25. Magrone T, Candore G, Caruso C, Jirillo E, Covelli V. Polyphenols from red wine modulate immune responsiveness: biological and clinical significance. Curr Pharm Des. 2008;14:2733–48.

26. Waterhouse AL, Walzem RL. Nutrition of grape phenolics. In: Rice-Evans CA, Packer L, editors. Flavonoids in health and disease. New York: Marcel Dekker; 1998. p. 359–86.
27. Halliwell B. Dietary polyphenols: good, bad, or indifferent for your health? Cardiovasc Res. 2007;73:341–7.
28. Bell JR, Donovan JL, Wong R, et al. (+)-catechin in human plasma after ingestion of a single serving of reconstituted red wine. Am J Clin Nutr. 2000;71:103–8.
29. Donovan JL, Bell JR, Kasim-Karakas S, et al. Catechin is present as metabolites in human plasma after consumption of red wine. J Nutr. 1999;129:1662–8.
30. Williamson G, Manach C. Bioavailability and bioefficacy of polyphenols in humans. II. Review of 93 intervention studies. Am J Clin Nutr. 2005;81:243S–55.
31. Manach C, Williamson G, Morand C, Scalbert A, Remesy C. Bioavailability and bioefficacy of polyphenols in humans. I. Review of 97 bioavailability studies. Am J Clin Nutr. 2005;81:230S–42.
32. Yu J, Smith G, Gross HB, Hansen RJ, Levenberg J, Walzem RL. Enzymatic o-methylation of flavanols changes lag time, propagation rate, and total oxidation during in vitro model triacylglycerol-rich lipoprotein oxidation. J Agric Food Chem. 2006;54:8403–8.
33. Hollman PC, Cassidy A, Comte B, et al. The biological relevance of direct antioxidant effects of polyphenols for cardiovascular health in humans is not established. J Nutr. 2011;141:989S–1009.
34. Koeth RA, Wang Z, Levison BS, et al. Intestinal microbiota metabolism of l-carnitine, a nutrient in red meat, promotes atherosclerosis. Nat Med. 2013;19:576–85.
35. Siri-Tarino PW, Sun Q, Hu FB, Krauss RM. Meta-analysis of prospective cohort studies evaluating the association of saturated fat with cardiovascular disease. Am J Clin Nutr. 2010;91:535–46.
36. Tang WH, Wang Z, Levison BS, et al. Intestinal microbial metabolism of phosphatidylcholine and cardiovascular risk. N Engl J Med. 2013;368:1575–84.
37. Wang Z, Klipfell E, Bennett BJ, et al. Gut flora metabolism of phosphatidylcholine promotes cardiovascular disease. Nature. 2011;472:57–63.
38. Khanna S, Tosh PK. A clinician's primer on the role of the microbiome in human health and disease. Mayo Clin Proc. 2014;89:107–14.
39. David LA, Maurice CF, Carmody RN, et al. Diet rapidly and reproducibly alters the human gut microbiome. Nature. 2014;505:559–63.
40. van Dorsten FA, Grun CH, van Velzen EJ, Jacobs DM, Draijer R, van Duynhoven JP. The metabolic fate of red wine and grape juice polyphenols in humans assessed by metabolomics. Mol Nutr Food Res. 2010;54:897–908.
41. van Duynhoven J, Vaughan EE, Jacobs DM, et al. Metabolic fate of polyphenols in the human superorganism. Proc Natl Acad Sci U S A. 2011;108 Suppl 1:4531–8.
42. Ley RE, Lozupone CA, Hamady M, Knight R, Gordon JI. Worlds within worlds: evolution of the vertebrate gut microbiota. Nat Rev Microbiol. 2008;6:776–88.
43. Smith MI, Yatsunenko T, Manary MJ, et al. Gut microbiomes of Malawian twin pairs discordant for kwashiorkor. Science. 2013;339:548–54.
44. Turnbaugh PJ, Ley RE, Mahowald MA, Magrini V, Mardis ER, Gordon JI. An obesity-associated gut microbiome with increased capacity for energy harvest. Nature. 2006;444:1027–31.
45. Dorrestein PC, Mazmanian SK, Knight R. Finding the missing links among metabolites, microbes, and the host. Immunity. 2014;40:824–32.
46. Thorburn AN, Macia L, Mackay CR. Diet, metabolites, and "western-lifestyle" inflammatory diseases. Immunity. 2014;40:833–42.
47. Muegge BD, Kuczynski J, Knights D, et al. Diet drives convergence in gut microbiome functions across mammalian phylogeny and within humans. Science. 2011;332:970–4.
48. Turnbaugh PJ, Ridaura VK, Faith JJ, Rey FE, Knight R, Gordon JI. The effect of diet on the human gut microbiome: a metagenomic analysis in humanized gnotobiotic mice. Sci Transl Med. 2009;1:6ra14.

49. Tuohy KM, Fava F, Viola R. 'The way to a man's heart is through his gut microbiota' – dietary pro- and prebiotics for the management of cardiovascular risk. Proc Nutr Soc. 2014;73:172–85.

50. Cani PD, Amar J, Iglesias MA, et al. Metabolic endotoxemia initiates obesity and insulin resistance. Diabetes. 2007;56:1761–72.

51. de La Serre CB, Ellis CL, Lee J, Hartman AL, Rutledge JC, Raybould HE. Propensity to high-fat diet-induced obesity in rats is associated with changes in the gut microbiota and gut inflammation. Am J Physiol Gastrointest Liver Physiol. 2010;299:G440–8.

52. Lin E, Freedman JE, Beaulieu LM. Innate immunity and toll-like receptor antagonists: a potential role in the treatment of cardiovascular diseases. Cardiovasc Ther. 2009;27:117–23.

53. Carbonero F, Benefiel AC, Alizadeh-Ghamsari AH, Gaskins HR. Microbial pathways in colonic sulfur metabolism and links with health and disease. Front Physiol. 2012;3:448.

54. Lundberg JO, Weitzberg E. Biology of nitrogen oxides in the gastrointestinal tract. Gut. 2013;62:616–29.

55. Rook GA, Lowry CA, Raison CL. Microbial 'old friends', immunoregulation and stress resilience. Evol Med Public Health. 2013;2013:46–64.

56. Rook GA, Raison CL, Lowry CA. Childhood microbial experience, immunoregulation, inflammation and adult susceptibility to psychosocial stressors and depression in rich and poor countries. Evol Med Public Health. 2013;2013:14–7.

57. Backhed F. Meat-metabolizing bacteria in atherosclerosis. Nat Med. 2013;19:533–4.

58. Chung SW, Chan BT. Trimethylamine oxide, dimethylamine, trimethylamine and formaldehyde levels in main traded fish species in Hong Kong. Food Addit Contam Part B Surveill. 2009;2:44–51.

59. Demarquoy J, Georges B, Rigault C, et al. Radioisotopic determination of l-carnitine content in foods commonly eaten in western countries. Food Chem. 2004;86:137–42.

60. Gregory JC, Buffa JA, Org E, et al. Transmission of atherosclerosis susceptibility with gut microbial transplantation. J Biol Chem. 2014.

61. Boehm G, Stahl B. Oligosaccharides from milk. J Nutr. 2007;137:847S–9.

62. Smilowitz JT, O'Sullivan A, Barile D, German JB, Lonnerdal B, Slupsky CM. The human milk metabolome reveals diverse oligosaccharide profiles. J Nutr. 2013;143:1709–18.

63. Bordiga M, Travaglia F, Meyrand M, et al. Identification and characterization of complex bioactive oligosaccharides in white and red wine by a combination of mass spectrometry and gas chromatography. J Agric Food Chem. 2012;60:3700–7.

64. Queipo-Ortuno MI, Boto-Ordonez M, Murri M, et al. Influence of red wine polyphenols and ethanol on the gut microbiota ecology and biochemical biomarkers. Am J Clin Nutr. 2012;95:1323–34.

65. Sharon G, Garg N, Debelius J, Knight R, Dorrestein PC, Mazmanian SK. Specialized metabolites from the microbiome in health and disease. Cell Metab. 2014;20:719–30.

66. Heinzmann SS, Merrifield CA, Rezzi S, et al. Stability and robustness of human metabolic phenotypes in response to sequential food challenges. J Proteome Res. 2012;11:643–55.

67. Kau AL, Ahern PP, Griffin NW, Goodman AL, Gordon JI. Human nutrition, the gut microbiome and the immune system. Nature. 2011;474:327–36.

68. Boto-Ordóñez M, Rothwell JA, Andres-Lacueva C, Manach C, Scalbert A, Urpi-Sarda M. Prediction of the wine polyphenol metabolic space: an application of the phenol-explorer database. Mol Nutr Food Res. 2014;58:466–77.

69. Loke WM, Jenner AM, Proudfoot JM, et al. A metabolite profiling approach to identify biomarkers of flavonoid intake in humans. J Nutr. 2009;139:2309–14.

70. Russell WR, Labat A, Scobbie L, Duncan SH. Availability of blueberry phenolics for microbial metabolism in the colon and the potential inflammatory implications. Mol Nutr Food Res. 2007;51:726–31.

71. Boto-Ordóñez M, Urpi-Sarda M, Queipo-Ortuño MI, et al. Microbial metabolomic fingerprinting in urine after regular dealcoholized red wine consumption in humans. J Agric Food Chem. 2013;61:9166–75.

72. Vazquez-Fresno R, Llorach R, Alcaro F, et al. (1)h-nmr-based metabolomic analysis of the effect of moderate wine consumption on subjects with cardiovascular risk factors. Electrophoresis. 2012;33:2345–54.

73. Forester SC, Waterhouse AL. Metabolites are key to understanding health effects of wine polyphenolics. J Nutr. 2009;139:1824S–31.

74. Stephanson N, Dahl H, Helander A, Beck O. Direct quantification of ethyl glucuronide in clinical urine samples by liquid chromatography-mass spectrometry. Ther Drug Monit. 2002;24:645–51.

75. Regueiroa J, Vallverdú-Queralta A, Simal-Gándara J, Estrucha R, Lamuela-Raventósa RM. Urinary tartaric acid as a potential biomarker for the dietary assessment of moderate wine consumption: a randomised controlled trial. Br J Nutr. 2014;111:1680–5.

76. Ahern PP, Faith JJ, Gordon JI. Mining the human gut microbiota for effector strains that shape the immune system. Immunity. 2014;40:815–23.

77. Huttenhower C, Kostic AD, Xavier RJ. Inflammatory bowel disease as a model for translating the microbiome. Immunity. 2014;40:843–54.

78. Clarke G, Grenham S, Scully P, et al. The microbiome-gut-brain axis during early life regulates the hippocampal serotonergic system in a sex-dependent manner. Mol Psychiatry. 2013;18:666–73.

79. Sudo N, Chida Y, Aiba Y, et al. Postnatal microbial colonization programs the hypothalamic-pituitary-adrenal system for stress response in mice. J Physiol. 2004;558:263–75.

80. Halpern GM. The case for pleasure and health. In: Proceedings of the 7th ARISE Symposium, Nice, France. 2001. London: ARISE.

81. Halpern GM. "We only eat what we like" or do we still? Flavour. 2012;1:17–9.

82. Halpern GM. We only eat what we like. www.beyondthirtynine.com. Accessed 28 Jan 2015.

83. Gibson EL. Emotional influences on food choice: sensory, physiological and psychological pathways. Physiol Behav. 2006;89:53–61.

84. Lupton D. Food, memory and meaning: the symbolic and social nature of food events. Soc Rev. 1994;42:664–85.

85. Stroebele N, De Castro JM. Effect of ambience on food intake and food choice. Nutrition. 2004;20:821–38.

86. Matthews T. The-abcs-of-wine-tasting. Wine Spectator, 1996. http://www.winespectator.com/webfeature/show/id/The-ABCs-of-Wine-Tasting_3217. Accessed 10 Jan 2015.

87. Costa VD, Lang PJ, Sabatinelli D, Bradley MM, Versace F. Emotional imagery: assessing pleasure and arousal in the brain's reward circuitry. Hum Brain Mapp. 2010;31:1446–57.

88. Clarke G, Grenham S, Scully P, et al. The microbiome-gut-brain axis during early life regulates the hippocampal serotonergic system in a sex-dependent manner. Mol Psychiatry. 2012;18:666–73.

89. Piombino P, Genovese A, Esposito S, et al. Saliva from obese individuals suppresses the release of aroma compounds from wine. PLoS One. 2014;9:e85611.

90. Poulsen MM, Jørgensen JO, Jessen N, Richelsen B, Pedersen SB. Resveratrol in metabolic health: an overview of the current evidence and perspectives. Ann N Y Acad Sci. 2013;1290:74–82.

Chapter 7
Cranberry Juice: Effects on Health

Diane L. McKay and Ted Wilson

Keywords Cranberry • *Vaccinium macrocarpon* • Urinary tract infection • Vasodilation • Heart disease • Cancer prevention • Proanthocyanidins • Fruit juice

Key Points

1. Cranberries have long been used as a part of traditional and folk medicine.
2. Most cranberry juice is consumed as a product containing 27 % v/v with sweeteners derived from other fruit juices or other sweeteners.
3. Cranberry juice contains a rich profile of phenolic compounds, especially proanthocyanidins or PAC, that appear to be responsible for an ability to prevent bacterial adhesions within the urinary tract.
4. Cranberry juice consumption may also protect against bacterial infections of the stomach and oral cavity, as well as cardiovascular disease and cancer.

D.L. McKay, Ph.D. (✉)
Friedman School of Nutrition Science and Policy, Jean Mayer USDA Human Nutrition
Research Center on Aging, Tufts University, 150 Harrison Avenue, Boston, MA 02111, USA
e-mail: diane.mckay@tufts.edu

T. Wilson, Ph.D.
Department of Biology, Winona State University, Winona, MN 54987, USA
e-mail: twilson@winona.edu

© Springer International Publishing Switzerland 2016
T. Wilson, N.J. Temple (eds.), *Beverage Impacts on Health and Nutrition*,
Nutrition and Health, DOI 10.1007/978-3-319-23672-8_7

Introduction

The American cranberry (*Vaccinium macrocarpon*) has been a part of the diet and folk medicine of North Americans for millennia. Native New Englanders used cranberries for food, fabric dye, and poultices to treat wounds and blood poisoning, and early American sailors, including whalers and mariners, consumed them as antiscorbutic agents [1, 2]. While *V. macrocarpon* cranberries are the variety most familiar to consumers in North America, close relatives of the cranberry, *V. oxyccos*, are also consumed in Northern Europe and Asia. In North America and Europe, cranberries are primarily processed and consumed in the form of cranberry juices, cranberry juice cocktails, and cranberry fruit drinks, with the oldest cranberry juice recipe dating back to 1683 [1].

Cranberries have only been cultivated for the last 150 years, thus relative to grape and other cultivated fruits, there is relatively little genetic diversity [3]. The typical annual crop size is approximately 850 million pounds, 95 % of which is processed into cranberry-based beverages, concentrates, sweetened dried cranberries, and sauces. Only 5 % of the total cranberry crop is sold and consumed as fresh fruit [4]. Cranberries are popular with consumers because of their tart taste and their purported health benefits. As one of the first functional foods in America, cranberry juice has been associated with protection from urinary tract infections (UTIs). More recently, studies also support a role for cranberry juice in improving oral and gastric health, promoting cardiovascular health, and inhibiting cancer development.

Cranberry Juice Consumption and Urinary Tract Infections

Urinary Tract Infections Are a Major Health Problem

UTIs occur when bacteria (primarily *Escherichia coli* or *E. coli*) adhere to the uroepithelial cells that line the bladder, kidney, or urethra and then multiply. Bacterial adhesion to uroepithelial cells requires the production of a set of structures called p-fimbriae on the cell walls of the colonizing bacteria. P-fimbriae are proteinaceous fibers that form adhesions to carbohydrates on the surface of uroepithelial cells permitting the adherence of bacteria within the urinary tract. Any bacteria that are unable to adhere to the epithelium are normally flushed out of the urinary tract during urination. Adhesion leads to colonization of the urinary tract epithelium and destruction of the lining of the bladder, as well as inflammation and rupturing of the underlying blood vessels, causing blood in the urine in some cases. The resultant inflammation promotes a painful burning sensation; persistent, untreated UTIs can lead to cystitis and pyelonephritis [5], which can eventually lead to the loss of one or both kidneys.

UTIs are very common, with about 60 % of American women being affected over a lifetime [6]. Persistent infections often require ongoing treatment with expensive antibiotics that necessitate visits to a physician and substantial costs to the health-care system. UTIs are most typically found in women but also occur in men and children. Persons at very high risk include the elderly, paraplegics, and quadriplegics, as well as those undergoing treatment for cancer of the prostate, bladder, or cervix. Folk medicine has long purported the use of cranberry juice for the treatment of UTIs. Furthermore, increasing clinical evidence supports the consumption of cranberry juice as a way for vulnerable populations to help prevent the onset or reduce the frequency of these infections.

Cranberry Juice Prevents Urinary Tract Infections

As mentioned, cranberry juice has been popular for many years for the treatment and prevention of UTIs. However, the first double-blind human clinical trial demonstrating the efficacy of cranberry juice was not published until 1994 [7]. In this trial, elderly women were randomized to 300 mL/day of a saccharine-sweetened 27 % cranberry beverage or a synthetic placebo drink that was indistinguishable in taste, appearance, and vitamin C content. Cranberry juice consumption led to significant reductions in the numbers of both bacteria and white blood cells in the urine over the 6-month study period.

Completion of UTI treatment does not always provide permanent protection from reinfection. UTIs reinfect approximately one-third of women within 1 year of initial treatment [8]. A Finnish study of UTI recurrence administered a 50 mL daily dose of a cranberry-lingonberry juice mixture to volunteers from a student health facility and an occupational health center [9]. Daily cranberry-lingonberry juice consumption for 6 months was associated with half the risk of UTI recurrence relative to a control group.

Recent studies have also shown a lower incidence of UTI relapse with regular, long-term consumption of cranberry juice or cranberry capsules in free-living adults age 20–79 years [10], older adults in long-term care facilities [11], and in children [12].

However, inconsistencies in other studies, most likely due to lack of a standardized dose, poor subject compliance, and the absence of a reliable, measurable biomarker of cranberry intake, have hampered efforts to unequivocally recommend cranberries as a preventive agent.

Early Hypotheses About Cranberries and UTI Prevention

There has been much speculation as to the mechanism by which cranberry products protect against UTIs. In the early 1900s, Blatherwick [13, 14] observed that consumption of 300–600 g of cranberry sauce per day could promote a short-term decrease in urine pH. It was hypothesized that this acidification was what prevented bacterial colonization of the urinary tract epithelium. While this theory was popular, subsequent studies were unable to demonstrate that the urine was always acidified postconsumption [15, 16]. However, because urinary hippuric acid excretion was also found to increase following cranberry consumption, that substance was suggested as being responsible for the protective effects. By the 1960s, it was determined that cranberry juice altered urine pH for only a short period of time, that the degree of acidification was not sufficient to provide bactericidal or bacteriostatic effects, and that neither acidification nor hippuric acid could be the primary mechanism [17].

In 1984, Sabota used *E. coli* isolates from UTI-afflicted humans to determine that cranberry juice contains a nondialyzable material that specifically inhibits the expression of the p-fimbriae of bacteria, hence preventing their attachment to and colonization of the urinary tract [18]. It was later determined that cranberry proanthocyanidins (PAC), a type of condensed tannin, is the active ingredient in cranberry that inhibits adherence of p-fimbriated *E. coli* to uroepithelial cells.

Other Bacterial Interactions with Cranberry Juice

Several reports have suggested that cranberry juice consumption may also have the capacity to affect bacterial populations outside the urinary tract. Adhesions similar to those produced on the p-fimbriae of uropathogenic *E. coli* are also required by bacteria that cause disease in the stomach and mouth. Gastric ulcers are largely caused by *Helicobacter pylori* (*H. pylori*) which require adhesion to the gastric epithelium for pathogenicity. Early in vitro studies by Burger et al. suggested that a high molecular weight constituent in cranberry juice inhibits the production of adhesions in *H. pylori* and that cranberry juice consumption may help prevent gastric ulcers [19]. More recent in vitro studies confirmed the inhibitory effects of cranberry on the adhesion of *H. pylori* to human mucus, erythrocytes, and gastric epithelial cells [20]. Clinical trials demonstrated that cranberry juice reduces *H. pylori* infection after 90 days of consumption [21].

Cranberries are also thought to promote good gum health by preventing bacterial adhesion within the oral epithelium and by preventing dental plaque buildup. Several in vitro studies have been conducted to assess whether cranberry components inhibit adhesion of oral bacteria to tooth surfaces and epithelial cells. Data from these studies support a beneficial effect of cranberry or its PAC constituents by blocking adhesion to and biofilm formation on target tissues of pathogens [20]. These studies have also shown that cranberry PACs may be potential therapeutic agents for the prevention and management of periodontitis, an inflammatory disease of bacterial origin affecting tooth-supporting tissues [22]. A clinical trial reported a significant reduction in total bacterial count in healthy volunteers who used a daily mouthwash supplemented with nondialyzable material from cranberries for 6 weeks when compared with a control group [23].

Table 7.1 Nutrient content of cranberries and selected cranberry products

Nutrient	Whole raw (1 c or 95 g)	Dried, sweetened (0.33 c or 40 g)	Juice, unsweetened (1 c or 253 g)	Juice (27 %) cocktail (1 c or 253 g)
Energy (kcal)	44	123	116	137
Water (g)	83	6	220	218
Protein (g)	0.37	0.03	0.99	0.00
Carbohydrate (g)	11.6	32.9	30.9	34.2
Total lipid (g)	0.12	0.55	0.32	0.25
Fiber (g)	4.4	2.3	0.3	0
Potassium (mg)	81	16	194	35
Sodium (mg)	2	1	4	5
Vitamin C (mg)	12.6	0.1	23.6	107.0

Adapted from McKay and Blumberg [2]

Cranberry Constituents and Their Biological Activities

Nutrients in Cranberries

Cranberries, like other whole fruits, are naturally low in calories, fat, and sodium, contain no cholesterol, and are a good source of dietary fiber (Table 7.1). Similarly, dried cranberries, cranberry juice, and juice cocktail contain little sodium and fat. Relative to other fruits, cranberries have low sugar content. Specific cranberry products, such as dried sweetened cranberries and cranberry juice cocktail (27 % juice), have been recognized by the American Heart Association as "heart healthy" based on their nutrient composition. One serving of either product contains <0.6 g total fat, <0.05 g saturated fat, and no cholesterol or *trans* fat. In addition, dried cranberries provide >10 % of the daily value of fiber, while cranberry juice cocktail contains >100 % of the daily value of vitamin C. Although vitamin C contributes to the high antioxidant activity of these foods, it is the phytochemicals in cranberries that are largely responsible for this effect.

Cranberry Phytochemicals and Pharmacokinetics

Cranberries contain a higher amount of total phenols per serving (507–709 mg gallic acid equivalents/100 g) than other common fruits including blueberries (258–531 mg/100 g), apples (185–347 mg/100 g), red grapes (175–370 mg/100 g), and strawberries (132–368 mg/100 g) [2].

Cranberries and cranberry juice are rich sources of phenolic compounds, particularly phenolic acids (including benzoic, hydroxycinnamic, and ellagic acids) and

Table 7.2 Phenolic phytochemicals in cranberry juice cocktail

Phenolic compound
Proanthocyanidins
Anthocyanins
Cyanidin-3-galactoside
Cyanidin-3-glucoside
Cyanidin-3-arabinoside
Peonidin-3-galactoside
Peonidin-3-glucoside
Peonidin-3-arabinoside
Flavonols
Hyperoside
Quercetin
Myricetin
Quercitrin
Avicularin
Phenolic acids
Benzoic acid
Chlorogenic acid
4-Hydroxycinnamic acid
3,4-Dihydroxybenzoic acid
Vanillic acid
Caffeic acid

Adapted from McKay and Blumberg, 2007 [2]

flavonoids (including flavonols, flavan-3-ols, anthocyanins, and PAC) (Table 7.2), and these phenolics appear responsible for their putative health benefits.

PAC, also called condensed tannins, is ubiquitous in plants, with fruits being the major source in the diet. Procyanidins, a subclass of proanthocyanidins, are mixtures of oligomers and polymers consisting of catechin and epicatechin units linked mainly through B-type bonds. In experimental studies, procyanidins possess a variety of activities, including antioxidant, antimicrobial, antiallergy, and antihypertensive actions. The procyanidins in cranberries contain more epicatechin than catechin (46.5 vs. 7.4 % of terminal units) which, unlike most other procyanidin-containing foods, are predominantly linked via A-type bonds. The A-type linkage is a structural feature that appears to be responsible for the unique antiadhesion action and some of the antioxidant properties of cranberries [2].

Little information is available regarding the pharmacokinetics of A-type PAC though their dimers, trimers, and tetramers have been found to be taken up by Caco-2 cells in vitro [24]. PAC-A2 were recently quantified in the urine of healthy volunteers following an acute dose of CJC [25]. The time to reach maximal concentration (T_{max}) of PAC-A2 at 11 h suggests that most of this compound was absorbed in the lower GI tract after being produced from oligomers and polymers via catabolism by gut microbiota. The measurement of PAC-A2 in urine suggests its potential as a biomarker of cranberry intake and compliance. In contrast to the A-type, B-type PACs have been readily detected in human plasma and urine after consumption of grape seed extracts and cocoa [26, 27].

While the bioavailability of phenolic compounds from other fruits has been reported in many studies, few human studies have examined the absorption and excretion of cranberry phenolic acids and flavonoids [28–31]. A recent pilot study by Singh et al. [32] suggests that quercetin-3-galactoside, a flavonol present at a relatively high level in cranberry fruit, is absorbed postprandially and could be a useful marker of cranberry consumption in humans. More recently, McKay et al. [25] reported that the sum total of phenolics, including phenolic acids, flavonols, and flavanols, detected in plasma reached a peak concentration at 8–10 h, while in urine the peak concentration of the sum appeared 2–4 h earlier. In plasma, protocatechuic acid, quercetin, and vanillic acid were the highest contributors to this total. In urine, the highest contributor was protocatechuic acid followed by 4-OH-phenylacetic acid. Anthocyanins, as well as anthocyanin glucuronides, were detected in urine, and their concentrations varied widely. Peonidin-3-galactoside was the predominant anthocyanin detected in both plasma and urine within 3 and 4 h, respectively, after consumption. Pronounced interindividual variability in the C_{max} and T_{max} of many compounds detected in both plasma and urine were observed, most likely due to individual differences in phase II enzyme polymorphisms as well as composition of GI microbiota.

Antioxidant Activity Following Cranberry Consumption

The effect of cranberry juices on antioxidant capacity in humans has been reported in numerous studies [25, 33–36]. Pedersen et al. [33] observed an increase in plasma total antioxidant capacity with acute cranberry juice consumption, assessed by reduction potential of plasma constituents, and attributed the effect to an increase in plasma vitamin C as well as total phenols. Vinson et al. [36] noted an increase in the ferric reducing ability of plasma (FRAP) assay following acute consumption relative to a control beverage. McKay et al. [25] reported plasma total antioxidant capacity assessed using the oxygen radical absorbance capacity (ORAC) and total antioxidant performance (TAP) assays following an acute dose of cranberry juice correlated with the appearance over time of individual metabolites, such as protocatechuic acid.

Ruel et al. [34] reported that cranberry juice consumption for 2 weeks decreased circulating oxidized LDL. Following an acute dose, McKay et al. [25] reported a 17.8 % increase in the resistance of LDL to Cu^{2+}-induced oxidation at 8 h compared to baseline. As with other markers of antioxidant activity reported in this study, the resistance of LDL against oxidation correlated with plasma protocatechuic acid.

Possible Effects of Cranberries on Cardiovascular Disease

Cranberry beverages are hypothesized to reduce cardiovascular risk by protecting LDL cholesterol particles from oxidative damage, lowering cholesterol, reducing inflammation, improving endothelial function and arterial stiffness, and by inhibiting platelet aggregation [2, 37–41]. Indeed, there is evidence that the polyphenolic components of cranberries favorably affect lipoprotein profiles, oxidative stress, inflammation, and endothelial function, as well as other cardiovascular risk factors, such as blood pressure and glucose metabolism. However, clinical evidence supporting the effects of cranberry products on biomarkers of cardiovascular risk is inconsistent.

For example, consumption of cranberry polyphenols improved lipid profiles in several animal models and in clinical trials with hypercholesterolemic, dyslipidemic, obese, and diabetic patients; however, no significant effects on plasma lipids were observed among healthy subjects or CVD patients following cranberry juice consumption [40]. Similarly, the anti-inflammatory effects of cranberry polyphenols were demonstrated by Ruel et al. [42] in a study of sedentary middle-aged subjects and by Zhu et al. [43] in hypercholesterolemic patients; however, several other human studies failed to show any significant effects on C-reactive protein, adhesion molecules, or biomarkers of inflammation.

The results of clinical studies to determine whether cranberry polyphenols, or bioactives, improve endothelial vasodilator function are promising. Cranberry juice appears to promote vasodilation in a manner similar to that associated with red wine and Concord grape juice [44, 45]. Using rat vessels, Maher et al. [46] demonstrated in vitro and in vivo that cranberry juice can dilate vessels at levels comparable to that of grape products and red wine. It appears that the effects of cranberry consumption on endothelial function in human are mostly acute. Although in one well-controlled study, a benefit on carotid-femoral pulse-wave velocity (PWV), a measure of arterial stiffness, was observed with chronic cranberry consumption [41].

Possible Effects of Cranberries on Cancer

In vitro studies demonstrate that *Vaccinium* fruit extracts can prevent or decrease a number of processes involved in carcinogenesis. The anticancer properties of *Vaccinium* fruit have been the subject of investigation since the late 1990s. The phytochemical constituents responsible for the observed anticancer activity of these fruits, including the flavonols, anthocyanins, PAC, various phenolic acids, triterpenoids (ursolic acid), and the stilbenes, are thought to act individually, additively, and synergistically. Studies using in vitro tumor models have shown that cranberry extracts and derived polyphenolic compounds can inhibit the growth and proliferation of breast, colon, prostate, and lung tumors. Possible mechanisms of action supported by this evidence include induction of apoptosis, decreased invasion and metastasis due to matrix metalloproteinase inhibition, decreased ornithine decarboxylase expression and activity, and inhibition of inflammatory processes including cyclooxygenase-2 (COX-2) activity [47, 48].

The first report of tumor growth inhibition by cranberry in vivo was from Ferguson et al. in 2006 [49]. They used mice with established xenografts of either U87 glioblastoma, HT-29 colon carcinoma, or DU145 prostate carcinoma cell lines. When compared with the control group, mice intraperitoneally injected with either a flavonoid-rich aqueous extract from cranberry press cake or a PAC fraction prepared from whole fruit extract had slower growth of the glioblastoma and prostate carcinoma and reduced volume of the colon tumor explants. In two of the treated animals, a complete regression of the tumors was observed.

In a later study, Prasain et al. [50] reported the antitumorigenic effects of a cranberry juice concentrate administered orally (via gavage). In this study, nitrosamine was used to induce bladder cancer in rats, and those that were treated with cranberry had a significant reduction in tumor weight and number of cancerous lesions when compared with the control group. The results of this study suggest that orally administered cranberry can provide metabolites present in sufficient quantity to inhibit tumorigenesis.

Cranberry Beverage Formulations Available to the Consumer

Cranberry beverage products can be marketed using several different designations related to the percentage of cranberry juice present in the beverage. The tartness of cranberry juice means that few people consume a 100 % cranberry or first press product. Products containing less than 100 % of the primary labeled ingredient must contain the words "beverage," "cocktail," or "drink" in the label. As mentioned in the chapter by Krasny:

> For multiple-juice beverages, whether diluted or single-strength, any juices in the product name must be listed in descending order of predominance by weight, unless a characterizing juice is declared as a flavor (e.g., raspberry-flavored apple and grape juice drink). There is also a mandatory percentage juice declaration requirement, based on the soluble solids content of expressed juice (not from concentrate), or minimum Brix levels (for reconstituted juice). When a beverage is made from concentrate, the product name must indicate that fact.

Variation in the amount of cranberry juice present in commercially available products is also a factor that makes it challenging to formulate dietary recommendations for optimal health benefits. While responsible for some of the popular aspects of cranberry palatability, the tartness (acidity) and polyphenolic content of cranberries also creates limits for manufacturers. A high polyphenolic content of a beverage can lead to a harmless brown precipitation, or what the consumer calls sedimentation, that tends to form on the store shelf. To help prevent this, manufacturers seldom add more than approximately 30 % v/v cranberry juice to their products and typically no more than 27 %; however, many products actually contain far less than this amount.

The tart taste of cranberries poses a challenge for both manufacturers and consumers; sweeteners are often used to improve cranberry juice palatability. Cranberry juice cocktails typically contain 27 % cranberry juice and are sweetened with added sugar in the form of cane sugar, beet sugar, or high fructose corn syrup. Artificial sweeteners are also used to improve palatability in many products and as a way to reduce the caloric content.

Another common method of sweetening cranberry products involves blending of cranberry juice with other high-sugar fruit juices such as pear or white grape because of consumer perceptions that beverages labeled "100 % juice" are healthier. Although the sugar and caloric content of a 100 % blended product may be approximately the same as one sweetened with high fructose corn syrup or cane sugar, the nutrient content of a 27 % cranberry juice cocktail that has the remaining 73 % volume consisting of fruit juice is obviously much greater than one with a high content of high fructose corn syrup and water. This fact has increased the consumer popularity of the "100 % juice" cranberry beverages.

For the consumer, determining the actual content of cranberry juice in commercially available products presents a potential source of confusion. For instance, in the clinical trial of Avorn et al. [7], participants consumed 300 mL/day of a product containing 27 % cranberry juice. However, if a consumer chose a cranberry drink containing only 10 % cranberry juice, they would theoretically need to consume over 800 mL/day to get the same amount of PACs and UTI prevention effects. Comparative clinical studies using different commercially available cranberry products are difficult to design and carry out and will remain difficult to evaluate. This relates to the nature of cranberry products and their palatability/manufacturing limitations. Moreover, the formulation (content of cranberry juice and of sweetener) changes frequently based on consumer preference and material costs of manufacturing.

Conclusion

Cranberry juice has been used in folk medicine for millennia. Recent clinical studies have confirmed its usefulness for the prevention of UTI. The active agents are PACs specific to cranberries which prevent bacterial adhesion to the urinary tract. These anti-adhesive effects may also be linked to possible health benefits with respect to oral and gastric health. There is emerging evidence to support a role for cranberries and their polyphenolic components in reducing the risk of cardiovascular diseases and certain cancers. However, our understanding of how cranberry juice affects human health remains challenging to determine in part because of the range of product formulations and the differences in the amount of cranberry juice actually present in the study of beverages.

References

1. Henig YS, Leahy MM. Cranberry juice and urinary-tract health: science supports folklore. Nutrition. 2000;16:684–7.
2. McKay DL, Blumberg JB. Cranberries (*Vaccinium macrocarpon*) and cardiovascular disease risk factors. Nutr Rev. 2007;65:490–502.
3. Roper TR, Vorsa N. Cranberry: botany and horticulture. Hortic Rev. 1997;21:215–49.
4. Alston JM, Medellín-Azuara J, Saitone TL. Economic impact of the North American cranberry industry. 2014. http://www.uscranberries.com/Images/News/GeneralFolder/EIReport20140814.pdf. Accessed 5 Feb 2015.
5. Dowling KJ, Roberts JA, Kaack MB. P-fimbriated *Escherichia coli* urinary tract infection: a clinical correlation. South Med J. 1987;80:1533–6.
6. Nicolle LE. Uncomplicated urinary tract infection in adults including uncomplicated pyelonephritis. Urol Clin North Am. 2008;35:1–12.
7. Avorn J, Monane M, Gurwitz JH, Glynn RJ, Choodnovskiy I, Lipsitz LA. Reduction of bacteriuria and pyuria after ingestion of cranberry juice. JAMA. 1994;271:751–4.
8. Ikaheimo R, Siitonen A, Heiskanen T, et al. Recurrence of urinary tract infection in a primary care setting: analysis of a 1-year follow-up of 179 women. Clin Infect Dis. 1996;22:91–9.
9. Kontiokari T, Sundquist K, Nuutinen M, Pokka T, Koskela M, Uhari M. Randomized trial of cranberry-lingonberry juice and lactobacillus GG drink for the prevention of urinary tract infections in women. BMJ. 2001;322:1571–84.
10. Takahashi S, Hamasuna R. A randomized clinical trial to evaluate the preventive effect of cranberry juice (UR65) for patients with recurrent urinary tract infection. J Infect Chemother. 2013;19:112–7.
11. Caljouw MAA, van den Hout WB, Putter H, Achterberg WP, Cools HJM, Gussekloo J. Effectiveness of cranberry capsules to prevent urinary tract infections in vulnerable older persons: a double-blind randomized placebo-controlled trial in long-term care facilities. J Am Geriatr Soc. 2014;62:103–10.
12. Salo J, Uhari M, Helminen M, Korppi M, Nieminen T, Pokka T, Kontiokari T. Cranberry juice for the prevention of recurrences of urinary tract infections in children: a randomized placebo-controlled trial. Clin Infect Dis. 2012;54:340–6.
13. Blatherwick ND. The specific role of foods in relation to the composition of urine. Arch Intern Med. 1914;14:409.
14. Blatherwick ND, Long ML. Studies of urinary acidity – the increased acidity by eating prunes and cranberries. J Biol Chem. 1923;57:815–8.
15. Fellers CR, Redmon BC, Parrott EM. Effect of cranberries on urinary acidity and blood alkali reserve. J Nutr. 1933;6:455–63.
16. Bodel PI, Cotrain R, Kass EH. Cranberry juice and the antibacterial action of hippuric acid. J Lab Clin Med. 1959;54:881–8.
17. Kahn HD, Panareillo VA, Saeji J, Sampson JR, Schwarz E. Effect of cranberry juice on urine. J Am Diet Assoc. 1967;52:251.
18. Sobota AE. Inhibition of bacterial adherence by cranberry juice: potential use for the treatment of urinary tract infections. J Urol. 1984;131:1013–6.
19. Burger O, Ofek I, Tabak M, Weiss E, Sharon N, Neeman I. A high molecular mass constituent of cranberry juice inhibits *Helicobacter pylori* adhesion to human gastric mucus. FEMS Immunol Med Microbiol. 2000;22:1–7.
20. Shmuely H, Ofek I, Weiss EI, Rones Z, Houri-Haddad Y. Cranberry components for the therapy of infectious disease. Curr Opin Biotechnol. 2012;3:148–52.
21. Zhang L, Ma J, Pan K, Go VL, Chen J, You WC. Efficacy of cranberry juice on *Helicobacter pylori* infection: a double-blind, randomized placebo-controlled trial. Helicobacter. 2005;10:139–45.
22. Feghali K, Feldman M, La VD, Santos J, Grenier D. Cranberry proanthocyanidins: natural weapons against periodontal diseases. J Agric Food Chem. 2012;60:5728–35.

23. Weiss EI, Kozlovsky A, Steinberg D, et al. A high molecular mass cranberry constituent reduces mutans streptococci level in saliva and inhibits in vitro adhesion to hydroxyapatite. FEMS Microbiol Lett. 2004;232:89–92.

24. Ou K, Percival SS, Zou T, Khoo C, Gu L. Transport of cranberry A-type procyanidin dimers, trimers, and tetramers across monolayers of human intestinal epithelial Caco-2 cells. J Agric Food Chem. 2012;60:1390–6.

25. McKay DL, Chen CY, Zampariello CA, Blumberg JB. Flavonoids and phenolic acids from cranberry juice are bioavailable and bioactive in healthy older adults. Food Chem. 2015;168:233–40.

26. Sano A, Yamakoshi J, Tokutake S, Tobe K, Kubota Y, Kikuchi M. Procyanidin B1 is detected in human serum after intake of proanthocyanidin-rich grape seed extract. Biosci Biotechnol Biochem. 2003;67:1140–3.

27. Holt RR, Lazarus SA, Sullards MC, et al. Procyanidin dimer B2 [epicatechin-(4beta-8)-epicatechin] in human plasma after the consumption of a flavanol-rich cocoa. Am J Clin Nutr. 2002;76:798–804.

28. Zhang K, Zuo Y. GC-MS determination of flavonoids and phenolic and benzoic acids in human plasma after consumption of cranberry juice. J Agric Food Chem. 2004;52:222–7.

29. Ohnishi R, Ito H, Kasajima N, et al. Urinary excretion of anthocyanins in humans after cranberry juice ingestion. Biosci Biotechnol Biochem. 2006;70:1681–7.

30. Milbury PE, Vita JA, Blumberg JB. Anthocyanins are bioavailable in humans following an acute dose of cranberry juice. J Nutr. 2010;140:1099–104.

31. Wang C, Zuo Y, Vinson JA, Deng Y. Absorption and excretion of cranberry-derived phenolics in humans. Food Chem. 2012;132:1420–8.

32. Singh AP, Vorsa N, Wilson T. Cranberry quercetin-3-galactoside in postprandial human plasma. Int J Food Nutr Sci. 2014;1:1–3.

33. Pedersen CB, Kyle J, Jenkinson AM, Gardner PT, McPhail DB, Duthie GG. Effects of blueberry and cranberry juice consumption on the plasma antioxidant capacity of healthy female volunteers. Eur J Clin Nutr. 2000;54:405–8.

34. Ruel G, Pomerleau S, Couture P, Lamarche B, Couillard C. Changes in plasma antioxidant capacity and oxidized low-density lipoprotein levels in men after short-term cranberry juice consumption. Metabolism. 2005;54:856–61.

35. Duthie SJ, Jenkinson AM, Crozier A, et al. The effects of cranberry juice consumption on antioxidant status and biomarkers relating to heart disease and cancer in healthy human volunteers. Eur J Nutr. 2006;45:113–22.

36. Vinson JA, Bose P, Proch J, Al Kharrat H, Samman N. Cranberries and cranberry products: powerful in vitro, ex vivo, and in vivo sources of antioxidants. J Agric Food Chem. 2008;56:5884–91.

37. Reed J. Cranberry flavonoids, atherosclerosis and cardiovascular health. Crit Rev Food Sci Nutr. 2002;42(3 Suppl):301–16.

38. Ruel G, Couillard C. Evidences of the cardioprotective potential of fruits: the case of cranberries. Mol Nutr Food Res. 2007;51:692–701.

39. Neto CC. Cranberry and blueberry: evidence for protective effects against cancer and vascular diseases. Mol Nutr Food Res. 2007;51:652–64.

40. Basu A, Rhone M, Lyons TJ. Berries: emerging impact on cardiovascular health. Nutr Rev. 2010;68:168–77.

41. Blumberg JB, Camesano TA, Cassidy A, et al. Cranberries and their bioactive constituents in human health. Adv Nutr. 2013;4:618–32.

42. Ruel G, Pomerleau S, Couture P, Lemieux S, Lamarche B, Couillard C. Low-calorie cranberry juice supplementation reduces plasma oxidized LDL and cell adhesion molecule concentrations in men. Br J Nutr. 2008;99:352–9.

43. Zhu Y, Ling W, Guo H, et al. Anti-inflammatory effect of purified dietary anthocyanin in adults with hypercholesterolemia: a randomized controlled trial. Nutr Metab Cardiovasc Dis. 2013;23:843–9.

44. Stein JH, Keevil JG, Wiebe DA, Aeschlimann S, Folts JD. Purple grape juice improves endothelial function and reduces the susceptibility of LDL cholesterol to oxidation in patients with coronary artery disease. Circulation. 1999;100:1050–5.
45. Chou EJ, Keevil JG, Aeschlimann S, Wiebe DA, Folts JD, Stein JH. Effect of ingestion of purple grape juice on endothelial function in patients with coronary heart disease. Am J Cardiol. 2000;88:553–5.
46. Maher MA, Mataczynski H, Stephaniak HM, Wilson T. Cranberry juice induces nitric oxide dependent vasodilation and transiently reduces blood pressure. J Med Food. 2000;3:141–7.
47. Neto CC, Amoroso JW, Liberty AM. Anticancer activities of cranberry phytochemicals: an update. Mol Nutr Food Res. 2008;52 Suppl 1:S18–27.
48. Neto CC. Cranberries: ripe for more cancer research? J Sci Food Agric. 2011;91:2303–7.
49. Ferguson PJ, Kurowska EM, Freeman DJ, Chambers AF, Koropatnick DJ. In vivo inhibition of growth of human tumor lines by flavonoid fractions from cranberry extract. Nutr Cancer. 2006;56:86–94.
50. Prasain JK, Jones K, Moore R, et al. Effect of cranberry juice concentrate on chemically-induced urinary bladder cancers. Oncol Rep. 2008;19:1565–70.

Chapter 8
Citrus Juices Health Benefits

Paul F. Cancalon

Keywords Orange • Grapefruit • Citrus juices flavanones • Signaling pathways • Inflammation • miRNA

Key Points

1. Orange and grapefruit juices contain vitamins, particularly vitamin C, and are high in potassium. They are also extremely low in sodium and lipids. These properties have been extensively examined.
2. Over the last few decades, attention has shifted toward the health properties of phytochemicals and among them polyphenols. Citrus fruit and juices are rich in polyphenols with the two more prominent being hesperidin in orange and naringin in grapefruit.
3. The most beneficial effects of citrus phytochemicals seem to involve the dampening of chronic inflammation which is considered to be at the root of most chronic diseases, including cardiovascular diseases, osteoporosis, dementia, and some forms of cancer.
4. Fruits and juices are not drugs, and measurable health effects can be expected to be mild relative to the more dramatic outcomes expected with pharmacological medications. It can be proposed that the main role of fruit and fruit juices is a disease risk reduction.
5. Some of these concepts are complex and would require extensive efforts to be made accessible to the general public.

P.F. Cancalon (✉)
Florida Department of Citrus, CREC,
700 Experiment Station Road, Lake Alfred, FL 33850, USA
e-mail: cancalon@ufl.edu

© Springer International Publishing Switzerland 2016
T. Wilson, N.J. Temple (eds.), *Beverage Impacts on Health and Nutrition*,
Nutrition and Health, DOI 10.1007/978-3-319-23672-8_8

Introduction

The health benefits of fruits are believed to be due, in large part, to phytochemicals and among them polyphenols. Citrus fruit and juices are rich in flavonoids, the two more prominent being hesperidin in oranges and naringin in grapefruit. Most beneficial effects of citrus phytochemicals seem to be generated by dampening of chronic inflammation. This slow debilitating process, sometimes referred to as "the silent killer," is considered to be at the root of most chronic diseases, including cardiovascular diseases (CVD), type 2 diabetes, osteoporosis, dementia, and some forms of cancer. Citrus juices have been reported by epidemiological, in vitro, animal, and clinical studies to have a beneficial influence on most of those diseases. The most convincing clinical evidence is associated with reduction of the risk of development of CVD and improving cognitive activities and functions. However, the benefits are mild and without the more dramatic effects expected with drug therapies. This review examines the beneficial health associations between citrus consumption and chronic diseases, particularly in the future area of epigenetics.

Citrus Juice Composition

Minerals and Vitamins

Orange and grapefruit contains nutrients, micronutrients, vitamins, and a mineral profile that is low or free of sodium while being high in potassium. Most citrus cultivars are free of lipids, contain high levels of vitamin C, and contain folate acid, thiamin, and to a lesser extent vitamin B6, niacin, and riboflavin [1, 2]. These properties fall within the guidelines of some of the generic FDA-approved health claims that are now allowed in the USA. The nutrient composition of grapefruit juice is not very different from that of orange. It is rich in vitamin C and potassium and low in sodium. Grapefruit juice contains a lower concentration of folate, thiamin, and niacin than orange juice. Citrus juices fortified with health-enhancing compounds not present in juices or present in small amounts have been developed. Substances added include calcium [3], vitamin D [4], and plant sterols [5]. Dietary fiber, found mainly in fruits, vegetables, whole grains, and legumes, can provide health benefits such as lowering the risk of diabetes and heart disease. Citrus juices have been reported in the past as containing little fiber but it seems that previous methods may have underestimated soluble fiber levels. However, the use of newer methods (AOAC 2009.01 and AOAC 2011.25) revealed that pulpy juice contain significantly more dietary fiber than pulp-free juice.

Phytochemicals

Recent attention has shifted toward the health properties of other compounds found in juice [6, 7]. Analyses of oranges have revealed the presence of 224 phytochemicals including 32 flavones, 13 flavanones, 6 flavanols, 9 anthocyanins, 15 carotenoids, and 4 coumarins. Research has focused mainly on the flavanones hesperidin and narirutin and to a lesser extent the carotenoid beta-cryptoxanthin and the polymethoxy flavones tangeretin and nobiletin [8]. Grapefruit also contains many phytochemicals including 13 polyphenols, mostly naringin and narirutin, and 20 carotenoids, particularly beta-carotene and lycopene, as well as limonoids, coumarins, and furanocoumarins (FCs) [8]. The main FCs include 6', 7'-dihydroxybergamottin, bergamottin, paradisins, and bergaptol. These compounds have been shown to interact with the cytochrome P450 3A4 (CYP3A4) to various extents and can increase the absorption of some drugs.

Juices, Modified Juices, and Drink Blends

It is now established that the health benefits of fruit juices are provided mainly by polyphenols as well as vitamins and other nutrients. To provide health benefits, a juice should contain significant amounts of these compounds; drinks with a low juice content should not be expected to provide significant benefits. Modifications of manufacturing procedures to increase polyphenol extraction and minimize subsequent processing decomposition are being developed for juices and other foods. A major juice processing company is promoting an orange extraction method that maximizes the extraction of phyto-compounds. The main problem with regard to citrus flavonoids is their low bioavailability, but several methods may be useful for helping to overcome this. Nielsen et al. [9] modified orange juice (OJ) flavonoids with a rhamnosidase to remove the terminal rhamnose of hesperidin and produce a hesperetin-7-glucoside (H-7-glc) juice. As a result, clinical studies showed that H-7-glc juice induces a doubling of the total plasma hesperetin as compared with untreated OJ, as well as a similar increase of the bone mineral density of ovariectomized rats [10]. Efforts have also lead to the development of customized fruit-juice drinks enriched in phytochemicals. Mullen et al. [11] prepared a low-calorie, polyphenol-rich drink, containing 168 mg of vitamin C and 51 kcal per 350 mL. Green tea flavan-3-ols, grape seed and pomace procyanidins, apple dihydrochalcones, procyanidins, chlorogenic acids, lemon flavanones, and grape anthocyanins were added to the 28 % juice beverage. The authors further showed that ingestion of such fruit-juice drink significantly reduced plasma levels of cholesterol and triglycerides [12]. Although over-the-counter drinks with specific phenolic additives are currently limited to only a few products, their use is likely to become more widespread in coming years.

Mechanisms of Action of Phytochemicals

Bioavailability and Metabolic Transformations In Vivo

The bioavailability and metabolism of polyphenols are the most critical steps in the mode of action of these compounds. Borges et al. [13] recently showed that some polyphenols absorbed from the small intestine appear in the circulatory system as glucuronidated, sulfated, and methylated metabolites. However, citrus flavonoids, in large part, travel to the large intestine where some are absorbed, while another fraction is transformed by colonic microflora generating low molecular weight phenolic and aromatic acids, which also enter the blood stream. Manach et al. [14] examined the bioavailability of hesperidin and narirutin, the main polyphenols in oranges. The concentrations of metabolites in the blood are very low, reaching μmol/L levels; the circulating forms for hesperidin were glucuronides (87 %) and sulfoglucuronides (13 %). More recently, the same group identified 61 metabolites following OJ absorption [15]. It is these final secondary metabolites and some degradation products that act on several pathways to promote health. Many of them have now been synthesized [16] for in vitro studies to determine their exact mode of action. Chanet et al. [17] investigated the impact of naringenin and hesperetin metabolites on monocyte adhesion to TNF-α-activated human umbilical vein endothelial cells and on gene expression. At the physiologically relevant concentration of 2 μm, hesperetin-3′-sulfate, hesperetin-3′-glucuronide, and naringenin-4′-glucuronide significantly decreased monocyte adhesion to TNF-α-activated endothelial cells by affecting the expression of related genes. In grapefruit, the two most abundant flavanones, naringin and narirutin, are both absorbed as the aglycone naringenin. Among their metabolites, naringenin-7-O-glucuronide and narigenin-4′-O-glucuronide are found in the largest amounts [14, 18].

Direct Antioxidant Theory

The first theory to explain the health benefits of fruit and fruit juices was based on their antioxidant potential. Oxidation is a chemical reaction that transfers electrons or hydrogen from a substance (antioxidant) to an electron acceptor (prooxidant) and by doing so becomes itself a prooxidant. Many fruit phytochemicals were shown, in vitro, to have significant antioxidant potential using such methods as the ORAC assay [19]. It was inferred that polyphenols present in the juices, once absorbed, would directly provide electrons to alleviate oxidative processes which cause cellular damage. Fruits and juices were classified according to their antioxidant content, implying a correlation with health benefits. Therefore, ORAC-based comparisons between fruits or juices were easy to generate and were used extensively for advertising purposes. The antioxidant theory was challenged by several groups, as early as 2004 [20]. The same year, Williams et al. [21] proposed that flavonoids, and their in vivo metabolites, do not act as conventional hydrogen-donating antioxidants but exert modulatory actions in cells through signaling pathways. These groups and many others concluded that the bioavailability of phytochemicals is limited because the amounts reaching the blood are too low to have a direct antioxidant effect. They also drew attention to the fact that phytochemicals present in the fruits and juices are extensively modified during the digestive process; many phenolic groups with antioxidant properties are neutralized by forming glucuronides and sulfates. As a consequence, the metabolites present in the blood often lose the antioxidant potential of the parent compound. These early studies laid down the foundation of the signaling theory. Today, it is generally agreed that phytochemicals do not provide significant health benefits by direct antioxidant mechanisms (for review, see [22]).

Inflammation Signaling Theory

The concept of inflammation can be defined as the reaction of the body to an injury; this phase is beneficial for helping the body to successfully repair itself (acute inflammation). If this initial phase cannot be completed, it becomes detrimental. The constant low-grade inflammation that ensues is referred to as chronic inflammation and is central to the etiology of CVD, insulin resistance, type 2 diabetes, osteoporosis, dementia, and some forms of cancer [23]. Inflammation is characterized by an increased production of a large number of pro-inflammatory molecules, among them the C-reactive protein, various cytokines, toll-like receptors, and transcription nuclear factors. These factors have different functions which have not all been clarified but are part of series of events leading to inflammatory pathway dysregulations resulting in chronic diseases [23]. The signaling theory proposes that the metabolites of several citrus juice bioactive compounds modulate these cascading pathways [24]. Dall'asta et al. [18] suggested that citrus flavonoid metabolites (naringenin-7-O-glucuronide and narigenin-4'-O-glucuronide), as well as naringenin, are able to perturb macrophage gene expression. Coelho et al. [25] reviewed the recent literature and concluded that the flavonoids (hesperidin, naringin) in OJ appear to play a role in the modulation of inflammatory markers and that the moderate consumption of OJ could have a beneficial effect in the prevention of inflammation and related chronic diseases.

Genomics Epigenetics

The signaling theory that seems to best explain the effects of juice phytochemicals is known, in many cases, to start with genetic alterations. Epigenetic modifications may be one of the major originating points of the cascading pathways regulating the activity of transcription factors that affect gene expression [26]. An epigenetic change is defined as a gene alteration that does not involve a change in the DNA sequence; it includes changes such as DNA methylation and miRNA modulations [27]. Very recent studies are starting to show that fruit and juice polyphenols can affect miR-NAs. An in vivo study demonstrated for the first time that citrus flavanones, hesperidin, and naringin at nutritional doses modulate the expression of miRNA in the liver of apolipoprotein E-deficient mice [28]. Hesperidin and naringin, at physiological doses for 2 weeks, affected the expression of 97 and 69 miRNAs, respectively. These data suggest that miRNA could also be potential targets of flavanones [28]. Such interaction could represent a major mechanism explaining the health benefits of citrus. Although still in their early stages, these studies seem to indicate that miRNAs are involved in the beneficial effects of citrus flavonoids. The mode of action appears to be a transient modification of the genes through epigenetic modifications. The effects have already been shown to last 18 to 24 h, but could possibly persist for up to a week, even when the all citrus juice metabolites have disappeared from the body [29]. These studies are particularly important since they may reveal the ultimate target of polyphenols. Epigenetics and particularly miRNA modifications may reveal beneficial alterations at the very onset of an ailment at a time when changes are not yet seen at the pathological level [30]. It may be possible to demonstrate that citrus juices induce cardiovascular protection long before clinical events can be diagnosed and that they play a role in limiting the onset of inflammation-related diseases.

Health Benefits of Citrus

As seen previously, most reported citrus health benefits are linked with chronic inflammation and associated diseases. Only a limited number of clinical studies have been performed; therefore, strong supporting evidence is often limited and much remains to be done. The best results have been obtained with cardiovascular protection but recently cognition data appear to be very promising.

Cardiovascular Health

The effects of citrus on cardiovascular health have been extensively reviewed by various groups [7, 31, 32]. The beneficial effects of vegetables, fruits, and fruit juices were initially revealed by epidemiological studies. As early as 1999, Joshipura et al. [33] showed that the lowest risk of ischemic stroke was associated with high consumption of cruciferous vegetables, citrus fruits, and vitamin C-rich fruits. One of the first clinical studies was performed by Kurowska et al. [34] who examined the effect of OJ on blood lipids in healthy men ($n=16$) and women ($n=9$) with elevated plasma total and LDL-cholesterol and normal plasma triglyceride concentrations. Consumption of 750 mL OJ daily for 17 weeks increased HDL-cholesterol concentrations by 21 % and triglyceride concentrations by 30 %; the first change would be predicted to reduce risk of CVD, while the latter will increase risk. Gorinstein's group ([35] and [7] for review) published several papers on the effects of citrus, mainly on patients with circulatory problems. The authors concluded that a diet supplemented with citrus positively influences serum lipid levels. Cesar et al. [36] reported decreased low-density lipoprotein cholesterol in 14 adults who consumed 750 mL/day of OJ for 60 days. The mechanism responsible for a decrease in blood lipids by citrus flavonoids remains to be elucidated. However, Kim et al. [37] hypothesized that citrus flavonoids may lower cholesterol levels by downregulating the expression of HMG-CoA reductase mRNA in a manner reminiscent of the mode of action of statins which inhibit the same enzyme. In a recent study, Kean et al. [38] examined the systolic blood pressure (SBP) in patients consuming 500 mL of OJ for 8 weeks and did not see a significant difference for the entire population. However, there was a significant drop in those with high SBP (>140 mmHg). Many of the studies discussed above have shown that positive results are observed mostly in patients who are at relatively high risk of CVD. Another common finding is that small volumes of juice seldom generate positive outcomes. It is now suggested that health benefits are only seen if the amount of flavonoids given exceeds a threshold dose, but that amount has not yet been determined. Morand et al. [39] studied the action of OJ in humans; they followed the effect starting from their genes, then to the biomarkers, and finally to the endpoint physiological results. In a 4-week study, volunteers consumed daily 500 mL of OJ, a control drink that contained hesperidin, or placebo. Results revealed a decrease in diastolic blood pressure and an improvement of the peripheral blood vessel resistance after both OJ and hesperidin. As part of this study, Milenkovic et al. [29] assessed nutrigenomic changes using microarray techniques and concluded that OJ may induce genomic changes that downregulate the events leading to the formation of atherosclerosis. In a follow-up study with grapefruit juice, the same group reported that consumption of grapefruit for 6 months was associated with stability in pulse wave velocity (PWV), a measure of arterial stiffness, while an increase in PWV was induced by the placebo [40]. The authors estimated that the magnitude of the changes could correspond to a small but significant 5 % reduction in the risk of CVD. Milenkovic and Morand [41] reported that consumption of the grapefruit juice for 6 months seems to modulate the expression of genes involved in the regulation of inflammation and the integrity of the vascular endothelium. The mechanisms responsible for flavanone action are not fully elucidated, and further research is needed to better evaluate and understand the protective effects of flavanones in CVD and possibly quantify these benefits.

Brain Health and Cognition

Several reports have pointed out that polyphenols have positive effects on brain activity (for review, see [42]). Polyphenols can affect brain activity and cognition because polyphenols such as naringin, quercetin, and their metabolites can cross the blood–brain barrier that shields this [43]. Several animal studies showed that naringin may protect rats against neuroinflammation induced by chemicals such as kainic acid [44]. It is only recently that the effects of citrus on cognitive functions have started to be examined clinically. Kean et al. [45] showed that 8 weeks of OJ supplementation (500 mL/day) was associated with benefits for executive function and memory in healthy older adults and generated a longer-lasting improvement in attention and working memory. The authors concluded that OJ rich in hesperidin attenuates cognitive decline in older adults. In a short-term study, Alharbi et al. [46] examined the effect of a flavonoid-rich orange juice and reported that the drink improved cognition processes in adults.

Cancer

The most compelling evidence of the influence of fruit and vegetable intake on the incidence of cancer has been provided by epidemiological studies. Franke et al. [47] pointed out that most studies on the effects of OJ on cancer were performed in vitro. Results from in vitro studies must be interpreted cautiously because the findings do not consider in vivo bioavailability and are difficult to extrapolate to the clinical area. In the future, stronger evidence may come from epigenetic analyses. Van den Berghe [48] reviewed the impact of polyphenols on cancer prevention and proposed that they may bring about the reversal of adverse epigenetic markers in cancer cells and could attenuate the progression of tumorigenesis. Use of epigenetics may provide probes to allow the monitoring of the anticarcinogenic properties of citrus juices.

Bone Health

Bone health is largely the result of equilibrium between osteoclast cells (that beak down bone) and osteoblasts (that build it). Several fruit phytochemicals, particularly hesperidin, may have a positive influence on bone health [49]. An interesting hypothesis was put forward by Uehara [50] who pointed out that hesperidin regulates hepatic cholesterol synthesis by inhibiting the activity of HMG-CoA reductase. Statins, which are cholesterol-lowering agents, also induce bone formation and inhibit bone resorption, both in vitro and in vivo. The author suggested that hesperidin may act on bone by the same mechanism as that of statins. Results accumulated so far have provided good indications that citrus may play a role in bone health. Although positive results have been provided by in vitro and animal studies, effects of citrus in humans remain to be demonstrated.

Sugar Metabolism and Insulin Resistance

The question of sugar in food and in fruit juices has become a very controversial subject [51]. This topic is also covered in greater detail in the chapter by White and Nicklas, as well as in a chapter by Temple and Alp. It is believed that excess consumption of calorie-rich foods is one of the main causes of rising obesity levels. Sugar-rich drinks have been especially stigmatized, and by extension the blame has also been extended to fruit juices. The polemic was exacerbated by the question of high-fructose corn syrup (HFCS), a primary sweetener of sodas, with opposite views being expressed [52]. Nicklas et al. [53] reported that the mean daily juice consumption was only 4.1 fl oz (116 g), which contributed a mean intake of only 58 kcal (3.3 % of total energy intake). The consumption of 500 mL a day of OJ for 4 weeks did not affect the weight of volunteers, and the authors reported food compensation during the study [39]. Daily consumption of 250 mL of OJ for 3 months was reported by Simpson et al. [54] not to adversely affect insulin sensitivity, body composition, or other indices of the metabolic syndrome. Furthermore, in vitro studies seem to indicate that naringin and hesperidin may interfere with glucose absorption. Using Caco-2 intestinal cell monolayers, Manzano and Williamson [55] reported that polyphenols inhibit glucose transport from the intestinal lumen into cells. Although still incomplete, these data appear to indicate that citrus compounds may positively influence sugar metabolism in humans by modulating glucose uptake.

The understanding of the effect of fruit juices and particularly citrus juices on sugar uptake and weight gain has been obscured by confusing definitions and poorly designed experiments. Recent results indicate that at moderate amounts of citrus juices do not have deleterious consequences on sugar and lipid metabolism and as a result do not promote weight gain.

Grapefruit–Drug Interaction

In 1991, Bailey et al. [56] discovered that the blood level of the drug felodipine was significantly higher in patients who had consumed grapefruit juice (GJ). The same phenomenon was also found to occur with various drugs and particularly some calcium channel blockers and some cholesterol-lowering drugs (statins). It was later shown, that the increase in drug bioavailability was due the elimination from the enterocytes lining the intestine of an enzyme called CYP3A4 of the P450 cytochrome family, by grapefruit furanocoumarins (FC). Following GJ ingestion, CYP3A4 is not replaced, and it is necessary to wait about 3 days for new enterocytes containing CYP3A4 to be formed. During that time, drugs metabolized by CYP3A4 are no longer partially destroyed by intestinal first-pass clearance and may reach the blood at increased concentrations.

Detailed information of the effect of grapefruit on most drugs can be obtained on a website established by Tufts University and the University of Florida [57]. The site reviews the drugs affected by grapefruit and classifies them as having a low or no interaction, a medium, or a high interaction. It reveals that for each class of drugs, there are some which are unaffected by grapefruit. The level of FCs in GJ is very variable and can be affected by various parameters ranging from cultivar to storage [58]. Through breeding, fruits have been developed which contain only traces of FCs; these appear to have no significant physiological effect. One such new grapefruit hybrid is called UF914; it is both a good quality fruit and seems to fulfill the low

FC requirements. The selection of grapefruits containing FCs in nonphysiological amounts should potentially resolve this drug interaction problem [59].

Conclusion

Some beneficial properties of citrus have been known for a long time, among those being low sodium, high potassium, absence of lipids, and the presence of vitamins—particularly folate and vitamin C. These attributes have given rise to several general food health claims. In recent years, research has focused on the health properties of polyphenols and especially the flavonoids hesperidin and naringin found in significant quantities only in citrus. A solid body of evidence supports the concept that these flavonoids act predominantly on various pathways leading to chronic inflammation. Results obtained to date have revealed several characteristics of the beneficial health impact associated with the consumption of citrus. Beneficial effects are usually mild and are seen mainly in subjects at risk for the health problem under investigation. Data to support citrus health benefits in people not noticeably exhibiting prior pathological symptoms is less clear. However, recent studies appear to indicate that citrus polyphenols may act through the modulation of epigenetic pathways and may have specific interactions at the level of miRNA regulation. If confirmed, this would suggest that consuming specific components found in citrus juices may provide a protective environment against inflammation-related ailments at the very onset of the process. Hopefully, future studies will confirm the protective role of citrus juices in reducing the risks of developing specific diseases.

References

1. McGill CR, Wilson AMR, Papanikolaou Y. Health benefits of citrus juices. In: Wilson T, Temple N, editors. Beverages in nutrition and Health. Totowa: Humana; 2004. p. 63–78.
2. Rampersaud GC, Valim MF. 100% Citrus juice: nutritional contribution, dietary benefits and association with anthropometric measures. Crit Rev Food Sci Nutr. 2015. doi:10.1080/104083 98.2013.862611.
3. Andon MB, Peacock M, Kanerva RL, De Castro JA. Calcium absorption from apple and orange juice fortified with calcium citrate malate (CCM). J Am Coll Nutr. 1996;15:313–6.
4. Tangpricha V, Koutkia P, Rieke SM, Chen TC, Perez AA, Holick MF. Fortification of orange juice with vitamin D: a novel approach for enhancing vitamin D nutritional health. Am J Clin Nutr. 2003;77:1478–83.
5. Devaraj S, Jialal I, Vega-López S. Plant sterol-fortified orange juice effectively lowers cholesterol levels in mildly hypercholesterolemic healthy individuals. Arterioscler Thromb Vasc Biol. 2004;24:e25–8.
6. Visioli F, De La Lastra CA, Andres-Lacueva C, et al. Polyphenols and human health: a prospectus. Crit Rev Food Sci Nutr. 2011;51:524–46.
7. Cancalon PF. Orange and grapefruit bioactive compounds: health benefits and other attributes. In: Skinner M, Hunter D, editors. Bioactives in fruit, health benefits and functional foods. Chichester: Wiley; 2013. p. 101–24.

8. Rothwell JA, Perez-Jimenez J, Neveu V, et al. Phenol-Explorer 3.0: a major update of the Phenol-Explorer database to incorporate data on the effects of food processing on polyphenol content. Database (Oxford). 2013;2013:bat070. doi:10.1093/database/bat070.

9. Nielsen IL, Chee WS, Poulsen L, et al. Bioavailability is improved by enzymatic modification of the citrus flavonoid hesperidin in humans: a randomized, double-blind, crossover trial. J Nutr. 2006;136:404–8.

10. Habauzit V, Nielsen IL, Gil-Izquierdo A, et al. Increased bioavailability of hesperetin-7-glucoside compared with hesperidin results in more efficient prevention of bone loss in adult ovariectomised rats. Br J Nutr. 2009;102:976–84.

11. Mullen W, Borges G, Lean ME, Roberts SA, Crozier A. Identification of metabolites in human plasma and urine after consumption of a polyphenol-rich juice drink. J Agric Food Chem. 2010;58:2586–95.

12. Peluso I, Villano DV, Roberts SA, et al. Consumption of mixed fruit-juice drink and vitamin C reduces postprandial stress induced by a high fat meal in healthy overweight subjects. Curr Pharm Des. 2014;20:1020–4.

13. Borges G, Lean ME, Roberts SA, Crozier A. Bioavailability of dietary (poly)phenols: a study with ileostomists to discriminate between absorption in small and large intestine. Food Funct. 2013;4:754–62.

14. Manach C, Morand C, Gil-Izquierdo A, Bouteloup-Demange C, Rémésy C. Bioavailability in humans of the flavanones hesperidin and naritutin after the ingestion of two doses of orange juice. Eur J Clin Nutr. 2003;57:235–42.

15. Manach C, Hubert J, Llorach R, Scalbert A. The complex links between dietary phytochemicals and human health deciphered by metabolomics. Mol Nutr Food Res. 2009;53:1303–15.

16. Khan MK, Rakotomanomana N, Loonis M, Dangles O. Chemical synthesis of citrus flavanone glucuronides. J Agric Food Chem. 2010;58:8437–43.

17. Chanet A, Milenkovic D, Claude S, et al. Flavanone metabolites decrease monocyte adhesion to TNF-α-activated endothelial cells by modulating expression of atherosclerosis-related genes. Br J Nutr. 2013;110:587–98.

18. Dall'Asta M, Derlindati E, Curella V, et al. Effects of naringenin and its phase II metabolites on in vitro human macrophage gene expression. Int J Food Sci Nutr. 2013;64:843–9.

19. Prior RL, Cao G, Prior RL, Cao G. Analysis of botanicals and dietary supplements for antioxidant capacity: a review. J AOAC Int. 2000;83:950–6.

20. Azzi A, Davies KJA, Kelly F. Free radical biology -terminology and critical thinking. FEBS Lett. 2004;558:3–6.

21. Williams RJ, Spencer JP, Rice-Evans C. Flavonoids: antioxidants or signaling molecules? Free Radic Biol Med. 2004;36:838–9.

22. Hollman PC. Unravelling of the health effects of polyphenols is a complex puzzle complicated by metabolism. Arch Biochem Biophys. 2014;559:100–5.

23. Laveti D, Kumar M, Hemalatha R, et al. Anti-inflammatory treatments for chronic diseases: a review. Inflamm Allergy Drug Targets. 2013;12:349–61.

24. Afman L, Milenkovic D, Roche HM. Nutritional aspects of metabolic inflammation in relation to health-insights from transcriptomic biomarkers in PBMC of fatty acids and polyphenols. Mol Nutr Food Res. 2014;58:1708–20.

25. Coelho RC, Hermsdorff HH, Bressan J. Anti-inflammatory properties of orange juice: possible favorable molecular and metabolic effects. Plant Foods Hum Nutr. 2013;68:1–10.

26. Pan MH, Lai CS, Wu JC, Ho CT. Epigenetic and diseases targets by polyphenols. Curr Pharm Des. 2013;19:6156–85.

27. Milenkovic D, Jude B, Morand C. miRNA as molecular target of polyphenols underlying their biological effects. Free Radic Biol Med. 2013;64:40–51.

28. Milenkovic D, Deval C, Gouranton E, et al. Modulation of miRNA expression by dietary polyphenols in apoE deficient mice: a new mechanism of the action of polyphenols. PLoS One. 2012;7:e29837.

29. Milenkovic D, Deval C, Mazur A, Morand C. Hesperidin displays relevant role in the nutrigenomic effect of orange juice on blood leukocytes in human volunteers: a randomized controlled cross-over study. PLoS One. 2011;6:e26669.

30. Joven J, Micol V, Segura-Carretero A, Alonso-Villaverde C, Menéndez JA, The Bioactive Food Components Platform. Polyphenols and the modulation of gene expression pathways: can we eat our way out of the danger of chronic disease? Crit Rev Food Sci Nutr. 2014;54:985–1001.
31. Chanet A, Milenkovic D, Manach C, Mazur A, Morand C. Citrus flavanones: what is their role in cardiovascular protection? J Agric Food Chem. 2012;60:8809–22.
32. Cancalon PF. Health impact of citrus and berry fruits F. Acta Hort (ISHS). 2014;1017:309–19.
33. Joshipura KJ, Ascherio A, Manson JE, et al. Fruit and vegetable intake in relation to risk of ischemic stroke. JAMA. 1999;282:1233–9.
34. Kurowska EM, Spence JD, Jordan J, et al. HDL-cholesterol-raising effect of orange juice in subjects with hypercholesterolemia. Am J Clin Nutr. 2000;72:1095–100.
35. Gorinstein S, Caspi A, Libman I, et al. Red grapefruit positively influences serum triglyceride level in patients suffering from coronary atherosclerosis: studies in vitro and in humans. J Agric Food Chem. 2006;54:1887–92.
36. Cesar TB, Aptekmann NP, Araujo M, Vinagre CC, Maranhao RC. Orange juice decreases low-density lipoprotein cholesterol in hypercholesterolemic subjects and improves lipid transfer to high-density lipoprotein in normal and hypercholesterolemic subjects. Nutr Res. 2010;30:689–94.
37. Kim HK, Jeong TS, Lee MK, Park YB, Choi MS. Lipid-lowering efficacy of hesperetin metabolites in high-cholesterol fed rats. Clin Chim Acta. 2003;327:129–37.
38. Kean RJ, Freeman J, Ellis JA, Butler LT, Spencer JPE. An investigation into the chronic effects of flavonoids in orange juice on cardiovascular health and cognition. Proc Nutr Soc. 2012;71(OCE2):E35.
39. Morand C, Dubray C, Milenkovic D, et al. Hesperidin contributes to the vascular protective effects of orange juice: a randomized cross-over study on healthy volunteers. Am J Clin Nutr. 2011;93:73–80.
40. Habauzit D, Milenkovic MA, Verny C, et al. Flavanones protect from arterial stiffness in postmenopausal women consuming grapefruit juice for 6 mo: a randomized, controlled, crossover trial. Am J Clin Nutr. 2015;102:66–74.
41. Milenkovic D, Morand C. Polyphenols and cardiovascular health: gene expression relationship. ICPH. 2013;6:23.
42. Lamport DJ, Dye L, Wightmanc JD, Lawton CL. The effects of flavonoid and other polyphenol consumption on cognitive performance: a systematic research review of human experimental and epidemiological studies. Nutr Aging. 2012;1:5–25.
43. El Mohsen MA, Marks J, Kuhnle G, et al. Absorption, tissue distribution and excretion of pelargonidin and its metabolites following oral administration to rats. Br J Nutr. 2006;95:51–8.
44. Golechha M, Chaudhry U, Bhatia J, Saluja D, Arya DS. Naringin protects against kainic acid-induced status epilepticus in rats: evidence for an antioxidant, anti-inflammatory and neuroprotective intervention. Biol Pharm Bull. 2011;34:360–5.
45. Kean RJ, Lamport DJ, Dodd GF, et al. Chronic consumption of flavanone-rich orange juice is associated with cognitive benefits: an 8-wk, randomized, double-blind, placebo-controlled trial in healthy older adults. Am J Clin Nutr. 2015;101:506–14.
46. Alharbi MH, Lamport DJ, Dodd GF. et al. Flavonoid-rich orange juice is associated with acute improvements in cognitive function in healthy middle-aged males. Eur J Nutr. 2015. doi:10.1007/s00394-015-1016-9.
47. Franke SI, Guecheva TN, Henriques JA, Prá D. Orange juice and cancer chemoprevention. Nutr Cancer. 2013;65:943–53.
48. Vanden Berghe W. Epigenetic impact of dietary polyphenols in cancer chemoprevention: lifelong remodeling of our epigenomes. Pharmacol Res. 2012;65:565–76.
49. Sacco SM, Horcajada MN, Offord E. Phytonutrients for bone health during ageing. Br J Clin Pharmacol. 2013;75:697–707.

50. Uehara M. Prevention of osteoporosis by foods and dietary supplements. Hesperidin and bone metabolism. Clin Calcium. 2006;16:1669–76.
51. Lustig RH, Schmidt LA, Brindis CD. Public health: the toxic truth about sugar. Nature. 2012;482:27–9.
52. Sievenpiper JL, de Souza RJ, Cozma AI, Chiavaroli L, Ha V, Mirrahimi A. Fructose vs. glucose and metabolism: do the metabolic differences matter? Curr Opin Lipidol. 2014;25:8–19.
53. Nicklas TA, O'Neil CE, Kleinman R. Association between 100% juice consumption and nutrient intake and weight of children aged 2 to 11 years. Arch Pediatr Adolesc Med. 2008;162:557–65.
54. Simpson EJ, Bennett IH, Macdonald IA. The effect of daily orange juice consumption on blood lipids, in overweight men. Ann Nutr Metab. 2013;63 suppl 1:181.
55. Manzano S, Williamson G. Polyphenols and phenolic acids from strawberry and apple decrease glucose uptake and transport by human intestinal Caco-2 cells. Mol Nutr Food Res. 2010;54:1773–80.
56. Bailey DG, Spence JD, Munoz C, Arnold JM. Interaction of citrus juices with felodipine and nifedipine. Lancet. 1991;337:268–9.
57. Center for Drug Interaction Research and Education. Grapefruit/grapefruit juice drug interaction information for patients. 2014. http://www.druginteractioncenter.org/. Accessed 10 Dec 2014.
58. Cancalon PF, Barros SM, Haun C, Widmer WW. Effect of maturity, processing and storage on the furanocoumarin composition of grapefruit and grapefruit juice. J Food Sci. 2011;76:C543–8.
59. Cancalon PF, Gmitter Jr FG. New grapefruit and pommelo cultivars with very little furanocoumarin contents are good candidate to provide a solution to the drug interaction problem. Fruit Process. 2013;4:126–9.

Part III
Health Effects of Milk: Dairy, Soy and Breast

Chapter 9
Effect of Cow's Milk on Human Health

Laura A.G. Armas, Cary P. Frye, and Robert P. Heaney

Keywords Milk • Chocolate milk • Milk consumption • Cardiovascular disease • Cancer • Body weight • Lactose intolerance • Osteoporosis • Type 2 diabetes

Key Points

1. Milk is a low-calorie source of calcium and other nutrients.
2. Observational studies of milk intake suggest a protective effect against cardiovascular disease, type 2 diabetes, and obesity.
3. Calcium (usually obtained via milk or dairy) is key in osteoporosis prevention.
4. Milk consumption has decreased over the past 60 years to an all-time low.
5. The milk industry has provided new milk flavors and individual serving sizes to boost consumption.
6. Milk promotion campaigns have increased milk awareness.

Introduction

Milk has been associated with good health and well-being for thousands of years. It is mentioned in the Bible several times ("…a land flowing with milk and honey…") as a metaphor for provision and abundance. For some peoples (i.e., nomadic pastoralists), milk was and is the principal source of all nutrients with consumption of 5–7 L daily.

L.A.G. Armas, M.D., M.S. (✉) • R.P. Heaney, M.D.
Creighton University, 601 N. 30th Street, Suite 4820, Omaha, NE, USA
e-mail: laura.armas@unmc.edu

C.P. Frye
International Dairy Foods Association, Washington, DC, USA

© Springer International Publishing Switzerland 2016
T. Wilson, N.J. Temple (eds.), *Beverage Impacts on Health and Nutrition*,
Nutrition and Health, DOI 10.1007/978-3-319-23672-8_9

With the focus on nutritional science, milk has been dissected into its component parts; calcium is "good for bones," fat is "bad for heart," but it's not so simple. In this overview, we will review the nutrient composition of milk, the health effects of milk, the trends in consumption, and the changes in the dairy industry and its responses to these forces.

Nutritional Value of Milk

The principal value of any food or beverage is that it nourishes and satisfies. Nutritional science takes this benefit apart, dissecting out individual nutrients for study and characterizing the roles they play in body metabolism. While this is necessary if we are to understand how nutrition works, it should be remembered that our bodies need adequate intakes of *all* nutrients for total health, that foods are almost always more than a sum of their parts, and that inadequate intakes of specific nutrients generally affect multiple body systems and organs, not just the ones involved in the index diseases classically connected to single nutrients.

Nutrient Density

Cow's milk is a nutrient-dense food, i.e., it has a high concentration of nutrients in relation to its energy (calorie) content [1, 2]. This is shown in Table 9.1. Note that two servings/day (a figure which characterized US milk intake through most of the twentieth century) provide less than 10 % of daily caloric requirements yet provide 50 % or more of the recommended intakes for phosphorus, calcium, riboflavin, and vitamins B_{12} and D. For all the other nutrients listed, milk provides substantially more per calorie than the average food in the diet. Precisely because of its rich nutrient content, cow's milk improves the overall nutritional quality of any diet into which it is incorporated [4, 5].

Specific Nutrients

Milk is a complex aqueous mixture containing nutrients in solution, suspension, and emulsion. It is roughly 90 % water by weight and, like all complete foods, contains protein, fat, carbohydrates, minerals, and vitamins. The specific quantity and type of each have been optimized over the course of evolution to provide all the nutrients needed for the early postnatal growth stages of all mammals.

Table 9.1 Contribution to recommended intakes for various nutrients from two servings of nonfat milk per day (mature adult)[a]

Nutrient	Content	Daily recommended intake[b] (%)
Protein	18 g	39
Phosphorus	510 mg	88
Calcium	632 mg	79
Vitamin D	232 IU	58
Potassium[c]	838 mg	18
Magnesium	74 mg	21/28
Riboflavin (B$_{12}$)	0.9 mg	82/100
Pyridoxine (B$_6$)	0.2 mg	18
Vitamin B$_{12}$	2.0 μg	100
Zinc	2.0 mg	21/29
Energy[d]	182 kcal	8

[a]Men or women aged 40–50; 70 kg weight if recommendation is weight based; as recommendations vary for different ages, so will percent daily recommended intakes [1, 3]
[b]First value is for men and second for women (where recommendations vary by sex)
[c]Potassium's daily reference value is 4700 mg/day
[d]Assuming 2200 kcal/day

Protein The principal proteins of milk are casein and whey (e.g., beta-lactoglobulin and alpha-lactalbumin). These are high-quality proteins, together containing in varying amounts all of the essential amino acids required for human growth and tissue maintenance. Because of its content of the amino acid tryptophan, milk is also an important source of niacin equivalents.

Carbohydrate The primary carbohydrate in cow's milk is lactose, a disaccharide. The principal importance of lactose in this context is that it is perceived to be a barrier to milk consumption because adults of some genetic backgrounds lose the mucosal enzyme lactase to a greater or lesser extent as they leave childhood (see also below "Lactose Intolerance").

Fat Fat in cow's milk contributes to its appearance, texture, and flavor. Milk fat is also a source of both energy and essential fatty acids. Furthermore, milk fat carries with it fat-soluble vitamins (A, D, E, K) and several health-promoting components such as conjugated linoleic acid (CLA), sphingomyelin, butyric acid, and myristic acid [2, 6, 7]. The fatty acids in milk fat are approximately 62 % saturated, 30 % monounsaturated, and 4 % polyunsaturated, with the remaining 4 % as other minor types of fatty acids [2]. Milk fat is unique among animal fats in that it contains a relatively high proportion of short-chain and medium-chain saturated fatty acids (i.e., those with 4–14 carbons in length). This is an important consideration because, in contrast to long-chain fatty acids, they are transported directly to the liver for metabolism, while long-chain fatty acids must be transported to the liver via chylomicrons. While cholesterol is a normal constituent of milk, its content is relatively low (i.e., less than 0.5 % of milk fat). One-cup servings (8 fluid oz) of whole, 2 %, and nonfat (skim) milk contain 24, 20, and 5 mg cholesterol, respectively [1].

Cow's milk is also an important source of many vitamins and minerals. Vitamin A in whole milk, added to lower-fat and fat-free milks in the USA and Canada, plays a key role in vision, cellular differentiation, and immunity [8]. Nearly all fluid milks in the USA and Canada are fortified with vitamin D to obtain the standardized amount of 400 IU/quart (100 IU per 250 mL) [9]. (Fortification is much lower, or nonexistent, in most European countries.) Vitamin D enhances the intestinal absorption of calcium and phosphorus and is essential for the maintenance of a healthy skeleton, among other still emerging effects. In addition to these fat-soluble vitamins, milk contributes appreciable amounts of water-soluble vitamins, such as riboflavin and vitamins B_6 and B_{12}.

In terms of minerals, cow's milk and other dairy foods are major sources of calcium and phosphorus [1]. All milks (unflavored and flavored), regardless of their fat content – whole, 2 % reduced-fat, 1 % low-fat, and nonfat milks – contain about 300 mg calcium per 8-oz serving and about 235 mg phosphorus [1]. Without including cow's milk (or other dairy foods) in the diet, it is difficult to meet calcium needs [10]. In fact, milk and other dairy foods have been recognized as the preferred source of calcium by several health professional organizations, as summarized by Miller et al. [11]. In addition to calcium and phosphorus, cow's milk contributes other essential minerals such as magnesium, potassium, and trace elements such as zinc [1], each of which supports skeletal and total body health. Potassium and magnesium also play a beneficial role in blood pressure regulation [2].

Health Effects of Milk

Until approximately 60 years ago, milk was synonymous with health which resulted in a US yearly consumption of whole milk averaging 134 L per person [12]. In 1953, Ancel Keys gained notoriety for his study correlating dietary fat intake and coronary heart disease (CHD) in seven countries [12]. Despite criticism at the time for his methods, this diet–disease hypothesis was well accepted by the general public and by the medical community. Milk and dairy products were demonized along with other sources of dietary fat because whole milk fat is mostly composed of saturated fatty acids as outlined previously. While certain saturated fats such as lauric acid, myristic acid, and palmitic acid *in isolation* increase low-density lipoprotein or LDL ("bad") cholesterol which is linked to cardiovascular disease (CVD), they are not eaten in the diet in isolation, and it would be unwise to consider their effects outside of the diet as a whole. Interestingly, the saturated fats in milk have been shown to increase high-density lipoprotein (HDL) ("good") cholesterol, thereby neutralizing the harmful effect of raised LDL cholesterol.

The overall effect of eliminating whole milk in favor of nonfat or reduced-fat milk was an overall decrease in milk consumption [12] over the next 50 years to almost half of its former consumption. Milk was replaced by carbonated beverages as the beverage of choice. The effect on the consumer has been remarkable. With the advent of the Internet as a means for disseminating information (regardless of fact) and its use by consumers in making daily health and nutrition decisions, the perception of milk on the "web" is important. A cursory Internet search on milk as a part of diet provides a view of drinking milk as anti-animal rights, dangerous, and unspiritual. In fact, nutrition as portrayed by many "nutritionists" on their websites and blogs is ideally dairy-free, fat-free, gluten-free, carb-free, meat-free, and grain-free as if ideal health is obtained through the elimination of entire food groups. This approach lies on the edge of disordered eating.

Importantly though, there has been more understanding of diet as a holistic whole rather than as a sum of disparate parts [13] and that using a methodology designed to elicit drug and medication effects is not ideal for testing diet components [14]. There has also been more understanding of the danger in using surrogate markers of disease as the only health outcome in a study design (e.g., cholesterol levels as a surrogate for CVD).

Cardiovascular Disease

The original link of milk to CVD was twofold. First, there was a link between dietary fat intake and CVD in 1953 which was tenuous at best and did not differentiate between types of fats or types of saturated fats. The second was the link between saturated fat effect on LDL as a marker of CVD without taking into account its effect on HDL. Although milk fat is a source of saturated fatty acids (albeit mostly of short-chain fatty acids), its stearic acid and short- and medium-chain fatty acids do not raise blood cholesterol levels. Moreover, individuals vary in their blood cholesterol responses to dietary fat and cholesterol as a result of diet–gene interactions [15]. In fact, in some individuals, a low-fat diet appears to increase the risk of CVD [16]. And while milk fat is a saturated fat, laboratory animal and in vitro studies indicate that CLA (conjugated linoleic acid) and sphingolipids, two of the components of milk fat, may themselves protect against heart disease [17].

To really understand the overall effect of milk on CVD, we need to step back from thinking of nutrients in isolation from the rest of the diet and also from thinking of them as drugs or medications. Instead, we must examine how people respond to dietary intake of foods over years and decades. Fortunately, there have been several papers published in recent years that have examined the relationship between dairy foods and hard outcomes such as CVD.

Elwood et al. [16] conducted a meta-analysis of six prospective cohort studies of milk and dairy intakes and risk of death, CHD, stroke, and type 2 diabetes. The six studies suggested a small reduction in all-cause mortality in the subjects with the highest dairy consumption (RR 0.87; 95 % CI: 0.77, 0.98). Data specifically on milk intake again showed a small but significant reduction in CHD in the group with the highest milk intake (RR 0.92; CI: 0.80, 0.99) [16]. Relative risk of stroke and type 2 diabetes was also similar with RRs of 0.79 (CI: 0.68, 0.91) and 0.85 (CI: 0.75, 0.96), respectively, for those with the highest dairy consumption [16]. The overall conclusion the authors reached was that milk effects on clinical outcomes were the complex effects of its lipids, calcium, magnesium, and potassium on blood lipids and blood pressure [16].

A meta-analysis by Soedamah-Muthu et al. [18] used a dose–response approach to characterize milk intake and found a small inverse association between amount of milk intake and all types of CVD. In recent years, increased attention has focused on the role of nonlipid risk factors such as blood pressure and weight in the development of CVD [19]. The American Heart Association, in its dietary guidelines, now emphasizes healthy eating patterns and behaviors rather than a narrow focus on dietary fat [20]. It is worth noting that while the AHA guidelines of 20+ years ago had virtually eliminated milk from a cardioprotective diet, the guidelines now recommend 2–4 servings of low-fat milk products as part of an overall healthy eating plan [20].

Overall, the most recent data and data analyses support that milk is not harmful and may actually be helpful in preventing CVD.

Hypertension and Stroke

The landmark DASH (Dietary Approaches to Stop Hypertension) study demonstrated that intake of a low-fat diet containing three or more servings of dairy foods, predominately low-fat milk, in combination with fruits and vegetables, significantly and quickly reduces blood pressure in persons with high blood pressure [21] and in patients with isolated systolic hypertension [22]. The blood pressure-lowering effect of the DASH combination diet containing dairy foods was significantly more effective in lowering blood pressure than the diet emphasizing fruits and vegetables alone. While the DASH diet has been noted for being low sodium, the effects on blood pressure were pronounced even when sodium intake was not lowered [23]. Other nutrients such as calcium, potassium, and magnesium are believed to contribute to the blood pressure-lowering effect of the diet.

Other studies, focusing specifically on stroke, reached the same conclusion. Massey's analysis of 30 studies [24] indicates that milk's nutrients, such as calcium, potassium, and magnesium, play a role in reducing the risk for stroke. Additional support for milk's beneficial effect against stroke is provided by a cohort study of over 3000 men of Japanese ancestry living in Hawaii. They were aged 55–68 years and were followed for 22 years [25]. In this study, non-milk drinkers experienced twice the rate of stroke as those who consumed two or more 8-oz glasses of milk per day [25]. A more recent prospective cohort study in the Netherlands with 10 years of follow-up on over 20,000 people found an inverse association between fermented full-fat milk and stroke mortality [26]. Other studies have associated calcium, potassium, and magnesium with reduced risk for stroke [2, 25]. The observation that calcium intake from dairy foods such as milk has a greater effect on reducing stroke risk than nondairy sources of calcium [27] suggests that the combination of nutrients found in dairy foods, or perhaps some other unknown factor, is probably responsible for the beneficial effect.

Osteoporosis

Consuming an adequate intake of milk and other calcium-rich foods throughout life helps to reduce the risk for osteoporosis, a bone-thinning disease affecting more than 28 million Americans, three-fourths of them women. Dairy foods constitute the principal source of calcium in the American diet [1]. Data from the third National Health and Nutrition Examination Survey (NHANES III) reported that more milk consumption in childhood was associated with higher bone mass and lower rates of fracture in older women [28]. A follow-up in the Framingham Offspring Study found a positive association between milk and yogurt intake in adults and hip bone mineral density [29]. A review found that in 50 of 52 controlled trials and metabolic studies, augmenting calcium intake increased bone gain during growth, reduced bone loss in later years, or lowered fracture risk. Further, a multicenter, randomized controlled trial found that drinking three servings of fat-free or low-fat milk each day improved indices of skeletal health in older adults [30]. Likewise, in a recent 2-year randomized controlled trial of 200 postmenopausal Chinese women, milk supplementation (800 mg calcium/day) reduced bone loss by more than 50 %, which is estimated to decrease lifetime fracture risk by 7–16 % [31].

Americans' low calcium intake is a major public health problem. A major cause of this is reduced intake of dairy products, such as milk, and substitution of low-calcium beverages, such as soft drinks [32, 33]. Whiting et al. [34] demonstrated that when low-nutrient beverages replace nutrient-rich milk, bone mass may be adversely affected. Adolescent girls who consumed more nutrient-free or nutrient-poor beverages, including soft drinks, juice drinks, and iced teas, had significantly lower bone mineral content than those with a lower intake of such beverages. Unsurprisingly, as consumption of nutrient-free or nutrient-poor beverages increased, milk consumption dropped. Recognizing children's low calcium intake, the American Academy of Pediatrics issued a policy statement stating that pediatricians should recommend that cow's milk (as well as cheese, yogurt, and other calcium-rich foods) be included in children's diets to help build bone mass and prevent rickets.

Cancer

Despite some reports to the contrary, it appears that intake of cow's milk may reduce the risk for certain cancers, such as the colon and breast. A cohort study from Sweden followed 45,306 men for almost 7 years during which time more than 400 men were diagnosed with colorectal cancer. The lowest risk was associated with the highest dairy intake, with milk having the strongest association [35]. Murphy et al. [36] reported similar findings in the EPIC study with dietary calcium from milk inversely associated with colorectal cancer risk regardless of the fat content of the milk. A recent meta-analysis of 19 studies of dairy products and colorectal cancer found consistent evidence of a protective effect [37].

Milk consumption is also associated with reduced risk for breast cancer, according to a 6-year cohort study of almost 49,000 premenopausal Norwegian women [38]. Compared to non-milk drinkers, women aged 34–39 years who consumed more than three 8-oz glasses (total of >680 g) of milk per day had a 44 % lower incidence of breast cancer. This relationship did not change after adjusting for other factors that could influence breast cancer risk, such as age, body mass index, and reproduction and hormonal factors. Whole, low-fat, and skim milks appeared to be equally protective [38]. The results of this study support earlier research findings also indicating a protective effect of cow's milk against breast cancer [39, 40].

Although more research is needed to determine how milk consumption may help reduce the risk of developing colon or breast cancer, several nutrients such as calcium and certain milk fat components (conjugated linoleic acid [CLA], sphingolipids, and butyric acid) can be identified tentatively as responsible for the benefit [2, 6]. In the case of colon cancer, a mechanism may be that calcium binds to bile and fatty acids in the gastrointestinal tract and thereby reduces damage to the mucosa.

Weight Control

For the past decade, research has supported a potentially beneficial role for cow's milk in weight control [41, 42]. In transgenic mice expressing the *agouti* gene in adipocytes, increasing dietary calcium from either supplements (calcium carbonate) or dairy foods (nonfat dry milk) reduced weight gain and body fat [42]. Further, weight gain was significantly lower in animals fed the high-dairy diet. In mice fed the diets supplemented with calcium or dairy foods, the expression and activity of adipocyte fatty acid synthase were inhibited, and stimulation of lipolysis was increased [42].

Observational studies on humans also link calcium/dairy intake to weight control. When data from the NHANES III were analyzed, an inverse association was found between intake of calcium/dairy foods and obesity, especially among adult women (see Fig. 9.1) [42]. Dairy/calcium intake has also been shown to

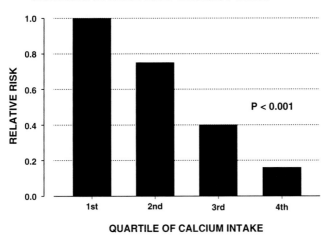

CALCIUM INTAKE AND OBESITY RISK*

Fig. 9.1 Relative risk of being in the highest body BMI quartile, expressed by quartile of calcium intake. Data are from NHANES III and are adjusted for age, sex, and energy intake, among other variables [42]

inversely correlate with weight in young children [43]. When the diets of 53 preschool children were analyzed over a 3-year period, lower body fat was found in children with higher dairy/calcium intakes. Also, when data from previously conducted clinical studies examining calcium and bone health (four observational and one double-blind, randomized, placebo-controlled trial, total $N = 780$) were reevaluated, a lower calcium intake was associated with a higher body fat at baseline and with less weight gain while under observation [41]. The conclusion from observational studies is that habitual diets high in dairy/calcium are associated with lower weight.

However, randomized controlled trials have had mixed results. Just adding dietary calcium to habitual diets does not always change body weight or fat mass as reported in a 1-year study in young women [44] (although at follow-up there was a decrease in fat mass accumulation [45]). It is easier to detect an effect on weight loss when calcium-rich foods are part of a calorie-deficient diet. This was demonstrated by Zemel et al. [46] who reported a significantly greater weight reduction in subjects on a ~1300 kcal weight-loss regimen when calcium was added and significantly more still when the calcium came from milk. Most impressively, the calcium-supplemented diets produced a much greater reduction in truncal obesity. Randomized controlled trials may not have a long-enough duration to observe a desired outcome. Observational studies may therefore be better suited for demonstrating the effects of habitual dairy intake.

Diabetes and Insulin Resistance

Increased body weight is causally linked to insulin resistance. In Zemel's study [46] of calcium and weight loss, dairy not only improved weight loss but also substantially improved glucose tolerance. Similar findings were made in the CARDIA study cohort (over 3000 black and white adults aged 18–30, followed for 10 years). The findings showed that dairy consumption was inversely associated with risk of developing each of the components of the insulin resistance syndrome (obesity, insulin resistance, and hyperinsulinemia in overweight individuals) [47]. Each daily serving of a dairy food was associated with a 21 % reduction in risk, and three servings per day reduced risk by over 60 %. The findings were the same for men and women, black and white.

Two cohort studies reported a lower risk of type 2 diabetes when comparing those with the highest dairy intake with the lowest. In the Women's Health Study, the relative risk was 0.79 (95 % CI 0.67–0.94, $p = 0.007$) [48], while in the Health Professionals Follow-up Study, carried out on men, the relative risk was 0.77 (CI 0.62–0.95, $p = 0.003$) [49]. In both studies, the reduction in risk was more pronounced with the low-fat than the high-fat dairy products.

Kidney Stones

The findings from two cohort studies suggest that consuming milk may help reduce the risk of kidney stones, specifically calcium oxalate stones (the most common type) [50, 51]. In both studies, food sources of calcium (mainly dairy) manifested an inverse association with kidney stones. A high calcium intake is thought to reduce risk by forming an insoluble calcium oxalate complex in the intestinal lumen, thereby decreasing the intestinal absorption and renal excretion of the oxalate found in foods (such as vegetables and whole grains) or produced by bacterial fermentation of fatty acids. When adults with a history of calcium oxalate kidney stones and normal urine calcium levels substituted 1.5 cups of skim milk for apple juice with meals, thereby increasing calcium intake from less than 400–800 mg/day, urine calcium levels increased, and urine oxalate levels decreased by an average of 18 % [52]. Similar findings came from a randomized trial of high and low calcium intakes (mostly from dairy sources) in stone-forming males. Higher calcium intakes resulted in both a 50 % reduction in stone risk and a reduction in urinary oxalate excretion [53]. This provides further support for both the protective effect of calcium and the underlying mechanism.

Others Because cow's milk is a major source of calcium in the diet, intake of this beverage may confer beneficial roles in other disorders associated with low calcium intakes, such as premenstrual syndrome, polycystic ovary syndrome, and periodontal disease [11, 54].

Lactose Intolerance

A barrier to increasing a person's dairy intake is lactose intolerance. Some individuals have difficulty digesting lactose because of reduced levels of the enzyme lactase, a condition called lactase nonpersistence. However, most persons with this condition can comfortably consume the amount of lactose in up to two or more cups of milk/day when taken with meals [2, 55]. Also, gradually increasing intake of milk improves tolerance to lactose. The reason is symbiosis between the intestinal flora and the human host. Just as vegetarians develop a flora that helps them digest the complex carbohydrates of beans, so milk drinkers develop a flora with lactase, which digests lactose for them. Symptomatic lactose intolerance thus develops only in lactase-nonpersistent individuals who do not regularly consume milk.

Trends in Cow's Milk Consumption

During the time period from 1900 to the 1940s, per capita consumption of fluid milk in the USA was stable at just under two servings per person per day. It then dropped slightly to approximately 1.3 servings per person per day (or 30 gal [114 L] per annum) during the period from 1950 to the 1970s. Fluid milk includes plain milk, flavored sweetened milks, buttermilk, and eggnog. Throughout the last three decades, fluid milk consumption has been on a consistent downward trend from 30.1 gal per capita in 1970 to 19.8 gal in 2012 (from about 1.32 to 0.87 servings per person per day) (Fig. 9.2) [56]. This decrease is attributed in large part to displacement of milk by beverages such as carbonated soft drinks, bottled water, fruit juices,

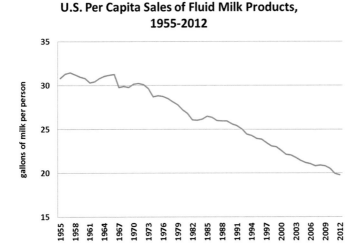

Fig. 9.2 Per capita total milk consumption (gallons) in the USA from 1955 to 2012 [56]

fruit drinks, and flavored teas and in more recent years by nondairy alternative milk beverages.

In 1945, Americans' milk intake was more than four times that of carbonated beverages [57]. By 1991, that relationship had partly reversed: intake of carbonated beverages was more than twice as great as milk consumption (Fig. 9.3) [57]. At the beginning of the twenty-first century, carbonated soft drink consumption began to wane at a faster pace than milk, as bottled water intake rose at a rapid rate. From 2000 to 2012, per capita annual milk consumption dropped almost 2 gal, but during the same time period, carbonated soft drink consumption decreased a total of 9.2 gal. Combined per capita consumption of bottled water and carbonated soft drinks was consistently three times greater than milk consumption from 2000 to 2012. The topic of soft drinks and bottled water are described in the chapters by Temple and Alp and by White. Another factor contributing to lower milk consumption is the growth of nondairy alternative beverages during the last decade [58], a topic discussed in the chapter by Woodside and colleagues.

Another pronounced trend in the USA is the shift away from whole milk to reduced-fat and nonfat milks [57, 59]. Between 1975 and 2012, annual consumption of plain whole milk decreased by 73 % to 5 gal per person (less than 2 oz per person per day). During this same period, 2 % reduced-fat milk increased by 34 % to 6.38 gal, 1 % low-fat milk increased by 112 %, and skim (nonfat) milk increased by 119 % (Fig. 9.4). Nevertheless, consumption of plain low-fat (1 % and skim) milks was still relatively low at 6.06 gal per person per year in 2012. Also noteworthy is the increase in sales of flavored (sweetened) milks, especially chocolate milk to 1.85 gal per annum. Similar to trends with plain milk, *whole* flavored milk

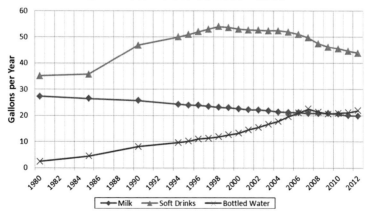

Fig. 9.3 Pattern of consumption of total milk, soft drinks, and bottled water from 1980 through 2012. Figure redrawn from data obtained from Putnam J. Major trends in US food supply, 1909–1999 [57]

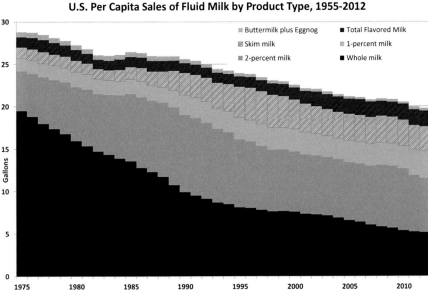

Fig. 9.4 US per capita sales of fluid milk by product type from 1955 to 2012. Calculations by International Dairy Foods Association

consumption has steadily declined to 12 % of flavored milk consumption, while lower-fat flavored milks have increased to make up 87 % of the total.

The modest growth in flavored milks, predominantly reduced-fat, low-fat, and nonfat chocolate varieties (Fig. 9.4) [60] may be explained by their taste and increased availability, as well as by the fact that an increasing number of consumers view flavored milk as a nutritious beverage. Flavored milk provides important contributions to the nutrient intakes of children and adolescents, offering the same nutritional benefits as unflavored milk. Both are nutrient-rich beverages, containing high proportions of nutrients in relation to calories. There are many types of flavored milk available today, ranging from low-fat and fat-free varieties to products that are similar to milk shakes. An 8-oz serving of low-fat flavored milk contains the same amount of total fat (2.5 g per cup) as unflavored low-fat milk. Flavored milks do contain added sugar, which adds about 60–70 kcal per 8-oz serving. The amount of added sugar in flavored milk is significantly less than the amount in sweetened, carbonated beverages. Approximately 40 % of the sugar in flavored milk is naturally occurring lactose (10 g per 8 oz).

Economic researchers have found that the steady decline of fluid milk sales and consumption since the 1970s reflects changes in frequency of fluid milk intake rather than changes in portion size. They analyzed USDA survey data collected between 1977 and 2008 and concluded that Americans are less apt to drink fluid milk with their midday and evening meals than in the earlier years, thus reducing the number of times per day that milk was consumed. In 2007–2008, consumption of fluid milk as a beverage, added to cereal or coffee, or used as an ingredient in selected coffee drinks accounted for 93 % of all fluid milk consumed. In 1977–1978, 39 % of adolescents and adults drank milk with a morning meal, 24 % consumed it at midday, and 21 % had fluid milk with their evening meal. By 2007–2008, these percentages had decreased to 28, 8, and 9 %, respectively [61].

Moreover, younger generations of Americans show a greater decline in consumption frequency. Those born in the 1990s consume fluid milk less often than those born in the 1970s, who in turn consume it less often than those born in the 1950s. Americans consumed less fluid milk in 2007–2008 than they did in 1977–1978 or 1994–1996. Over the 30 years between 1977–1978 and 2007–2008, the proportion of individuals not consuming milk on a given day rose from 12 to 24 % among preadolescent children and from 41 to 54 % among adolescents and adults. Thus, if all other factors remain constant, this research suggests that as new generations replace older generations, the population's average level of milk consumption will continue to decline.

Industry Efforts to Increase Milk Consumption

Faced with growing food and beverage choices for consumers, the dairy industry's response to declining per capita milk consumption includes offering products that are intended to be tasty, affordable, interesting to consumers, and readily available, as well as creating innovative marketing campaigns so that consumers choose it over other products [62].

To meet consumers' demands for lower-fat foods, the dairy industry developed and promoted a variety of reduced-fat (2 % fat), low-fat (1 % fat), and nonfat (skim) milks fortified with nutrients such as vitamins A and D. Additionally, nonfat milks have added nonfat dried milk, or milk protein, and thickeners such as gums and whiteners, which enhance mouthfeel and create opacity of the milk. This makes the taste and appearance similar to higher-fat milk but with more protein and no added fat. For occasional milk drinkers who have lactase nonpersistence, lactose-reduced (70 % less lactose) and lactose-free (0 % lactose) milks were made available. Americans purchased 79.6 million gallons of lactose-free and lactose-reduced milk in 2013 at a cost of $600 million dollars [58].

With consumers seeking foods and beverages that offer additional nutrients, milk products have been introduced that are fortified with protein, calcium, vitamins C and E, and omega-3 fatty acids (eicosapentaenoic acid [EPA], docosahexaenoic acid [DHA], or α-linolenic acid [ALA]) for heart and brain health and plant sterols for heart health. Fluid milk is also an excellent carrier for probiotic cultures or health-promoting bacteria [63]. A variety of health benefits have been attributed to specific strains of lactic acid bacteria (e.g., *Lactobacillus, Bifidobacterium*) or foods such as cultured milks containing these probiotic cultures.

The dairy industry has introduced a wide variety of flavored milks (e.g., chocolate, strawberry, vanilla, mocha, banana, cappuccino) of varied fat content (whole, low fat, and nonfat). Chocolate milk in lower-fat and nonfat varieties is the most popular flavored milk [64]. As of 2013, schools accounted for the highest proportion (by volume) of flavored milk sold (50 %), followed by retail stores (31 %) and food-service establishments (19 %). A recent trend is school wellness plans and new nutrition criteria for milk sold in schools that only permit nonfat flavored milk. This has spurred new product development efforts. As a result, new products are now available, namely, nonfat flavored milk with reduced sugars and fewer calories. In 2012, a survey of milks offered at schools found that flavored milk averaged 122 kcal per 8-oz serving, which was a 27 % reduction (44 kcal) from milk offered over the previous 6 years. Added sugar declined by 45 % (7.5 g per serving) over the same time period [65]. The reduction of sugar content for flavored milk sold at schools was achieved by reducing the amount of caloric sweetener (e.g., sucrose, high-fructose corn syrup, or regular corn syrup) used, choosing alternate sweeteners with higher sucrose equivalence, or selecting types of cocoa and flavorings that are less bitter [66]. Nonnutritive sweeteners (e.g., sucralose, aspartame, or acesulfame-K) are occasionally used to reduce the sugar content and calories of flavored milk sold at retail, but are not typically used for school milk due to local school district policies.

Increasing children's milk intake is particularly important given the high percentage of children not meeting their daily calcium recommendations. As many as 78 % of girls and 85 % of boys at ages 9–13 and nearly 90 % of girls and almost 58 % of boys at ages 14–18 fall short of meeting their calcium needs [67]. Like unflavored milks, flavored milks contain about 300 mg of calcium per 8-oz serving or about one-third to one-half of the daily calcium recommendation for children [1, 8]. Offering flavored milk as part of school meal programs has been demonstrated to increase milk and nutrient intake [68]. A study of a representative sample ($N = 3888$) of children ages 12–17 found that those who consumed flavored milk drank more milk and had higher calcium intakes than the nondrinkers of flavored milk [69]. Moreover, research demonstrates that school-aged children who drink flavored milk do not have higher added sugar intakes compared to children who are nondrinkers of the beverage [69]. In addition, children who drink flavored milk have higher total milk intakes compared to those who drink exclusively plain milk, and milk drinkers (including both plain and flavored) do not have higher BMIs compared to nondrinkers [70].

In response to consumers' demand for convenience, the dairy industry is offering milk products in attractive packaging, such as resealable single-serve plastic containers (e.g., 10, 12, 16 oz), with extended shelf life, and in more locations such as convenience stores and food-service establishments. The availability of single-serve bottles has driven the increase in flavored milk consumption. To increase opportunities for fluid milk consumption, dairy processors are also applying new technologies to extend milk's shelf life. These include thermal processing (e.g., ultra-high-temperature pasteurization), packaging (e.g., retort and aseptic), and physical manipulation (e.g., ultrafiltration).

Dairy producers represented by the National Dairy Promotion and Research Board and milk processors who make up the Milk Processor Education Program (MilkPEP) have supported high-profile advertising and promotions such as the "Got Milk?" and "Milk Mustache" campaigns to improve milk's image and "reason to believe" in and consume this beverage. Some of the promotional campaigns to increase milk consumption target specific groups such as children, teens, mothers, or African-Americans and Hispanics, whereas other campaigns focus on the contribution of milk's nutrients to health (e.g., reduced risk for osteoporosis or hypertension). New efforts by MilkPEP are focused on marketing and promoting milk for two prime usage occasions, namely, breakfast at home and refueling with chocolate milk post-workout.

The breakfast-at-home promotion features milk as a "great tasting, affordable, and convenient" breakfast beverage providing an important source of protein. An 8-oz glass of milk has 8 g of high-quality protein, which is more protein than in an egg [71]. Launched in 2008, the generic milk campaign also promotes the benefits of chocolate milk as a recovery beverage for athletes. More than 20 scientific studies, including athletes from sports spanning running, cycling, and soccer, support the advantages of drinking chocolate milk after strenuous exercise. As part of a regular recovery routine, it is an ideal way to help athletes refuel, rebuild, and reshape their bodies with high-quality protein scientifically shown to help repair and rebuild muscles. In fact, according to recent research, drinking chocolate milk after a tough workout may give athletes a performance edge. Runners ran 23 % longer in their next run and saw a 38 % increase in signs of muscle building when they drank fat-free chocolate milk after their run, compared to a typical sports drink [72]. Other research suggests that regularly recovering with chocolate milk could help athletes gain muscle tone. Milk and milk's high-quality protein have been shown to help athletes gain more lean muscle and lose more fat compared to drinking carbohydrate-only or soy protein beverages, as part of a regular workout and recovery routine [73].

Efforts have also been made to encourage positive role modeling for consumption of milk. Findings reveal that the milk consumption patterns of mothers influence the amount and type of milk consumed by their children [74, 75]. This suggests that milk promotion efforts targeted to one group (e.g., women to prevent osteoporosis) may have a farther reaching impact (e.g., by increasing milk consumption by children and adolescents).

Conclusion

Because cow's milk is a nutrient-dense, inexpensive food, its consumption improves the overall nutritional quality of the diet. Accumulating evidence indicates that consumption of cow's milk is actually associated with numerous health benefits including reduced risk for osteoporosis, CVD, hypertension, some cancers, stroke, and kidney stones, as well as better weight control and less risk of type 2 diabetes.

Over the past 40 years, intake of cow's milk has changed dramatically. Consumption of total milk, whole milk, and reduced-fat milk has decreased, whereas intake of low-fat and nonfat milks has increased. The decline in total milk consumption is contributing to the growing problem of Americans' low calcium intake.

To help increase intake of cow's milk and improve Americans' overall nutritional status and health, the dairy industry has introduced an increasing variety of milks. In addition to milks of varied fat content, other varieties of milk are also available including flavored milks, fortified milks, specialty milks (e.g., low or reduced in lactose), and milks with extended shelf life. Milks are increasingly being offered in visually attractive resealable single-serve containers and in more settings such as convenience stores and food-service establishments. Milk's nutritional and health benefits, increased accessibility, and effective advertising and promotion campaigns targeted at increasing consumption during specific usage occasions are helping to make milk a more competitive beverage.

References

1. US Department of Agriculture. USDA nutrient database for standard reference. Nutrient Data Laboratory. December 7, 2011. Report No.: Release 14.
2. Miller G, Jarvis J, McBean L, editors. Handbook of dairy foods and nutrition. 3rd ed. Boca Raton: CRC; 2006.
3. National Academy of Sciences, Institute of Medicine, Food and Nutrition Board. Dietary reference intakes: recommended intakes for individuals. US Department of Agriculture; Report No: November 4, 2013. http://fnic.nal.usda.gov/dietary-guidance/dietary-reference-intakes/dri-tables. Accessed 17 Oct 2014.
4. Johnson R, Panely C, Wang M. The Association between noon beverage consumption and the diet quality of school-age children. J Child Nutr Manag. 1998;22:95–100.
5. Barr SI, McCarron DA, Heaney RP, et al. Effects of increased consumption of fluid milk on energy and nutrient intake, body weight, and cardiovascular risk factors in healthy older adults. J Am Diet Assoc. 2000;100:810–7.
6. Parodi P. Cow's milk components with anti-cancer potential. Aust J Dairy Technol. 2001;56:65–73.
7. Molkentin J. Occurrence and biochemical characteristics of natural bioactive substances in bovine milk lipids. Br J Nutr. 2000;84 Suppl 1:S47–53.
8. Standing Committee on the Scientific Evaluation of Dietary Reference Intakes. Dietary reference intakes for calcium, phosphorus, magnesium, vitamin D, and fluoride. Washington, DC: National Academy Press; 1997.
9. Ross C, Taylor CL, Yaktine AL, Del Valle HB. DRI dietary reference intakes for calcium and vitamin D. Washington, DC: Institute of Medicine of the National Academies; 2011.
10. Weaver CM, Proulx WR, Heaney R. Choices for achieving adequate dietary calcium with a vegetarian diet. Am J Clin Nutr. 1999;70:543S–8.
11. Miller GD, Jarvis JK, McBean LD. The importance of meeting calcium needs with foods. J Am Coll Nutr. 2001;20:168S–85S.
12. Bauman D, Lock A. Update: milk fat and human health – separating fact from fiction. WCDS Advances in Dairy Technology; 2012.
13. Jacobs D, Tapsell L, Temple N. Food synergy: the key to balancing the nutrition research effort. Public Health Rev. 2011;33:509–31.
14. Heaney RP. Nutrients, endpoints, and the problem of proof. J Nutr. 2008;138:1591–5.
15. Williams PT, Krauss RM. Low-fat diets, lipoprotein subclasses, and heart disease risk. Am J Clin Nutr. 1999;70:949–50.
16. Elwood PC, Pickering JE, Givens DI, Gallacher JE. The consumption of milk and dairy foods and the incidence of vascular disease and diabetes: an overview of the evidence. Lipids. 2010;45:925–39.

17. Kritchevsky D, Tepper SA, Wright S, Tso P, Czarnecki SK. Influence of conjugated linoleic acid (CLA) on establishment and progression of atherosclerosis in rabbits. J Am Coll Nutr. 2000;19:472S–7S.
18. Soedamah-Muthu SS, Ding EL, Al-Delaimy WK, et al. Milk and dairy consumption and incidence of cardiovascular diseases and all-cause mortality: dose-response meta-analysis of prospective cohort studies. Am J Clin Nutr. 2011;93:158–71.
19. McGill HC, McMahan CA, Zieske AW, et al. For the Pathobiological Determinants of Atherosclerosis in Youth (PDAY) Research Group. Effects of nonlipid risk factors on atherosclerosis in youth with a favorable lipoprotein profile. Circulation. 2001;103:1546–50.
20. Krauss RM, Eckel RH, Howard B, et al. AHA Dietary Guidelines. Revision 2000: a statement for healthcare professionals from the Nutrition Committee of the American Heart Association. Circulation. 2000;102:2284–99.
21. Appel LJ, Moore TJ, Obarzanek E, et al. A clinical trial of the effects of dietary patterns on blood pressure. DASH Collaborative Research Group. N Engl J Med. 1997;336:1117–24.
22. Moore TJ, Conlin PR, Ard J, Svetkey LP. DASH (dietary approaches to stop hypertension) diet is effective treatment for stage 1 isolated systolic hypertension. Hypertension. 2001;38:155–8.
23. Bray GA, Vollmer WM, Sacks FM, Obarzanek E, Svetkey LP, Appel LJ. A further subgroup analysis of the effects of the DASH diet and three dietary sodium levels on blood pressure: results of the DASH-Sodium Trial. Am J Cardiol. 2004;94:222–7.
24. Massey LK. Dairy food consumption, blood pressure and stroke. J Nutr. 2001;131:1875–8.
25. Abbott RD, Curb JD, Rodriguez BL, Sharp DS, Burchfiel CM, Yano K, The Honolulu Heart Program. Effect of dietary calcium and milk consumption on risk of thromboembolic stroke in older middle-aged men. Stroke. 1996;27:813–8.
26. Goldbohm RA, Chorus AM, Galindo Garre F, Schouten LJ, van den Brandt PA. Dairy consumption and 10-y total and cardiovascular mortality: a prospective cohort study in the Netherlands. Am J Clin Nutr. 2011;93:615–27.
27. Iso H, Stampfer MJ, Manson JE, et al. Prospective study of calcium, potassium, and magnesium intake and risk of stroke in women. Stroke. 1999;30:1772–9.
28. Kalkwarf HJ, Khoury JC, Lanphear BP. Milk intake during childhood and adolescence, adult bone density, and osteoporotic fractures in US women. Am J Clin Nutr. 2003;77:257–65.
29. Sahni S, Tucker KL, Kiel DP, Quach L, Casey VA, Hannan MT. Milk and yogurt consumption are linked with higher bone mineral density but not with hip fracture: the Framingham Offspring Study. Arch Osteoporos. 2013;8:119.
30. Heaney RP, McCarron DA, Dawson-Hughes B, et al. Dietary changes favorably affect bone remodeling in older adults. J Am Diet Assoc. 1999;99:1228–33.
31. Lau EM, Woo J, Lam V, Hong A. Milk supplementation of the diet of postmenopausal Chinese women on a low calcium intake retards bone loss. J Bone Miner Res. 2001;16:1704–9.
32. US Department of Agriculture, US Department of Health and Human Services. Nutrition and your health: dietary guideline for Americans. Washington, DC: US Government Printing Office; 2000. Report No.: Bulletin 232.
33. NIH Consensus Development Panel on Osteoporosis Prevention, Diagnosis, and Therapy. Osteoporosis prevention, diagnosis, and therapy. JAMA. 2001;285:785–95.
34. Whiting SJ, Healey A, Psiuk S, Mirwald R, Kowalski K, Bailey DA. Relationship between carbonated and other low nutrient dense beverages and bone mineral content of adolescents. Nutr Res. 2001;21:1107–15.
35. Larsson SC, Bergkvist L, Rutegard J, Giovannucci E, Wolk A. Calcium and dairy food intakes are inversely associated with colorectal cancer risk in the Cohort of Swedish Men. Am J Clin Nutr. 2006;83:667–73.
36. Murphy N, Norat T, Ferrari P, et al. Consumption of dairy products and colorectal cancer in the European Prospective Investigation into Cancer and Nutrition (EPIC). PLoS One. 2013;8:e72715.
37. Aune D, Lau R, Chan DS, et al. Dairy products and colorectal cancer risk: a systematic review and meta-analysis of cohort studies. Ann Oncol. 2012;23:37–45.

38. Hjartaker A, Laake P, Lund E. Childhood and adult milk consumption and risk of premenopausal breast cancer in a cohort of 48,844 women - the Norwegian women and cancer study. Int J Cancer. 2001;93:888–93.
39. Knekt P, Jarvinen R, Seppanen R, Pukkala E, Aromaa A. Intake of dairy products and the risk of breast cancer. Br J Cancer. 1996;73:687–91.
40. Jarvinen R, Knekt P, Seppanen R, Teppo L. Diet and breast cancer risk in a cohort of Finnish women. Cancer Lett. 1997;114:251–3.
41. Davies KM, Heaney RP, Recker RR, et al. Calcium intake and body weight. J Clin Endocrinol Metab. 2000;85:4635–8.
42. Zemel MB, Shi H, Greer B, Dirienzo D, Zemel PC. Regulation of adiposity by dietary calcium. FASEB J. 2000;14:1132–8.
43. Carruth BR, Skinner JD. The role of dietary calcium and other nutrients in moderating body fat in preschool children. Int J Obes Relat Metab Disord. 2001;25:559–66.
44. Gunther CW, Legowski PA, Lyle RM, et al. Dairy products do not lead to alterations in body weight or fat mass in young women in a 1-y intervention. Am J Clin Nutr. 2005;81:751–6.
45. Eagan MS, Lyle RM, Gunther CW, Peacock M, Teegarden D. Effect of 1-year dairy product intervention on fat mass in young women: 6-month follow-up. Obesity (Silver Spring). 2006;14:2242–8.
46. Zemel M, Thompson W, Zemel P, et al. Dietary calcium and dairy products accelerate weight and fat loss during energy restriction in obese adults. Am J Clin Nutr. 2002;75:342S–3S.
47. Pereira MA, Jacobs Jr DR, Van Horn L, Slattery ML, Kartashov AI, Ludwig DS. Dairy consumption, obesity, and the insulin resistance syndrome in young adults: the CARDIA Study. JAMA. 2002;287:2081–9.
48. Liu S, Choi HK, Ford E, et al. A prospective study of dairy intake and the risk of type 2 diabetes in women. Diabetes Care. 2006;29:1579–84.
49. Choi HK, Willett WC, Stampfer MJ, Rimm E, Hu FB. Dairy consumption and risk of type 2 diabetes mellitus in men: a prospective study. Arch Intern Med. 2005;165:997–1003.
50. Curhan GC, Willett WC, Rimm EB, Stampfer MJ. A prospective study of dietary calcium and other nutrients and the risk of symptomatic kidney stones. N Engl J Med. 1993;328:833–8.
51. Curhan GC, Willett WC, Speizer FE, Spiegelman D, Stampfer MJ. Comparison of dietary calcium with supplemental calcium and other nutrients as factors affecting the risk for kidney stones in women. Ann Intern Med. 1997;126:497–504.
52. Massey LK, Kynast-Gales SA. Substituting milk for apple juice does not increase kidney stone risk in most normocalciuric adults who form calcium oxalate stones. J Am Diet Assoc. 1998;98:303–8.
53. Borghi L, Schianchi T, Meschi T, et al. Comparison of two diets for the prevention of recurrent stones in idiopathic hypercalciuria. N Engl J Med. 2002;346:77–84.
54. Heaney RP. Ethnicity, bone status, and the calcium requirement. Nutr Res. 2002;22:153–78.
55. Suarez FL, Savaiano D, Arbisi P, Levitt MD. Tolerance to the daily ingestion of two cups of milk by individuals claiming lactose intolerance. Am J Clin Nutr. 1997;65:1502–6.
56. USDA. Economic Research Service. Fluid milk sales by product [homepage on the Internet]. 2014. http://www.ers.usda.gov/data-products/dairy-data. Accessed 15 June 2014.
57. Putnam J. Major trends in US food supply, 1909–1999. Food Rev. 2000;23:8–15.
58. DMI Dairy Management, Inc. Total U.S. multi-outlet: retail monthly milk snapshot. 2013. www.midwestdairy.com/download_file.cfm?FILE_ID=3505. Accessed 15 July 2014.
59. Putnam J, Kantor L, Allshouse J. Per capita food supply trends: progress toward dietary guidelines. Food Rev. 2000;23:2–14.
60. International Dairy Foods Association. Dairy facts [homepage on the Internet]. 2014. http://www.idfa.org/resource-center/industry-facts/. Accessed 17 Oct 2014.
61. Stewart H, Dong D, Carlson A. Why are Americans consuming less fluid milk? A look at generational differences in intake frequency. USDA; 2013. Report No.: 149.
62. Vivien Godfrey and the Challenges Facing MilkPEP [homepage on the Internet]. FoodBev. com Sept 27, 2012. http://www.foodbev.com/index.php/news/vivien-godfrey-and-the-challenges-facing. Accessed 17 Oct 2014.

63. National Dairy Council. Functional foods: an overview. Dairy Council Digest. 1999;70:31–6.
64. International Dairy Foods Association. Milk facts. Washington, DC: International Dairy Foods Association; 2000.
65. Prime Consulting Group. 2012–2013 school milk product profile, MilkPEP school channel survey. 2013.
66. National Dairy Council: Dairy Management, Inc. Formulating reduced calorie/reduced sugar flavored milks [homepage on the Internet]. May 2007. http://www.innovatewithdairy.com/SiteCollectionDocuments/DMI%20Formulating%20Flavored%20Milk.pdf. Accessed 17 Oct 2014.
67. US Department of Agriculture. Report of the dietary guidelines advisory committee on the dietary guidelines for Americans. August 2010.
68. Guthrie HA. Effect of a flavored milk option in a school lunch program. J Am Diet Assoc. 1977;71:35–40.
69. Johnson RK, Frary C, Wang MQ. The nutritional consequences of flavored-milk consumption by school-aged children and adolescents in the United States. J Am Diet Assoc. 2002;102:853–6.
70. Murphy MM, Douglass JS, Johnson RK, Spence LA. Drinking flavored or plain milk is positively associated with nutrient intake and is not associated with adverse effects on weight status in US children and adolescents. J Am Diet Assoc. 2008;108:631–9.
71. US Department of Agriculture. USDA national nutrient database for standard reference. 2013. Report No.: Release 25.
72. Lunn WR, Pasiakos SM, Colletto MR, et al. Chocolate milk and endurance exercise recovery: protein balance, glycogen, and performance. Med Sci Sports Exerc. 2012;44:682–91.
73. Hartman JW, Tang JE, Wilkinson SB, et al. Consumption of fat-free fluid milk after resistance exercise promotes greater lean mass accretion than does consumption of soy or carbohydrate in young, novice, male weightlifters. Am J Clin Nutr. 2007;86:373–81.
74. Fisher J, Mitchell D, Smiciklas-Wright H, Birch L. Maternal milk consumption predicts the tradeoff between milk and soft drinks in young girls' diets. J Nutr. 2001;131:246–50.
75. Johnson RK, Panely C, Wang M. Associations between the milk mothers drink and the milk consumed by their school-aged children. Fam Econ Nutr Rev. 2001;13:27–36.

Chapter 10
Are Soy-Milk Products Viable Alternatives to Cow's Milk?

Jayne V. Woodside, Sarah Brennan, and Marie Cantwell

Keywords Soy milk • Soy protein • Isoflavones • Phytoestrogens • Breast cancer • Cardiovascular disease

Key Points

1. Soy milk is increasingly consumed as an alternative to cow's milk.
2. Compared with cow's milk, it is lower in fat and a comparable source of protein and contains high levels of isoflavones.
3. Soy intake may have a role in the development of endocrine-responsive cancers, such as breast cancer, but its influence on bone health and cardiovascular-related outcomes is unclear.
4. Carefully designed studies which take into account the heterogeneous nature of the effect of soy products are necessary in order to clarify the associations between soy intake and health outcomes.

Introduction

In recent years, there has been a growth in the popularity of alternatives to cow's milk. These include milk substitutes manufactured from soy, rice, and almond sources. Surprisingly, little research has been carried out on the health benefits of rice, coconut, or almond milk, so this chapter concentrates on the health implications of soy beverages with respect to conditions such as lactose intolerance, osteoporosis, cancer, cardiovascular disease (CVD), and menopausal symptoms, as well

J.V. Woodside, Ph.D. (✉) • S. Brennan, Ph.D. • M. Cantwell, Ph.D.
Centre for Public Health, Institute of Clinical Science B, Queens University Belfast,
Grosvenor Road, Belfast BT12 6BJ, Northern Ireland
e-mail: j.woodside@qub.ac.uk

© Springer International Publishing Switzerland 2016   151
T. Wilson, N.J. Temple (eds.), *Beverage Impacts on Health and Nutrition*,
Nutrition and Health, DOI 10.1007/978-3-319-23672-8_10

Table 10.1 Nutritional content of soy milk (per 100 g) in comparison with cow's milk (whole, semi-skimmed, and skimmed)

	Soya, nondairy alternative to milk, unsweetened	Soya, nondairy alternative to milk, sweetened, calcium enriched	Whole (average)	Semi-skimmed (average)	Skimmed (average)
Protein (g)	2.4	3.1	3.3	3.4	3.4
Fat (g)	1.6	2.4	3.9	1.7	0.2
Carbohydrate (g)	0.5	2.5	4.5	4.7	4.4
Energy (kcal)	26	43	66	46	32
Calcium (mg)	13	89	118	120	122

Data taken from McCance and Widdowson's The Composition of Foods [1]

as discussing whether these products are nutritionally equivalent to cow's milk. Soy milk has attracted interest because it is a reasonably good source of protein and is lower in fat than cow's milk (Table 10.1). However, soy protein has a lower absorption ratio in the gut and a poorer biologic value relative to cows' milk protein. In addition, the amino acid patterns of the two milk sources differ (soy milk contains lower amounts of methionine, branched chain amino acids lysine and proline, and higher quantities of aspartate, glycine, arginine, and cysteine than cow's milk) [2], and such differences could be important, particularly when used for infant feeding.

Soy milk is also a major source of isoflavones. These compounds are found predominantly in legumes (peas, beans, lentils, and peanuts). They form one class of a wider group of chemicals known as phytoestrogens. Soybeans and soy products, such as soy milk, are perhaps the most common food source of isoflavones. Those foods contain large amounts of the isoflavones genistein and daidzein. However, other legumes, especially clovers, contain higher total levels and, in addition to genistein and daidzein, also contain formononetin and biochanin. The amount of phytoestrogen found in each soy protein depends on the processing technique used and its relative abundance in the specific soy product of interest. The secondary soy products (milk or flour) contain lower amounts of the isoflavones than the primary products. Different brands of soy milk can therefore vary in isoflavone content; examples from the USDA database [3] are shown in Table 10.2. The isoflavones are covalently bound to glucose, and when ingested by humans, these glyconated isoflavones are enzymatically cleaved in the gut to the active forms.

Consumption of plant-based milks has increased in recent years. In the USA, retail sales of dairy-alternative beverages reached $1.33 billion in 2011 [4], although in the context of milk sales overall, this represents approximately 4.7 % of the 2.28 billion gallons of dairy milk [5]. Dairy-alternative beverages tend to be primarily consumed by vegans/vegetarians and those with cow's milk allergies or lactose intolerance [4], and the popularity of such products has led to the inclusion of calcium-fortified nondairy milks in the USDA "My Plate" dietary recommendations [6]. Soy products are the most commonly consumed nondairy alternatives [4], although consumption varies substantially worldwide. Consumption of these products in the USA has increased significantly in recent years, with soy food sales

Table 10.2 Isoflavone content (mg/100 g, edible portion) of soy milk

Isoflavone	Soy milk (all flavors), low fat, with added calcium, vitamins A and D	Soy milk (all flavors), nonfat, with added calcium, vitamins A and D
Daidzein	1.01	0.30
Genistein	1.51	0.41
Glycitein	0.04	0.00
Total isoflavones	2.56	0.70

Data taken from the USDA Database on the Isoflavone Content of Foods, Release 2.0 [4]. Each estimation is based on one value

increasing from $1 billion to $5.2 billion between 1996 and 2011 [7], with a dramatic increase in sales observed after health claims were approved by the Food and Drink Administration in 1999. The increase in consumption may also be attributable to the increasing range of soy products available, although soy milk is the most commonly consumed soy product in the US population. Findings published in 2002 reported that soy dairy substitutes were also the most commonly consumed soy product overall in Western Europe [8]. However, evidence from data collected between 2005 and 2010 suggests that soy product sales are ever-changing within Europe [9]; for example, overall volume sales for soy-based products in Western Europe increased, although soy drinks and milk sales decreased in Germany, the Netherlands, and the UK during this period. Therefore, consumption rates are subject to change, and this is a factor which is important to keep in consideration when categorizing exposure to soy intake in future studies. In Asian countries, by contrast, the soy products typically consumed are the more traditional ones [8].

The research carried out into the health effects of phytoestrogens has utilized a variety of food sources, including soy milk, soy protein, and extracted isoflavones. Few of these studies focused on the health effects of soy milk specifically. All these studies provide relevant evidence and will therefore be included for discussion in later sections.

Nutritional Comparison of Soy and Cow's Milk

Giving a general estimate of the nutritional value of soy milk is difficult as it varies considerably from brand to brand. Those brands labelled as "extra" or "fortified" have more calcium, vitamins A and D, and other nutrients, while flavored soy milk usually contains more calories and sugar. Nutritionists recommend that those who substitute soy milk for dairy milk should follow the recommended 2–3 servings per day and use milk that has at least 30 % of the daily requirement of calcium per serving.

For infant milk formulas, the content of nutrients in soy protein formulas is similar to that found in cow-milk formulas. Several clinical studies have shown that feeding soy protein formulas to full-term infants is associated with normal growth, nutritional status, and bone mineralization.

Lactose Intolerance

Lactose, a disaccharide of glucose and galactose, is a sugar peculiar to mammalian milk and milk products. Its universal presence in milk means that all newborn mammalian species have the appropriate enzyme, lactase, to digest it. However, after weaning, lactase activity declines rapidly in all species, including humans. In the absence of lactase, milk drinking may produce diarrhea, abdominal pain, and distension. Lactose intolerance, although difficult to quantify accurately, is common in adult populations worldwide, except for adults with a northern European genetic background. Even among this population, it is estimated that 5–15 % may be alactasic [10]. For those who are lactose intolerant, soy milk can provide an alternative to cow's milk. The chapter by Friel and Qasem examines human breast milk and infant formula in greater detail.

Cow-milk allergy (CMA) induces a large spectrum of clinical manifestations in infants and children. These mainly affect the gastrointestinal tract, skin, and, more rarely, the respiratory tract. It has been estimated that CMA occurs in ≤2 % of all children in the first 3 years of life [11]. Soy protein formula is a potential alternative food for children with IgE-mediated CMA as it has lower immunogenicity and allergenicity than cow-milk formula and better palatability than hydrolyzed formulas [11]. However, concerns have been expressed about the nutritional adequacy of soy protein formula and about the long-term effects of high phytoestrogen intake on later reproductive and sexual development, immune function, and thyroid disease [2]. In response to these concerns, American and European guidelines recommend that soy protein formulas should only be considered in exceptional circumstances [2] and that even for CMA, extensively hydrolyzed protein formula should be considered because 10 to 14 % of these infants will also have a soy protein allergy [12].

Cancer

Soy milk and, more generally, soy protein intake have been examined in relation to their association with cancers at various sites. Most observational studies have examined soy protein intake, but extracted isoflavone supplements have been used in intervention studies.

Interest has focused on soy and breast cancer due to the relatively low breast cancer mortality rates in Asian countries where soy foods are commonly consumed and intake of isoflavone is high. This relationship was reported a quarter century ago [13]. It had been reported several times that when people whose diets are traditionally high in soy foods move to a Western lifestyle (including diet), this has led to an increase in breast cancer incidence.

Many epidemiological studies have been conducted of soy intake and risk of breast cancer. These studies suggest that soy intake may be associated with a small reduction in breast cancer risk [14]. An association with a reduced risk of breast cancer recurrence has also been suggested [15, 16], although not in all studies [17,

18]. The strengths of the associations observed may depend on menopausal status and, for recurrence and survival, on receptor status. In the most recent meta-analysis, the protective effect of soy on risk was only observed among studies conducted in Asian populations, but not in Western populations, while no dose–response relationship was seen [19]. Epidemiologic evidence therefore suggests a protective association between increased soy milk and, more generally, soy food intake and reduced breast cancer risk, particularly among Asian populations. Some studies have suggested that it is early life exposure to soy that may be most protective, which may explain why some epidemiological studies, focusing on adult intake, have only shown weak associations. Of particular note, soy foods do not appear to be associated with a detrimental effect on survival. It must be emphasized that observational evidence can only test associations and not infer causality, while the likelihood of residual confounding in these studies remains high.

A limited amount of evidence has come from experimental studies. These studies, the majority of which investigated isolated isoflavones, have produced conflicting results and raised some safety concerns, particularly in Western populations [20]. In vitro studies have reported that genistein may inhibit the growth and metastatic activity of breast cancer cell lines [21]. Findings using animal models observed that supplementation with isoflavones prevents mammary tumors induced by chemical carcinogens [22]. Isoflavone supplementation has previously been shown to have hormonal effects. A number of supplementation studies conducted in the 1990s suggested a stimulatory effect of such supplementation on breast tissue in that epithelial proliferation was increased as was progesterone receptor expression [23, 24]. More recent studies have examined the effect of isoflavone supplementation on breast density. No effect was observed in postmenopausal women, but a modest increase was seen in premenopausal women which points to an increase in breast cancer risk [25]. A recent phase II trial examined proliferation and signs of atypia in fine-needle aspirates collected from the breasts of healthy women before and after 6 months of supplementation with soy isoflavone. Epithelial cell proliferation increased in the soy-treated premenopausal participants, but not in those who were postmenopausal [26]. The heterogeneity of response to isoflavone exposure depends on gut microflora activity and particularly on whether an individual produces equol, an end metabolite formed in the biotransformation of dietary soy. Clearly, further well-designed research is required to fully elucidate the role of soy milk in breast cancer etiology.

Limited work examining other types of cancer also suggests a possible role for soy foods in cancer prevention. Meta-analyses of observational studies have suggested an association between increased soy food intake and reduced prostate cancer risk [27, 28]. However, a 1-year intervention with a soy isoflavone drink had no effect on prostate-specific antigen levels in healthy older men [29]. A meta-analysis of observational studies concluded that soy consumption was associated with a 21 % reduction in colorectal cancer risk in women but not men [30]. The evidence is somewhat mixed for lung cancer with one meta-analysis observing a reduction in risk with increasing soy food intake [31], while a more recent meta-analysis suggested only a borderline reduction in risk, particularly in nonsmokers [32]. Only a few individual studies have examined gastric cancer and results have been mixed. A similar lack of a definite association has been observed for endometrial and ovarian cancers.

Osteoporosis

Estrogen replacement therapy is highly effective at reducing the rate of bone loss and can also enhance the replacement of lost bone. The influence of cow's milk on bone health is examined in greater detail in the chapter "Effect of Cow's Milk on Human Health." Epidemiological data suggest that osteoporosis is about one third as common in Japanese women (who consume a diet rich in soy products) compared with those on a Western diet [33]. However, there are many confounding factors distinguishing Asian women from Western women (lifestyle, sociocultural, and morphological factors), while the extent to which this difference is genetic is unknown.

A number of randomized controlled trials have tested the effect of soy protein and isolated isoflavones on bone health. Meta-analyses of these studies suggest that soy isoflavone intervention significantly attenuates bone loss of the spine [34], decreases urinary deoxypyridinoline (DPD, a marker of bone resorption), and increases serum bone-specific alkaline phosphatase (a marker of bone formation). However, most studies published since these meta-analyses have tended to show no effect of such supplementation on bone-related endpoints [35–38]. One study, however, did demonstrate an effect on whole-body bone loss [39]. Two meta-analyses were recently published that looked at the impact of soy isoflavone supplementation on bone mineral density (BMD) [40, 41], but only one reported a beneficial outcome [40]. Another meta-analysis confirmed effects on DPD, but not on markers of bone formation [42]. A systematic review of meta-analyses suggests that soy isoflavones may help prevent postmenopausal osteoporosis and improve bone strength but that further work is required to examine drug interactions and changes in other biomarkers of bone health and BMD at specific skeletal sites [43]. Similarly, it has been suggested that the action of isolated soy protein or purified or concentrated soy isoflavones may differ to that of soy milk or whole soy foods within a traditional Asian diet [42, 44]. However, few studies have formally examined the influence of different components of soy.

In summary, these studies indicate that isoflavones appear to have some potential to prevent bone loss under experimental conditions. However their effect, and that of soy milk, must be confirmed by larger long-term studies, with a careful choice of the intervention/food/component to be tested and with suitable endpoints.

Cardiovascular Disease

The protective role of a diet rich in soy milk or soy protein on coronary heart disease (CHD) has been hypothesized based on the relatively low incidence of the disease in Asian countries. However, it must again be remembered that Asian lifestyles are distinct from Western lifestyles in a number of ways, e.g., their diet is much lower in saturated fat and higher in fiber [44].

A number of studies have examined the associations between dietary isoflavone and/or soy intake, on the one hand, and CVD risk factors and CVD risk, on the other hand [45–48]. Such studies have usually shown an inverse association between soy intake and risk factors or risk, suggesting that diets rich in soy protein or isoflavones have effects that decrease the risk of CVD.

Isoflavones in the form of soy milk may affect CHD risk by a number of mechanisms. They can act as antioxidants; early studies suggested that such a biological effect may be important in reducing CVD risk through the inhibition of LDL oxidation. However, studies have been conflicting in terms of whether such an antioxidant effect can be demonstrated in vivo, although a recent study in Indonesia did demonstrate that isoflavone supplementation decreases oxidative stress in postmenopausal women after 6 and 12 months of treatment [49].

The hypolipidemic effects of soy protein and its constituents have been more thoroughly examined. Early meta-analyses concluded that soy protein, compared with animal protein, significantly decreases serum concentrations of total cholesterol, LDL cholesterol, and triglycerides and increases HDL cholesterol, with this effect being dose responsive and occurring in adults with or without hypercholesterolemia [50, 51]. A further meta-analysis reported similar findings in type 2 diabetics [52]. In contrast, the Nutrition Committee of the American Heart Association (AHA) assessed 22 randomized trials of isolated soy protein published since 1999. The dose of soy protein ranged from 25 to 135 g/day, and a small effect (approximately −3 %) on LDL cholesterol was observed, but not on other lipids, and there was no dose–response effect [53]. This review also carried out a similar analysis of studies examining isolated isoflavones and reported no change in lipid levels. Further interventional studies have also produced conflicting results regarding changes in blood lipid levels [54–58]. These meta-analyses and systematic reviews are interesting, and some positive findings have appeared, but such contrasting results require careful examination of the data; dose and initial lipid status may or may not be important [53]. The food matrix should also be considered; a recent study made a direct comparison and observed that whole soy lowers LDL cholesterol but daidzein does not [57].

The effect of isoflavones and/or soy protein on other CVD risk factors has also been examined. The Scientific Committee of the AHA reviewed the evidence and concluded that increased consumption of soy protein with isoflavones does not affect blood pressure [53]. However, a later meta-analysis reported a significant decrease in blood pressure in hypertensive, but not normotensive, subjects after treatment with soy isoflavones [59]. A recent study demonstrated no effects of either soy protein or isolated isoflavones on blood pressure over 6 months in postmenopausal women, although there was some evidence of benefit in those who were initially hypertensive [60].

The effect of soy protein on inflammatory markers, such as interleukin-6, endothelial cytokines, and endothelial function, has also been examined, but again with mixed results [58, 60, 61]. The data are similarly mixed for levels of glucose and insulin. More studies are required that examine both inflammatory and diabetes-related endpoints, giving careful consideration to the type and amount of soy and/or isoflavones to be tested, the endpoints used, and the characteristics of the participants.

Early studies suggested that isoflavones could affect the arterial wall and improve systemic arterial compliance. A limited number of more recent studies have examined whether increased intake of soy protein or isoflavone intake affects circulating markers of endothelial activation or function, and, again, results have been conflicting [49, 60]. Neither soy nor isolated daidzein supplementation over 6 months in equol producers showed an effect on carotid intima–media thickness (IMT) [57], while, overall, no effect of soy protein isolate on vascular function was demonstrated over 3 months in men and postmenopausal women [62]. However, in an observational study of patients at high risk of cardiovascular events, a higher intake of isoflavone was associated with better vascular endothelial function and lower carotid atherosclerotic burden [63].

Further work is required on the effects of soy protein and its constituents on CHD risk. There are several possible mechanisms by which soy could help prevent CHD. Substituting soy protein for animal protein may indirectly benefit cardiovascular health by reducing intake of saturated fat and increasing intake of polyunsaturated fat, fiber, vitamins, and minerals; however, the possible importance of this is not known.

"Heart-smart" health claims, such as "cholesterol-free" and "heart healthy," have, in recent years, been approved by the Food and Drug Administration and appear on soy-milk products in the USA. However, the inconsistent evidence surrounding soy product intake and cardiovascular health to date has not met the stricter criteria of the European Food Safety Authority regarding health claims on food products.

Menopausal Symptoms

The use of phytoestrogen supplements as potential natural hormone replacement therapy and for the relief of menopausal symptoms became popular during the 1990s, but since then a meta-analysis of 25 trials has revealed that soy phytoestrogens do not reduce hot flushes or other menopausal symptoms [64].

Other Nondairy Milks

Numerous varieties of nondairy milks have become available in recent years. Some of the most common varieties are described here, although current knowledge regarding their effects on health is limited.

Grain milks, made from fermented grains such as rice, oats, spelt, rye, einkorn wheat, or quinoa, are increasingly used as substitutes for cow's milk in adults. These milks are lower in fat than cow's milk and tend to be sweeter and thinner as they contain more carbohydrate and less protein [65]. Grain milks are often fortified with calcium and other vitamins and minerals.

Oat milk is composed of a well-balanced mixture of fat, protein, complex carbohydrates, vitamins, and minerals and is especially high in vitamin E and folate [66, 67].

It reduces LDL cholesterol in healthy and hypercholesterolemic subjects [66, 67]; this is thought to be due to its high levels of soluble fiber, which is rich in beta-glucan, although the exact mechanism has not been established [68].

Almond milk is derived from ground almonds and is also lower in protein and calcium than cow's milk and contains no saturated fat or cholesterol [65]. In 2011, this milk was consumed by approximately 9 % of US consumers [4]. It is commonly fortified with vitamins and minerals including vitamins A, D, and E [65]. It comes in a variety of flavors with low-fat varieties also being available.

Coconut milk is the aqueous product extracted from coconut endosperm. It has a very high oil content, most of which is saturated fat. Although there is insufficient evidence to date, it has been suggested that the high levels of lauric acid, a saturated fatty acid, may decrease the total-to-HDL cholesterol ratio because of an increase in HDL cholesterol [69]. However, as coconut milk contains a variety of saturated fatty acids with differing, and possibly detrimental, effects on blood lipid levels, it is not recommended for regular use [70].

Conclusion

Alternatives to cow's milk continue to gain popularity. Soy milk, along with other foods containing soy protein which are rich in isoflavones, has attracted interest as potential health-promoting foods. Such foods may have a role to play in endocrine-responsive cancers, osteoporosis, and CVD prevention, but existing data are largely inconsistent or simply inadequate at present to support such suggested health benefits. The effects of these foods may be heterogeneous, depending on individual metabolic response to increased intake (equol status), the population being studied (Asian or Western), the background level of intake of that population, the health status of that population, the timing of the exposure, the menopausal status of female participants, and the soy product being tested (soy milk, soy protein, or extracted isoflavones). Consideration of such factors will be required when designing future studies to allow a more scientifically credible evaluation of the health effects of intake of these foods.

References

1. McCance and Widdowson's The Composition of Foods – Integrated Dataset. http://tna.europarchive.org/20110116113217/http://www.food.gov.uk/science/dietarysurveys/dietsurveys/. Accessed 10 Feb 2014.
2. Agostini C, Axelsson I, Goulet O, et al. Soy protein infant formulae and follow-on formulae: a commentary by the European Society for Paediatric Gastroenterology Hepatology and Nutrition Committee on Nutrition. J Pediatr Gastroenterol Nutr. 2006;42:352–61.
3. http://www.ars.usda.gov/SP2UserFiles/Place/12354500/Data/isoflav/Isoflav_R2.pdf. Accessed 10 Feb 2014.

4. http://www.packagedfacts.com/Soy-Milk-Dairy-6504961. Accessed 5 June 2014.
5. http://www.foodnavigator-usa.com/Markets/Almond-milk-catching-up-with-soy-as-favorite-non-dairy-milk-alternative. Accessed 5 June 2014.
6. http://www.choosemyplate.gov/food-groups/dairy-tips.html#nomilk. Accessed 5 June 2014.
7. http://www.soyfoods.org/soy-products/sales-and-trends. Accessed 27 May 2014.
8. Keinan-Baker L, Peeters PHM, Mulligan AA, et al. Soy product consumption in 10 European countries: the European Prospective Investigation into Cancer and Nutrition (EPIC) study. Public Health Nutr. 2002;5:1217–26.
9. Agriculture and Agri-Food Canada. Soy-based products in Western Europe. Ottawa: Agriculture and Agri-Food Canada; 2011. http://www.ats-sea.agr.gc.ca/eur/6062-eng.htm. Accessed 29 May 2014.
10. Turner GK. Lactose intolerance and irritable bowel syndrome. Nutrition. 2000;16:665–6.
11. Businco L, Bruno G, Giamietro PG. Soy protein for the prevention and treatment of children with cow-milk allergy. Am J Clin Nutr. 1998;68:1447S–52S.
12. Bhatia J, Greer F, American Academy of Pediatrics Committee on Nutrition. Use of soy protein-based formulas in infant feeding. Pediatrics. 2008;121:1062–8.
13. Adlercreutz H. Western diet and Western diseases: some hormonal and biochemical mechanisms and associations. Scand J Clin Lab Invest. 1990;201:S3–23.
14. Nagata C, Mizoue T, Tanaka K, et al. Soy intake and breast cancer risk: an evaluation based on a systematic review of epidemiologic evidence among the Japanese population. Jpn J Clin Oncol. 2014;44(3):282–95.
15. Chi F, Wu R, Zeng Y-C, Xing R, Liu Y, Xu Y-G. Post-diagnosis soy food intake and breast cancer survival: a meta-analysis of cohort studies. Asia Pac J Cancer Prev. 2013;14:2407–12.
16. Nechuta SJ, Caan BJ, Chen WY, et al. Soy food intake after diagnosis of breast cancer and survival: an in-depth analysis of combined evidence from cohort studies of US and Chinese women. Am J Clin Nutr. 2012;96:123–32.
17. Boyapati SM, Shy XO, Ruan ZX, Dai Q, Cai Q, Gao YT, Zheng W. Soyfood intake and breast cancer survival: a follow-up of the Shanghai Breast Cancer Study. Breast Cancer Res Treat. 2005;92:11–7.
18. Conroy SM, Maskarinec G, Wilkens LR, Henderson BE, Kolonel LN. The effects of soy consumption before diagnosis on breast cancer survival: the Multiethnic Cohort Study. Nutr Cancer. 2013;65:527–37.
19. Dong J-Y, Qin L-Q. Soy isoflavone consumption and risk of breast cancer incidence or recurrence: a meta-analysis of prospective studies. Breast Cancer Res Treat. 2011;125:315–23.
20. Trock BJ, Hilakivi-Clarke L, Clarke R. Meta-analysis of soy intake and breast cancer risk. J Natl Cancer Inst. 2006;98:459–71.
21. Kousidou OC, Mitropoulou TN, Roussidis AE, Kletsas D, Theocharis AD, Karamanos NK. Genistein suppresses the invasive potential of human breast cancer cells through transcriptional regulation of metalloproteinases and their tissue inhibitors. Int J Oncol. 2005;26:1101–9.
22. Hamdy SM, Latif AK, Drees EA, Soliman SM. Prevention of rat breast cancer by genistin and selenium. Toxicol Ind Health. 2012;28:746–57.
23. Petrakis NL, Barnes S, King EB, Lowenstein J, Wiencke J, Lee MM, Miike R, Kirk M, Coward L. Stimulatory influence of soy protein isolate on breast secretion in pre- and postmenopausal women. Cancer Epidemiol Biomarkers Prev. 1996;5:785–94.
24. McMichael-Phillips DF, Harding C, Morton M, Roberts SA, Howell A, Potten CS, Bundred NJ. Effects of soy-protein supplementation on epithelial proliferation in the histologically normal human breast. Am J Clin Nutr. 1998;68:1431–5.
25. Hooper L, Madhavan G, Tice JA, Leinster SJ, Cassidy A. Effects of isoflavones on breast density in pre- and post-menopausal women: a systematic review and meta-analysis of randomised controlled trials. Hum Reprod Update. 2010;16:745–60.
26. Khan SA, Chatterton RT, Michel N, et al. Soy isoflavone supplementation for breast cancer risk reduction: a randomised phase II trial. Cancer Prev Res. 2012;5:309–19.
27. Yan L, Spitznagel EL. Soy consumption and prostate cancer risk in men: a revisit of a meta-analysis. Am J Clin Nutr. 2009;89:1155–63.

28. Hwang YW, Kim SY, Jee SH, Kim YN, Nam CM. Soy food consumption and risk of prostate cancer: a meta-analysis of observational studies. Nutr Cancer. 2009;61:598–606.
29. Adams KF, Chen C, Newton KM, et al. Soy isoflavones do not modulate prostate-specific antigen concentrations in older men in a randomised controlled trial. Cancer Epidemiol Biomarkers Prev. 2004;13:644–8.
30. Yan L, Spitznagel EL, Bosland MC. Soy consumption and colorectal cancer risk in humans: a meta-analysis. Cancer Epidemiol Biomarkers Prev. 2010;19:148–58.
31. Yang W-S, Va P, Wong M-Y, Zhang H-L, Xiang Y-B. Soy intake is associated with lower lung cancer risk: results from a meta-analysis of epidemiologic studies. Am J Clin Nutr. 2011;94:1575–83.
32. Wu SH, Liu Z. Soy food consumption and lung cancer risk: a meta-analysis using a common measure across studies. Nutr Cancer. 2013;65:625–32.
33. Cooper C, Campion G, Melton LJ. Hip fractures in the elderly – a world-wide projection. Osteoporos Int. 1992;2:285–9.
34. Ma D-F, Qin L-Q, Wang P-Y, Katoh R. Soy isoflavone intake increases bone mineral density in the spine of menopausal women: meta-analysis of randomised controlled trials. Clin Nutr. 2008;27:57–64.
35. Kenny AM, Mangano KM, Abourizk RH, et al. Soy proteins and isoflavones affect bone mineral density in older women: a randomised controlled trial. Am J Clin Nutr. 2009;90:234–42.
36. Levis S, Strickman-Stein N, Ganjet-Azar P, Xu P, Doerge DR, Krischer J. Sot isoflavones in the prevention of menopausal bone loss and menopausal symptoms. Arch Intern Med. 2011;171:1363–9.
37. Tai TY, Tsai KS, Tu ST, et al. The effect of soy isoflavone on bone mineral density in post-menopausal Taiwanese women with bone loss: a 2 year randomised double-blind placebo-controlled study. Osteoporos Int. 2012;23:1571–80.
38. Brink E, Coxam V, Robins S, Wahala K, Cassidy A, Branca F. Long term consumption of isoflavone-enriched foods does not affect bone mineral density, bone metabolism, or hormonal status in early postmenopausal women: a randomised, double-blind, placebo-controlled study. Am J Clin Nutr. 2008;87:761–70.
39. Wong WW, Lewis RD, Steinberg FM, et al. Soy isoflavone supplementation and bone mineral density in menopausal women: a 2-y multicenter clinical trial. Am J Clin Nutr. 2009;90:1433–9.
40. Taku K, Melby MK, Takebayashi J, et al. Effect of soy isoflavone extract supplements on bone mineral density in menopausal women: meta-analysis of randomised controlled trials. Asia Pac J Clin Nutr. 2010;19:33–42.
41. Ricci E, Cipriani S, Chiaffarino F, Malvezzi M, Parazzini F. Soy isoflavones and bone mineral density in perimenopausal and postmenopausal Western women: a systematic review and meta-analysis of randomised controlled trials. J Womens Health. 2010;19:1609–17.
42. Taku K, Melby MK, Kurzer MS, Mizuno S, Watanabe S, Ishimi Y. Effect of soy isoflavone supplements on bone turnover markers in menopausal women: systematic review and meta-analysis of randomised controlled trials. Bone. 2010;47:413–23.
43. Taku K, Melby MK, Nishi N, Omori T, Kurzer MS. Soy isoflavones for osteoporosis: an evidence-based approach. Maturitas. 2011;70:333–8.
44. Reinwald S, Akabas SR, Weaver CM. While versus the piecemeal approach to evaluating soy. J Nutr. 2010;140:2335–43S.
45. Goodman-Gruen D, Kritz-Silverstein D. Usual dietary isoflavone intake is associated with cardiovascular disease risk factors in postmenopausal women. J Nutr. 2001;131:1202–6.
46. Zhang X, Gao Y-T, Yang G, et al. Urinary isoflavonoids and risk of coronary heart disease. Int J Epidemiol. 2012;41:1367–75.
47. Zhang X, Shu XO, Gao Y-T, et al. Soy food consumption is associated with lower risk of coronary heart disease in Chinese women. J Nutr. 2003;133:2874–8.
48. Yu D, Zhang X, Xiang Y-B, et al. Association of soy food intake with risk and biomarkers of coronary heart disease in Chinese men. Int J Cardiol. 2014;172(2):e285–7.
49. Pusparini MD, Dharma R, Suyatna FD, Mansyur M, Hidajat A. Effect of soy isoflavone supplementation on vascular endothelial function and oxidative stress in postmenopausal women: a community randomised controlled trial. Asia Pac J Clin Nutr. 2013;22:357–64.

50. Anderson JW, Johnstone BM, Cook-Newell ME. Meta-analysis of the effects of soy protein intake on serum lipids. N Engl J Med. 1995;332:276–82.
51. Reynolds K, Chin A, Lees KA, Nguyen A, Bujnowski D, He J. A meta-analysis of the effect of soy protein supplementation on serum lipids. Am J Cardiol. 2006;98:633–40.
52. Yang B, Chen Y, Xu T, et al. Systematic review and meta-analysis of soy products consumption in patients with type 2 diabetes mellitus. Asia Pac J Clin Nutr. 2011;20:593–602.
53. Sacks FM, Lichtenstein A, van Horn L, Harris W, Kris-Etherton P, Winston M. Soy protein, isoflavones and cardiovascular health: an American Heart Association Science Advisory for Professionals from the Nutrition Committee. Circulation. 2006;113:1034–44.
54. Crouse JR, Morgan T, Terry TG, Ellis J, Vitolins M, Burke GL. A randomised trial comparing the effect of casein with that of soy protein containing various amounts of isoflavones on plasma concentrations of lipids and lipoproteins. Arch Intern Med. 1999;159:2070–6.
55. Bakhtiary A, Yassin Z, Hanachi P, Rahmat A, Ahmad Z, Jalali F. Effects of soy on metabolic biomarkers of cardiovascular disease in elderly women with metabolic syndrome. Arch Iran Med. 2012;15:462–8.
56. Ma L, Grann K, Li M, Jiang Z. A pilot study to evaluate the effect of soy isolate protein on the serum lipid profile and other potential cardiovascular risk markers in moderately hypercholesterolaemic Chinese adults. Ecol Food Sci Nutr. 2011;50:473–85.
57. Liu Z, Ho SC, Chen Y, et al. Whole soy, but not purified daidzein, had a favourable effect on improvement of cardiovascular risks: a six-month randomised, double-blind, and placebo-controlled trial in equol-producing postmenopausal women. Mol Nutr Food Res. 2014;58:709–17.
58. Mangano KM, Hutchins-Wiese HL, Kenny AM, et al. Soy proteins and isoflavones reduce interleukin-6 but not serum lipids in older women: a randomised controlled trial. Nutr Res. 2013;33:1026–33.
59. Liu XX, Li SH, Chen JZ, et al. Effect of soy isoflavones on blood pressure: a meta-analysis of randomised controlled trials. Nutr Metab Cardiovasc Dis. 2012;22:463–70.
60. Liu Z-M, Ho SC, Chen Y-M, Woo J. Effect of soy protein and isoflavones on blood pressure and endothelial cytokines: a 6-month randomised controlled trial among postmenopausal women. J Hypertens. 2013;31:384–92.
61. Azadbakht L, Kimiagar M, Mehrabi Y, Esmaillzadeh A, Hu FB, Willett WC. Soy consumption, markers of inflammation and endothelial function. Diabetes Care. 2007;30:967–73.
62. Teede HJ, Dalais FS, Kotsopoulos D, Liang Y-L, Davis S, McGrath BP. Dietary soy has both beneficial and potentially adverse cardiovascular effects: a placebo-controlled study in men and postmenopausal women. J Clin Endocrinol Metab. 2001;86:3053–60.
63. Chan Y-H, Lau K-K, Yiu K-H, et al. Isoflavone intake in persons at high risk of cardiovascular events: implications for vascular endothelial function and the carotid atherosclerotic burden. Am J Clin Nutr. 2007;86:938–45.
64. Krebs EE, Ensrud KE, MacDonald R, Wilt TJ. Phytoestrogens for treatment of menopausal symptoms: a systematic review. Obstet Gynecol. 2004;104:824–36.
65. Holzmeister LA. Supermarket smarts. Nondairy milks. Diabetes Self Manag. 2007;24:75–83.
66. Onning G, Akesson B, Oste R, Lundquist J. Effects of consumption of oat milk, soya milk, or cow's milk on plasma lipids and antioxidative capacity in healthy subjects. Ann Nutr Metab. 1998;42:211–20.
67. Onning G, Wallmark A, Persson M, Akesson B, Elmståhl S, Oste R. Consumption of oat milk for 5 weeks lowers serum cholesterol in free-living men with moderate hypercholesterolemia. Ann Nutr Metab. 1999;43:301–9.
68. Bell S, Goldman VM, Bistrian BR, Arnold AH, Ostroff G, Forse RA. Effect of β-glucan from oats and yeast on serum lipids. Crit Rev Food Sci Nutr. 1999;39:189–202.
69. Cunningham E. Is there science to support claims for coconut oil? J Am Diet Assoc. 2011;111:786.
70. American Dietetic Association. Position of the American Dietetic Association and Dietitians of Canada: dietary fatty acids. J Am Diet Assoc. 2007;107:1599–611.

Chapter 11
Human Milk and Infant Formula: Nutritional Content and Health Benefits

James K. Friel and Wafaa A. Qasem

Keywords Human milk • Infant formula • Bioactive compounds • Breast-feeding

Key Points

1. Breast milk is acknowledged as the superior source of nutrition for infants.
2. Breast-feeding has been recommended by many professional organizations as an adequate and natural way to feed the growing infant due to its wide health benefits.
3. Infant formula is the only acceptable alternative to breast milk when breast-feeding is contraindicated.
4. Breast milk contains complete well-balanced macro-/micronutrients to match the growth the infant.
5. Cytokines immune factors, growth factors, hormones, antimicrobial agents, nucleotides, antioxidants, and enzymes are the mixture of bioactive components of the breast milk that have been shown to influence the health of infants.

J.K. Friel, Ph.D. (✉) • W.A. Qasem, M.D.
Department of Human Nutritional Sciences, Faculty of Agricultural and Food Sciences,
University of Manitoba, Winnipeg, MB, Canada
e-mail: James.Friel@umanitoba.ca

© Springer International Publishing Switzerland 2016
T. Wilson, N.J. Temple (eds.), *Beverage Impacts on Health and Nutrition*,
Nutrition and Health, DOI 10.1007/978-3-319-23672-8_11

Introduction: What Is the Best Milk for an Infant?

Recommendations from Authoritative Bodies

Current recommendations by Health Canada and the American Academy of Pediatrics (AAP) are to exclusively breast-feed for the first 6 months of life with human milk being the primary source of milk [1–3]. Formula feeding is recommended for those who choose not to breast-feed. The consumption of whole or reduced fat cow's milk is not recommended during the first year of life [4]. As of 2010, about 75 % of mothers in the USA initiate breast-feeding and 13 % continue to exclusively breast-feed to 6 months [5]. In Canada, the rate of initiation of breast-feeding is 90.3 %, while the rate of exclusive breast-feeding at 3 months is 51.7 %. Six months after birth, the proportions of exclusively breast-fed infants further fall to 14.4 % [6].

The first year of life is a time of more rapid growth, development, and maturation than any subsequent year. Growth of the body and development of the nervous system depends on an appropriate intake of calories and essential nutrients. The joint publication by the American and Canadian nutrition working groups, sponsored by the American Institute of Medicine, defines infancy as the period from birth to 12 months of age, divided into two 6-month periods [7]. The determination of the adequate intake (AI) during the first 6 months of life for every nutrient is based on the average intake by full-term infants born to healthy well-nourished mothers and exclusively fed human milk. The mean intake of a nutrient was calculated based on the average concentration of the nutrient from 2 to 6 months of lactation and assuming an average volume of milk intake of 780 mL/day [8]. In the second 6 months of infancy, AIs are based on nutrients available from 600 mL/day of human milk and that provided by the usual intake of complementary foods. Exclusive human milk feeding is the preferred method of feeding normal full-term infants for the first 4–6 months of life as recommended by most health professionals [1, 2]. While there are national regulations for upper and lower limits of nutrient content of infant formulas, specific Dietary Reference Intakes (DRIs) to meet the needs of formula-fed infants were not proposed. This was an error since, as a percentage of the total kinds of milk consumed during the first year of life [9], formula is the milk food most consumed (Fig. 11.1). To omit setting recommendations is to penalize infants whose parents have chosen not to breast-feed or have switched to formula.

Breast-feeding is rarely contraindicated [2]. Infants who have galactosemia, or whose mother uses illegal drugs, has untreated active tuberculosis, or has been infected with HIV should not breast-feed [2]. However, smoking, environmental contaminants, moderate alcohol consumption, or the use of most prescription and over-the-counter drugs should preclude breast-feeding.

With all the best intentions and technological expertise, "humanized" infant formulas do not compare to mother's own milk. Therefore, it is logical and appropriate for health professionals to encourage the consumption of human milk whenever

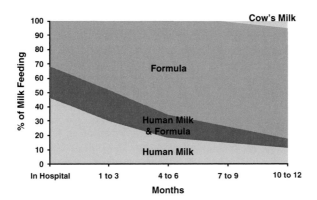

Fig. 11.1 Percentage of the total kinds of milk consumed during the first year of life. Adapted from Ross Labs, LLC (Edmonds, WA, USA)

possible. However, once the information is presented, there is no justification for attempting to coerce women into making a feeding choice [9].

Sometimes a formula-fed child and rarely a breast-fed infant develop a sensitivity to cow's milk, either cow's milk allergy (CMA) or lactose intolerance. The prevalence of CMA has been estimated to occur at 2.2–2.8 % [10]. Secondary lactase deficiency does occur in infancy, usually following a gastrointestinal disorder.

While human milk is "uniquely superior" for infant feeding and is species specific, the most acceptable alternative is commercial formulas. Manufacturers do their utmost to mimic human milk. At present all substitute feedings differ markedly from human milk [2]. A "formula" is just an equation that is proprietary, consisting of a composite mix of nutrients, emulsifiers, and stabilizers that will differ between manufacturers. Recently, polyunsaturated fatty acids such as arachidonic acid (ARA) and docosahexaenoic acid (DHA) acid have been added to infant formula due to their potential beneficial effects on the brain development of infants. More recently, probiotics have begun to emerge as a possible new ingredient added to some brands of infant formula [11]. Formulas in North America that are marketed for term infants are either (a) cow milk based (casein or whey predominant), (b) soy protein based, or (c) protein hydrolysate based. The use of soy-based formulas, speciality formulas, or formulas for the feeding of the premature infant is beyond the scope of this review.

The success of formula manufacturers is due to (a) aggressive marketing; (b) lack of support for breast-feeding from family, friends, and the medical profession; (c) cultural and public perception; (d) convenience; and (e) some government programs giving infant formula away for free. With the increase in working mothers, formula feeding becomes a practical and attractive alternative. Guidelines for formula composition have evolved over the years to provide not only what must be in a formula but minimum and maximum levels as well. Standards may vary between countries.

Developing Countries

Historically, breast-feeding has been the preferred method of feeding in all countries. The introduction of formula feeding in developing countries has been extremely controversial. In 1981 the WHO/UNICEF "International Code of Marketing of Breast-milk Substitutes" [12] was endorsed by many countries worldwide. The code seeks to prevent formula promotion at the expense of breast-feeding. It does not ban infant formula but outlines inappropriate marketing practices. This is important because marketing techniques can be very subtle. Organizations such as the Infant Feeding Action Coalition (INFACT) promote and protect breast-feeding. They believe that if the WHO code is properly implemented, breast-feeding rates would increase and infant health would improve. Unfortunately, these goals have been difficult to achieve. One reason for this is that the implementation of the WHO code may have a negative impact on the profits made by formula manufacturers.

Nutrient Content of Breast Milk and Infant Formula

Specific nutrient requirements are expressed as the amount of nutrient needed per 100 kcal of total food intake. This reflects nutrient interaction and can be applied to feeds of different caloric concentration. Human milk has a caloric density of 670 kcal/L. Most term formulas are designed to have the same caloric density.

The composition of a formula depends on many factors and differs between manufacturers. For example, cholesterol exists in human milk but is not added to formula because the public perceives cholesterol as "bad." Low-iron formulas are marketed even though health professionals do not recommend their use as a standard feed. They remain on the market because the public and some health professionals perceive them as beneficial in dealing with problems such as colic and constipation. As well, companies will not remove their low-iron formula until "the other guy does" and as long as substantial consumer demand exists. To facilitate marketing, manufacturers in the USA use the label Generally Recognised As Safe (GRAS) for any new ingredient added to infant formula.

The composition of human milk changes during feeding so that most of the fat appears in the latter part of feeding, probably saturating the infant and providing a signal for terminating feeding. This does not occur in the formula-fed infant as the composition of formula is constant. It appears that the infant who is breast-fed has more control over the amount consumed at a feeding than does the formula-fed infant [9]. Furthermore, frequent feedings with small amounts at each feeding, as is seen in infants who are breast-fed ad libitum, may lead to favorable changes in metabolism [13]. These differences may affect feeding habits later in life.

Macronutrients: Protein, Lipids, and Carbohydrate

The protein content of human milk is high during early lactation (colostrum) and then gradually declines to a low level of 0.8–1 % in mature milk. The high protein concentration of colostrum is largely due to very high concentrations of secretory IgA and lactoferrin. These proteins provide protection against bacteria giving benefits in early life beyond the role of building blocks for tissue synthesis. Indeed, human milk is truly the first and foremost "functional food."

Milk proteins are separated into various classes, mainly caseins (10–50 % of total) and whey (50–90 % of total) proteins [14]. Milk fat globule membrane proteins and protein derived from cells present in milk comprise 1–3 %. For some years, manufacturers prepared their formula with either a whey or casein base. For the term infant, there appears to be no advantage nutritionally of whey-predominant over casein-predominant formulas. Interestingly, digested fragments of human casein, but not bovine casein, which is less well digested, may exert physiological effects, such as enhancing calcium uptake by cells and playing a role in infant sleeping patterns [14]. Little is known about the role of hormones that are present in human milk and that may play a role in the developing infant.

Human milk contains significant amounts of linoleic acid (18:2, n–6; 10–12 %), linolenic acid (18:3, n–3; 1–2 %), and a small but significant amount of long-chain (n–6 and n–3) fatty acids [15]. While the level of total polyunsaturated fatty acids (PUFA) in human milk varies with the intake of the mother, it is generally 13–20 %. The marketed formulas contain 0.15 and 0.40 % of DHA and ARA, respectively [11].

The primary carbohydrate source in human milk is lactose with very small amounts of other sugars. This is also the principle carbohydrate of formulas. No minimum or maximum level of carbohydrate is set for North America. Corn syrup solids and/or maltodextrin may be used in certain formulas.

Micronutrients: Minerals and Vitamins

Minerals

Minerals can be divided broadly into macro (calcium, phosphorus, magnesium, sodium, potassium, chlorine, and sulfur) and micro (iron [Fe], zinc [Zn], copper [Cu], molybdenum [Mo], manganese [Mn], rubidium [Rb], cobalt [Co], iodine [I], and selenium [Se]). Lead and aluminum [16] are present in human milk and may ultimately prove to be essential in trace amounts for humans, as has been shown in other species; however, in excess, they are problematic for human health. Our study of 19 women who gave birth to full-term infants demonstrated that mineral concentrations differed in human milk over the first 3 months of lactation [17]. Zn, Cu, Rb, and Mo decreased with time. As with Zn and Cu, the decline in Mo suggests homoeostatic regulation, implying possible essentiality for human infants. Cerium, cesium, lanthanum, and tin have not been shown to be essential, and no consistent pattern in our data occurred that would indicate either maternal or dietary regulation. In general, the mineral content of human milk is not influenced by maternal diet, parity, maternal age, time of milk collection, different breasts, or socioeconomic status [18].

The ultra-trace elements [<1 μg/g dry diet] exist naturally in human milk but depend on protein sources in formulas where they occur as contaminants. Although many of these elements have no specified human requirement, we believe that recommendations for ultra-trace elements need to be established. Our concern is that as preparation techniques for making more purified ingredients becomes available, less of these elements will occur in the normal diet of the formula-fed infant. A particular example is Mo which is not usually added to infant formula but appears to be essential [19].

Vitamins

Human milk has all the vitamins required by the infant but is low in vitamins D and K. Vitamin K is given to all infants at birth, and vitamin D (also considered to be a hormone) is usually recommended as a supplement for breast-fed infants. Minimum and maximum levels of vitamins are regulated for formulas so that they are complete. The AAP and Health Canada recommend a daily dose of 400 IU of vitamin D supplementation for breast-fed infants and infants receiving less than 1 L of formula [3, 20]. Formula labels state the amount of all nutrients, including vitamins, that must be present when the shelf life expires. Because of this, "overage" is necessary as some vitamins will break down over time. Thus, as much as 60 % over label claim might be present for different nutrients, primarily vitamins [21].

Supplements

The use of supplements for infants fed with human milk is controversial. Some see supplements as undermining the integrity of human milk and implying that it is not adequate. Suggesting that human milk can be improved upon is "....like entering a minefield, one must tread carefully" [22]. Nonetheless, human milk is neither a perfect nor a complete food [23]. There is good data to support the administration of vitamin K soon after birth to prevent hemorrhagic disease of the newborn and vitamin D supplements during early infancy to prevent rickets [3, 20, 23].

Iron is a contentious infant formula ingredient because the amount of fortification required is not yet certain. Current practice is for iron supplements to be deferred until 4–6 months of age, but formulas with a low content (<4 mg/L) may lead to anemia. In the USA, the AAP recommends iron supplementation of 1 mg/kg/day for the exclusively breast-fed infants at 4 months of age until weaning is commenced with iron-rich foods [1]. Unpublished data from our laboratory support this recommendation as we found a significant increase in iron status in these infants receiving a modest iron supplement (7.5 mg/day). It was believed that consuming iron-fortified formulas would result in intolerance and gastrointestinal distress, theories which have been discredited [24]. Fluoride supplements, once recommended for all infants, are no longer recommended during the first year of life [1]. Formulas that conform to specification of Canadian/American guidelines do not require supplementation with any minerals or vitamins as they are complete. For a review of regulations for the nutrient content of infant formulas, see Fomon [9].

Maternal Influences on Milk Content

In general, the content of protein, lipid, carbohydrate, energy, minerals, and most water-soluble vitamins in human milk is not affected by poor maternal nutrition [25]. Fat-soluble vitamins and fatty acids are affected by the maternal diet [26]. It appears that there are mechanisms to ensure constant supply and quality of nutrients to the breast-fed infant. The major difference between a breast-fed and a formula-fed infant is that many of the components of human milk also facilitate the absorption of nutrients and have a function beyond nutrient requirements. Adding more of a nutrient to formula is not necessarily as good as having a bioactive component in human milk even if present in small amounts (e.g., lactoferrin for both iron absorption and as a bactericide). There are many properties of human milk that attend to such detail for the benefit of the infant.

Bioactivity of Human Milk and Formulas

Bioactive Compounds in Human Milk: An Overview

Human milk is "alive," that is, it has functional components that have a role beyond simply the provision of essential nutrients. According to Dorland's Medical Dictionary, a tissue is "an aggregation of similarly specialized cells united in the performance of a single function." Human milk could be classified as a "tissue" which would alter the perspective on how human milk is viewed. There are active and functional ingredients in human milk whose role is evident and others for whom no clear role has been defined.

Bioactive compounds in human milk can be divided into several broad categories: (a) those compounds involved in milk syntheses, nutritional composition, and bioavailability and (b) compounds that aid in protection and subsequent development of the infant. To date many bioactive compounds have been identified in human milk including cytokines immune factors, growth factors, hormones, antimicrobial agents, nucleotides, antioxidants, and enzymes (see reference 27 for a review). Hormones, enzymes, cytokines for immunity, and cells present in milk have physiologically active roles in other tissues so that it is reasonable to assume they play a role in infant growth and development [11]. Indeed, many bioactive compounds can survive the environment of the neonatal gut, thereby potentially exerting important physiological functions [27, 28].

The composition of human milk can vary. Nutrient content changes over time so that the makeup of colostrum, transitional milk, and mature milk is quite different. Nutrient content also changes within the same feed, whereas formula clearly content does not. This appears to be of importance to infant regulation of food intake.

Early postnatal exposure to flavor passed into human milk from the mother's own diet can predispose the young infant to respond to new foods. The transition from the breast-feeding period to the initiation of a varied solid food diet can be made easier if the infant has already experienced these flavors. Cues from breast milk can influence food choices and make safe new foods with flavors already experienced in breast milk [29]. Again this does not happen with formula feeding.

A variety of cells exist in human milk. Macrophages, polymorphonuclear leucocytes, epithelial cells, and lymphocytes have been identified in human milk and appear to have a dynamic role to play within the infant gut. These cells may offer systemic protection after transport across the "leaky gut," particularly in the first week of life [30]. Antiviral and antibacterial factors exist in human milk with secretary IgA produced in the mammary gland being one of the major milk proteins [14]. There may even be a pathway from the infant back to the mother which tailors production of antibodies against microbes to which the infant has been exposed.

Enzymes

Enzymes serve to catalyze reactions and need be present only in small amounts to be effective. Hamosh [27] classifies enzymes in human milk into three categories: (a) those that function in the mammary gland, e.g., lipoprotein lipase, phosphoglucomutase, and antiproteases; (b) enzymes that might function in the infant, e.g., proteases, α-amylase (facilitates digestion of polysaccharides), and lysozyme (bactericidal); and (c) enzymes whose function is unclear, namely, lactate dehydrogenase, DNase, and RNase. It is only recently that the physiological significance of enzymes in human milk has become appreciated. More than just protein, and not present at all in infant formulas, enzymes are another example of why human milk must be seen as alive. The enzymes in human milk appear to have a more highly organized tertiary structure than enzymes from other tissues, which may be to protect function by resisting denaturation in the gut [27]. For example, in human milk, the enzyme catalase has been found to protect against bacterial breeches of the intestinal barrier [31]. We think that as well as serving an immediate function in the intestine, some enzymes may be transported across the gut or act within the body to offer protection to the infant.

Interestingly, amylase digests polysaccharides that are not present in human milk. Amylase is important after the initiation of such starch supplements as cereals [27]. It is as if the mammary gland is "thinking ahead" and assisting the infant gut in the transition to weaning. Milk digestive lipase assists the newborn whose endogenous lipid digestive function is not well developed at birth.

Glutathione peroxidase (GHSPx) activity appears to correlate with milk selenium concentration [32]. It may be related to fatty acid function or maintain milk integrity by neutralizing free radicals. We measured both GHSPx and superoxide dismutase over 3 months in full-term milk and found high activity of both enzymes [33]. Since there are at least 44 enzymes whose substrates could be lipid peroxides or hydrogen peroxide [27], it may be that these enzymes protect the infant's gut.

Antioxidants

Recent interest has focussed on the antioxidant properties of human milk. Several groups have reported the ability of colostrum [34] and mature milk [35] to resist oxidative stress, using a variety of end points. This ability in human milk appears to be heterogeneous rather than attributable to a specific compound. Infant formulas appear to be less resistant to oxidative stress than is human milk. This is noteworthy since formulas always have considerably more vitamins E and C, considered to be two of the more important antioxidants, than is found naturally in human milk [36]. Some have suggested that the attainment of adult levels of some antioxidants during infancy is dependent on human milk feeding [21].

Effects on Microbiome

The gut microbiome is a complex ecosystem consisting of more than 1000 species of live bacteria which play major roles in nutrition and in the development of the immune system [37]. It has been shown that there are variations in the gut microbiome composition between formula-fed and breast-fed infants. The microbiome of breast-fed infants is predominated by the beneficial *Bifidobacterium* and *Lactobacillus* bacteria. In contrast, *Enterococci*, *Clostridium*, and *Escherichia* are the abundant bacteria observed in the microflora of formula-fed infants [38]. The predominance of these unfavorable bacteria may lead to a less acidic gut environment, which will further promote the growth of pathogenic-type bacteria. Colonic bacterial imbalance has long-term implications as a result of inflammation which is the key pathophysiological factor in gastrointestinal disorders such as inflammatory bowel disease [39].

Health Benefits of Human Milk

Overview

The health benefits of human milk are significant. Breast-feeding protects against a wide variety of illnesses, particularly incidence and severity of diarrhea, otitis media, upper respiratory illnesses, botulism, and necrotizing enterocolitis [1]. Prior to advancements in hygiene, infants who were not breast-fed did not fare well and mortality rates could be as high as 90 % [7, 26]. Even with the use of current formulas, breast-fed infants have a lower incidence of many illnesses and are generally sicker for shorter times [40] than formula-fed infants. Breast-fed infants are reported to have decreased incidence of diabetes, cancer, and cardiovascular disease later in life [2]. However, the recent findings from the National Longitudinal Survey of Youth (NLSY) suggested that longer duration of breast-feeding may not necessarily result in long-term healthier childhood and well-being [41].

Growth

Growth is the most practical measure of the overall health and well-being of infants. One would expect that with all the advantages of human milk, a breast-fed baby would gain weight faster [42]. It is a puzzling phenomenon that growth of the exclusively breast-fed infant is lower in weight-for-age than a formula-fed infant. The average difference at 12 months is 600 to 650 g, with no difference in height so that a breast-fed infant is leaner. There is probably more energy intake by a formula-fed infant. The relevance of less growth in breast-fed infants is questionable as no negative effects on functional outcomes have been observed. We found that infants who had consumed home formulas made of evaporated milk grew more than either formula-fed or breast-fed babies [43]; however, they did not perform as well as infants fed with human milk on tests of visual function [44].

Cognitive Development

There is controversy in this area as it is difficult to carry out the ideal study. Breast-fed infants appear to have enhanced cognitive and neurological outcomes in comparison to formula-fed infants [45]. Results from the largest clinical trial of breast-feeding (Promotion of Breastfeeding Intervention Trial) provided evidence that former breast-fed infants scored higher in intelligence scores than formula-fed infants [46]. Increased duration of breast-feeding has been linked with higher verbal IQ scores. Increasing the period of exclusive breast-feeding appears to enhance infant motor development [47]. We found enhanced visual acuity in full-term breast-fed infants compared to formula-fed infants; this is related to blood fatty acid levels [44]. The explanation for these consistent observations is highly controversial. Possibly there are components of human milk that enhance cognitive development. Other factors that may be responsible are the act of breast-feeding itself, maternal education, and social class.

A paper by Allan Lucas reporting improved neurological development in infants fed with human milk sparked much debate concerning which factors really explain the increased cognitive development in the human milk-fed infant [48]. It is reasonable to assume that breast milk, as it contains long-chain PUFA, enzymes, hormones, trophic factors, peptides, and nucleotides, may enhance brain development and learning ability. Further, it would be sensible to feed human milk whenever possible if any or all of the above differences turn out to be true. Whether an infant fed with human milk has better development because of maternal factors or biological factors does not lessen the value of enhanced development to the infant.

International Aspects of Breast-Feeding

Overview

The WHO attributes seven of ten childhood deaths in developing countries to just five main causes: pneumonia, diarrhea, measles, malaria, and malnutrition. All of them can be prevented, some specifically by breast-feeding [49].

In nonindustrialized countries, the advantages of feeding human milk are easily seen and the use of a commercially available or home-prepared formula is not recommended [9]. Home-prepared formulas are usually poorly designed and nutritionally inadequate. These problems are aggravated when there is an absence of a safe water supply, hygienic conditions, and adequate storage facilities.

Evidence from developing countries indicates that infants breast-fed for less than 6 months or not at all have a mortality rate 5 to 10 times higher in the second 6 months of life than those breast-fed for 6 months or more [12]. Improper marketing of breast milk substitutes still occurs and can lead to inappropriate feeding practices, resulting in malnutrition, illness, and death in developing countries [50].

The Economics of Breast-Feeding

It has been estimated that $13 billion would be saved each year in the USA if 90 % of mothers exclusively breast-feed for 6 months [51]. Benefits of breast-feeding include reduced health-care costs, reduced employee absenteeism, and savings on the cost of formula. The impact of savings on formula purchase is more pronounced in developing countries. In fact, formula has gotten so expensive that it may not be an option in poorer countries. In countries "in transition," this may be more of an issue.

The Politics of Breast-Feeding

Historically, most human infants have been breast-fed. To enhance infant feeding practices, WHO and UNICEF launched the Baby-Friendly Hospital Initiative in 1992. This policy encourages exclusive breast-feeding in hospital soon after birth, with no other food or drink to be given unless medically indicated. This was done to encourage exclusive breast-feeding and discourage the introduction of supplementary formula feeding. It is known that women who receive a "discharge pack" when leaving hospital, containing a breast pump rather than infant formula, will breast-feed longer [52].

"Exclusive" breast-feeding is defined as no other food or drink, not even water, except breast milk for at least 4 and if possible 6 months after birth. Using this criterion, rates for exclusive breast-feeding for the first 6 months is 33 % in African countries. In Europe, the rate is 24 %. Where the advantages of breast-feeding have been widely publicized, breast-feeding rates are increasing, e.g., Australia, Canada, and the USA (http://apps.who.int/gho/data/view.main.NUT1710?lang=en).

In underdeveloped countries, breast-feeding is so ingrained into the many cultures and traditions of society that the pressure to breast-feed is intense. In fact a woman can be ostracized from her community for formula feeding. This is why "free samples" are so insidious. If the milk supply dries up and a woman is forced to formula feed, she may become an outcast. HIV has altered perception on formula feeding as even UNICEF, who have been stanch supporters of breast-feeding, at one time considered providing formula to HIV-positive mothers in order to protect the infant. This idea has since been dropped. How this issue will be dealt with has not been decided.

If milk is not continually removed from the mother's breast, the ability to secrete milk is lost within one to two weeks. It is common practice to offer an occasional bottle of formula. A better alternative would be for a mother to acquire a breast pump in order to have milk frozen for those times she is unable to feed.

Conclusion

There is no doubt that human milk is the best food for a human infant. The reasons are endless and convincing. Nonetheless, it is a challenge for the formula industry to make the best suitable alternative to human milk. There are, were, and always will be some women who are unable or choose not to follow recommendations to breast-feed for whatever reason (http://www.who.int/topics/breastfeeding/en/index. html). We have a responsibility to those mothers and their infants to produce a formula that meets their needs. Future changes in infant formulas are likely to be designed to have a positive effect on physical, mental, and immunological outcomes [53]. Our hope is that formula will include bioactive ingredients that perform some of the same functions found in that exemplary fluid, human milk.

References

1. Gartner LM, Morton J, Lawrence RA, et al. Breastfeeding and the use of human milk. Pediatrics. 2005;115:496–506.
2. American Academy of Pediatrics. Section on breastfeeding. Breastfeeding and the use of human milk. Pediatrics. 2012;129:827–41.
3. Health Canada. Nutrition for healthy term infants: recommendations from birth to six months. Can J Diet Pract Res. 2012;73:204.
4. American Academy of Pediatrics. The use of whole cow's milk in infancy. Pediatrics. 1992;89:1105–7.
5. U.S. Department of Health and Human Services. Maternal, infant, and child health. Healthy People 2020. http://healthypeople.gov/2020/topicsobjectives2020/overview. aspx?topicid%3D26. Accessed 28 Dec 2013.
6. Chalmers B, Levitt C, Heaman M, O'Brien B, Sauve R, Kaczorowski J. Breastfeeding rates and hospital breastfeeding practices in Canada: a national survey of women. Birth. 2009;36:122–32.
7. Fomon SJ. Infant feeding in the 20th century: formula and breast. J Nutr. 2001;131:409S–20.
8. Institue of Medicine. Dietary reference intakes for vitamin A, vitamin K, arsenic, boron, chromium, copper, iodine, iron, manganese, molybdenum, nickel, silicon, vanadium, and zinc. 2001. http://www.iom.edu/Activities/Nutrition/SummaryDRIs/DRI-Tables.aspx. Accessed 17 Dec 2013.
9. Fomon SJ. Nutrition of normal infants. St. Louis: Mosby; 1993. p. 455–8.
10. Saarinen KM, Juntunen-Backman A, Jarvenpaa AL, et al. Supplementary feeding in maternity hospitals and the risk of cow's milk allergy: a prospective study of 6209 infants. J Allergy Clin Immunol. 1999;104:457–61.
11. Institute of Medicine. Infant formula: evaluating the safety of new ingredients. http://www.iom.edu/~/media/Files/Report Files/2004/Infant-Formula-Evaluating-the-Safety-of-New-Ingredients/infantformula.pdf. Accessed 4 Jan 2014.
12. International Organization of Consumers Unions. In: Annelies A, editor. Protecting infant health. Penang: International Organization of Consumers Unions; 1986. p. 36–9.
13. Jenkins DJA, Wolever TMS, Vinson U, et al. Nibbling vs gorging: metabolic advantages of increased meal frequency. N Engl J Med. 1989;321:929–34.
14. Lonnerdal B, Atkinson S. Nitrogenous components of milk. A. Human milk proteins. In: Jensen UG, editor. Handbook of milk composition. San Diego: Academic; 1995. p. 351–68.

15. Redenials WAN, Chen ZY. Trans, n-2, and n-6 fatty acids in Canadian human milk. Lipids. 1996;31:5279–82.
16. Quarterman J. Lead. In: Mertz W, editor. Trace element in human and animal nutrition. Orlando: Academic; 1986. p. 281–317.
17. Friel JK, Longerich H, Jackson S, Dawson B, Sutrahdar B. Ultra trace elements in human milk from premature and term infants. Biol Tr Elem Res. 1999;67:225–47.
18. Lonnerdal B. Regulation of mineral and trace elements in human milk: exogenous and endogenous factors. Nutr Rev. 2000;58:223–9.
19. Friel JK, Simmons B, MacDonald AC, Mercer CN, Aziz K, Andrews WL. Molybdenum requirements in low birth weight infants receiving parenteral and enteral nutrition. J Par Ent Nutr. 1999;23:155–9.
20. Wagner CL, Greer FR. Prevention of rickets and vitamin D deficiency in infants, children, and adolescents. Pediatrics. 2008;122:1142–52.
21. Friel JK, Bessie JC, Belkhode SL, et al. Thiamine riboflavin, pyridoxine, and vitamin C status in premature infants receiving parenteral and enteral nutrition. J Ped Gastro Ent Nutr. 2001;33:64–9.
22. Godel JC. Breast-feeding and anemia: let's be careful. CMAJ. 2000;162:343–4.
23. Fomon SJ, Straus UG. Nutrient deficiencies in breast-fed infants. N Engl J Med. 1978;299:355–7.
24. Nelson SE, Ziegler EE, Copeland AM, et al. Lack of adverse reaction to iron-fortified formula. Pediatrics. 1988;81:360–4.
25. Lonnerdal B. Effects of maternal dietary intake on breast milk composition. J Nutr. 1986;116:499–513.
26. Lonnerdal B. Breast milk: a truly functional food. Nutrition. 2000;16:509–11.
27. Hamosh M. Enzymes in human milk. In: Jensen UG, editor. Handbook of milk composition. San Diego: Academic; 1995. p. 388–427.
28. L'Abbe MR, Friel JK. Enzymes in human milk. In: Huang V-S, Sinclair A, editors. Recent advances in the role of lipids in infant nutrition. Champaign: AOCS; 1998. p. 133–47.
29. Mennella JA, Jagnow CP, Beauchamp GK. Prenatal and postnatal flavour learning by human infants. Pediatrics. 2001;107:1–6.
30. Weaver LT, Lalver MF, Nelson R. Intestinal permeability in the newborn. Arch Dis Child. 1984;59:236–41.
31. Lindmark-Mansson H, Akesson B. Antioxidative factors in milk. Br J Nutr. 2000;84:S103–10.
32. Mannan S, Picciano MF. Influence of maternal selenium status on human milk selenium concentration and glutathione peroxidase activity. Am J Clin Nutr. 1987;46:95–100.
33. L'Abbe M, Friel JK. Glutathione peroxidase and superoxide dismutase concentrations in milk from mothers of premature and full-term infants. J Ped Gastro Ent Nutr. 2000;31:270–4.
34. Buescher ES, McIllherhan SM. Antioxidant properties of human colostrum. Pediatr Res. 1988;24:14–9.
35. Friel JK, Martin SM, Langdon M, Herzberg G, Buettner GR. Human milk provides better antioxidant protection than does infant formula. Pediatr Res. 2002;51:612–8.
36. Ross Products Division. Ross Ready Reference. Columbus: Abbott Laboratories; 1999.
37. Lee YK, Mazmanian SK. Has the microbiota played a critical role in the evolution of the adaptive immune system? Science. 2010;330:1768–73.
38. Bezirtzoglou E, Tsiotsias A, Welling GW. Microbiota profile in feces of breast- and formula-fed newborns by using fluorescence in situ hybridization (FISH). Anaerobe. 2011;17:478–82.
39. Xavier RJ, Podolsky DK. Unravelling the pathogenesis of inflammatory bowel disease. Nature. 2007;448:427–34.
40. Dewey KG, Heinig MJ, Nommsen-Rivers LA. Differences in morbidity between breast-fed and formula-fed infants. J Pediatr. 1995;126:696–702.
41. Colen CG, Ramey DM. Is breast truly best? Estimating the effects of breastfeeding on long-term child health and wellbeing in the United States using sibling comparisons. Soc Sci Med. 2014;109:55–65.

42. Dewey KG, Heinig MJ, Nommsen LA, Pearson JM, Lonnerdal B. Growth of breast-fed and formula-fed infants from 0 to 18 months: the DARLING study. Pediatrics. 1992;89:1035–41.
43. Friel JK, Andrews WL, Simmons BS, Mercer C, Macdonald A, McCloy U. An evaluation of full-term infants fed on evaporated milk formula. Acta Paediatr. 1997;86:448–53.
44. Courage ML, McCloy U, Herzberg G, et al. Visual acuity development and fatty acid composition of erythrocytes. J Dev Behave Paediatr. 1997;19:9–17.
45. Friel JK. Cognitive development in breast-fed infants. J Hum Lact. 1999;15:97–8.
46. Kramer MS, Aboud F, Mironova E, et al. Breastfeeding and child cognitive development: new evidence from a large randomized trial. Arch Gen Psychiatry. 2008;65:578–84.
47. Dewey KG, Cohen RJ, Brown KH, Rivera LL. Effects of exclusive breast feeding for four versus six months on maternal nutritional status and infant motor development. J Nutr. 2001;131:262–7.
48. Lucas A, Morley R, Cole TJ, Lister G, Leeson-Payne C. Breast milk and subsequent intelligence quotient in children born preterm. Lancet. 1992;339:261–4.
49. World Health Organization. Newborns: reducing mortality. http://www.who.int/mediacentre/factsheets/fs333/en/index.html. Accessed 5 Jan 2014.
50. World Health Organization. Country Implementation of the international code of marketing of breast-milk substitutes: status report. 2011. http://apps.who.int/iris/bitstream/10665/85621/1/9789241505987_eng.pdf. Accessed 5 Jan 2014.
51. Bartick M, Reinhold A. The burden of suboptimal breastfeeding in the United States: a pediatric cost analysis. Pediatrics. 2010;125:1048–56.
52. Dunghy CI, Christensen-Syalonski J, Losch M, Russel D. Effect of discharge samples on duration of breast-feeding. Pediatrics. 1992;90:233–7.
53. Ryan AS, Benson JD, Flammang AM. Infants formulas and medical foods. In: Schmidt MK, Labuza TP, editors. Essentials of functional foods. Gaithersburg: Aspen; 2000. p. 137–63.

Part IV
Beverage Health Effects on Energy Balance, Diabetes, and in Older Adults

Chapter 12
Beverages, Satiation, Satiety, and Energy Balance

James H. Hollis

Keywords Beverages • Satiety • Satiation • Obesity • Physical form

Key Points

1. Beverages have weaker satiation or satiety properties than solid food equivalents.
2. Increased consumption of beverages may increase risk of weight gain.
3. Dietary compensation for the energy in beverages occurs but is not complete.
4. The physical and chemical characteristics of beverages could influence the effect on energy balance.

Introduction

The high medical, social, and economic costs make reducing the number of overweight or obese individuals a leading public health goal throughout the world. To better understand how the obesity epidemic arose and to aid the development of new strategies to curb the obesity epidemic, there has been an increased focus on understanding how food characteristics influence energy balance. A better understanding of this relationship would be useful to (a) improve effective weight management strategies, (b) assist the food industry in food product reformulations that aid weight management, and (c) guide government policy relating to the food industry. One

J.H. Hollis, Ph.D. (✉)
Department of Food Science and Human Nutrition, Iowa State University,
220 Mackay Hall, Ames, IA 50011, USA
e-mail: jhollis@iastate.edu

© Springer International Publishing Switzerland 2016
T. Wilson, N.J. Temple (eds.), *Beverage Impacts on Health and Nutrition*,
Nutrition and Health, DOI 10.1007/978-3-319-23672-8_12

salient food characteristic that has recently come under considerable scrutiny is its physical form (liquid or solid). The reason for this interest is that the putative weak satiation/satiating properties of energy-yielding beverages are a potential contributor to the obesity epidemic.

When considering the effect of beverages on energy balance and body weight, it must be recognized that beverages are a diverse group of foods that includes sugar-sweetened beverages, fruit/vegetable juices, milk, smoothies, tea/coffee, alcoholic beverages, energy drinks, and meal replacement drinks. These beverages differ substantially in terms of their macronutrient content, viscosity, taste intensity, energy density, bioactive content, and mouthfeel, each of which could influence the effect on energy balance. Moreover, beverages are also consumed in a variety of contexts (e.g., as a snack, an accompaniment to a meal, or a meal replacement) which may also influence their impact on energy balance. Consequently, beverages are likely to differ markedly in their effects on energy balance and some may be more problematic than others.

This chapter will describe satiation, satiety, and diet-induced thermogenesis (DIT) before briefly reviewing the literature regarding the effect of beverages on these components of energy balance. This chapter will also discuss the mechanisms that may potentially explain why beverages have a weak effect on satiation and satiety.

Satiation, Satiety, Thermogenesis, and Energy Balance

Satiation and satiety are important concepts in the understanding of appetite control and food intake. Satiation occurs during a meal and contributes to the cessation of eating, whereas satiety begins at the end of a meal and inhibits further eating episodes. Differences in the satiation or satiety response could influence energy balance by altering meal size or meal patterning to influence overall energy intake. While there is a physiological aspect to satiation and satiety overall, food intake is determined by a complex interaction between environment (e.g., food availability, constraints on food access) and physiology that is still not well understood [1].

Most studies of satiation or satiety use the preload design where a test meal (this may be a solid or liquid meal) is provided and the effect on appetite and food intake is monitored over the following 15 min to several hours. These studies have several limitations which must be considered when interpreting the data provided. First, these studies are generally short term and measure satiation or satiety at a single meal or over a limited timespan (<24 h). Consequently, it is not possible to know from these studies if participants compensate for the effect of the test food on food intake by eating more or less at subsequent meals over a period of several days to compensate for the perturbation in energy balance. Moreover, these studies do not allow time for the impact of psychological behaviors that influence on eating to be expressed (e.g., the reduction of food intake due to noticeable weight gain). Second, eating or drinking behavior in the laboratory may not reflect eating behavior in a free-living situation. For example, in the laboratory participants are generally provided with free food in excess of what could usually be expected to be eaten. Consequently, caution should be used when extrapolating from these studies to free-living individuals. Despite these limitations, short-term studies provide useful mechanistic data to support observations made from epidemiological studies or randomized control trials. At this time, short-term studies have provided a substantial amount of data regarding the role of beverages on energy balance and have been useful in forming the hypothesis that the regular consumption of energy-yielding beverages contributes to weight gain.

Diet-induced thermogenesis refers to the obligatory increase in energy expenditure, above the resting metabolic rate, required to absorb, metabolize, and store ingested food. A commonly used estimate of DIT is 10 % of caloric intake. However, the DIT also depends on factors such as macronutrient content or palatability of the meal and therefore may be manipulated to increase total energy expenditure [2].

The Effect of Beverages on Energy Balance

The introduction of beverages into the habitual diet or a change in the type of beverages consumed could influence energy balance in several ways. First, if beverages possess weak satiation properties, their energy may add to the amount of energy provided by a meal rather than replacing calories from other parts of the meal. In addition, there may not be a compensatory response by eating less at subsequent meals. Second, beverages consumed during the inter-meal interval may not result in a reduction in food intake at subsequent meals thus increasing the number of eating occasions and food intake. Third, there may be a reduction in DIT as beverages require less processing than solid foods. However, this effect may be mitigated if the beverage contains certain bioactive compounds (e.g., caffeine) that increase energy expenditure.

Beverage Macronutrient Content and Satiation/Satiety

Beverages generally provide carbohydrate, protein, and/or fiber; as the majority of studies have concentrated on these food components, they will be the focus of this section. While beverages typically provide negligible amounts of fat, the recent increase in consumption of specialty coffees, such as lattes, that contain cream may provide significant amounts of fat in a beverage form. The influence of such beverages on energy balance warrants further research. A notable exception is milk. Full-fat milk contains 3.3 % fat and efforts have been made to encourage consumers to switch to milk that contains 2 or 1 % fat to aid weight management. However, it is not clear that consuming full-fat milk contributes to obesity, and a recent study suggests that consumption of full-fat milk is associated with lower body weight [3]. It is not clear why consuming full-fat milk would be associated with reduced body weight but may be due to an effect on satiety or bioactive compounds contained in the fat fraction. Further research is required to clarify the effect of full-fat milk on energy balance.

Evidence from studies using solid foods generally supports a hierarchical effect of macronutrients on satiation and satiety (protein > CHO > fat; [4]). However, this difference in satiety may not always be sufficiently large to influence food intake [5]. The effect of fiber on satiation and satiety has not been well established due to the large number of different types of fiber used in studies [6].

Beverage Macronutrient Content, Energy Balance, Satiation, and Satiety

Satiation

In an early study, it was found that replacing sugar in a beverage with aspartame reduced the amount of energy consumed at that meal [7]. Consequently, replacing sugar-sweetened beverages (SSBs) with diet versions may be a useful method to aid weight management. Expanding on these results, later studies have found that the effect on energy intake is not specific to beverages containing carbohydrate and consuming any energy-yielding beverage with a meal adds to the amount of energy consumed. In one study, participants reported to the laboratory on five separate occasions to consume a meal accompanied by one of five different beverages (360 mL of water, diet cola, regular cola, fruit juice, or 1 % milk). Despite the extra volume and energy provided by the beverages, there was no effect on the amount of solid food eaten, and as a result, total caloric intake (solid food plus beverage) was significantly increased when an energy-yielding beverage accompanied the meal [8]. Similar findings were provided by a later crossover study where participants consumed a beverage (water, diet cola, regular cola, 1 % milk, or orange juice) with a meal [9]. It is frequently suggested that drinking water with a meal will aid weight management by increasing satiation and reducing the amount eaten. However, it has been reported that drinking water with a meal has no effect on meal size [10]. The portion size of the beverage may also be important, and providing larger portions of energy-yielding beverages with a meal increases energy intake further [11]. These data suggest that consuming an energy-yielding beverage with a meal, regardless of the predominant macronutrient, increases overall energy intake at that meal.

Satiety

Specific Macronutrients: Carbohydrates

SSBs are the largest single source of sugar in the diet [12]. Multiple lines of evidence converge to produce a persuasive, although arguably not compelling, case that the regular consumption of SSBs leads to modest weight gain. While studies report a temporal relationship between the increase in SSB consumption and obesity [13], this association is confounded by an increase in sedentary behavior, higher overall energy intake, and a change in other eating patterns that have occurred over the same period. Moreover, there has been a reduction in the consumption of SSBs over the past decade that has not been accompanied by a fall in obesity rates although obesity rates have flattened in some segments of the population [14]. Cross-sectional studies have shown a link between consumption of SSBs and body weight [15] although reverse causality cannot be discounted (i.e., overweight/obesity individuals consume more SSBs rather than high consumption of SSB causes overweight/obesity). While several large prospective cohort studies have found a statistically significant association between consumption of SSBs and obesity, the effect size is arguably quite modest. An example is provided by a meta-analysis of three large prospective cohort studies that found that consumption of SSBs and fruit juice was associated with increased body weight [16]. However, the observed effects were rather modest with the authors estimating that replacing one serving of SSB each day with water is associated with 0.49 kg less weight gain over a 4-year period, while replacing one serving of fruit juice with water results in 0.35 kg less weight gain over the same period. A meta-analysis of randomized control trials in children and adults also reported an association between SSB and weight gain although, again, the effects size was relatively modest [17].

One potential strategy to prevent the weight gain attributed to the regular consumption of SSBs is to replace the caloric sweetener products with a noncaloric equivalent. Recently, three long-term randomized control trials have investigated the effect of replacing SSBs with diet or noncaloric beverages. In a study of overweight or obese adults, Tate et al. [18] found that replacing caloric beverages with water or diet beverages resulted in weight loss of 2–2.5 % over a 6-month period, although these results were not statistically significant. Conversely, during a 1-year intervention study, children reduced consumption of SSBs from an average of 1.7 servings a day to nearly zero which resulted in a statistically significant weight loss of 1.9 kg. Similar results were reported by de Ruyter et al. [19]. At this time, it appears that replacing SSBs with a noncaloric equivalent would result in a modest, but likely clinically significant, reduction in weight gain.

Specific Macronutrients: Protein

Studies of solid foods indicate that protein is the most satiating macronutrient. However, high-protein solid foods typically provide an amount of protein in excess of what is provided by a beverage. It has been suggested that there is a threshold level of protein that needs to be consumed before there is an effect on satiation/satiety, and it is not clear that the amount of protein in a beverage reaches this amount [20]. Still, some studies have found that proteins in beverages increase satiety although the results are not consistent.

Mourao and Mattes [21] reported that a beverage containing protein was not as satiating as its solid equivalent and did not elicit a compensatory response. However, Poppitt et al. [22] found that increasing the protein content of a beverage reduced postprandial hunger compared to water although not sufficiently to reduce food intake at a test meal eaten 2 h later. This possibly weak effect of protein in beverages on appetite was also reported by Panahi et al. [23] who found that drinking chocolate milk or infant formula reduces food intake at a meal consumed 30 min later, although when the duration between drinking the beverage and eating the test meal was increased to 2 h, there was no effect on food intake.

Some studies have shown that the type of protein provided by a beverage may cause differential effects on satiation/satiety. For instance, Hall et al. [24] found that individuals who consumed a beverage containing whey protein consumed significantly less at a buffet meal compared to people who ingested an equivalent beverage containing casein. Other studies have found that adding whey to a beverage increases postprandial satiety and reduces food intake in normal weight adults [25] or suppresses the secretion of ghrelin which is a hormone related to hunger [26].

Specific Macronutrients: Fiber

Adding fiber to beverages has been promoted as a way to increase fiber intake and also potentially improve appetite control. Studies have shown that adding certain soluble fibers to beverages can increase satiety without increasing the viscosity or taste of the beverage [27]. Similar results were provided by another study that found that drinking a beverage containing soluble fiber, caffeine, and green tea catechins suppressed appetite and reduced food intake at a subsequent meal [28].

Fiber can also be used to increase the viscosity of a beverage. Due to differences in the physical and chemical characteristics (e.g., acid stability, gelling strength, fermentation) of these fibers, it is difficult to compare beverages that use different fibers as viscosity agents as the physiological response likely differs due the multiple mechanisms through which fiber can influence appetite. Moreover, many studies do not adequately report the chemical and physical properties of the fibers and often do not characterize the viscosity of the beverage (e.g., viscosity at a variety of sheer rates). The data examining the effect of viscosity on satiation and satiety is currently inconsistent and a more systematic examination of viscous fibers on appetite is warranted.

Mattes and Rothacker [29] found that increasing the viscosity of a beverage using microcrystalline cellulose had a greater and prolonged suppression of postprandial hunger, but this had no effect on food intake over the following 24 h. Lyly et al. [30] compared the effect of beverages thickened with guar gum, wheat bran, and oat beta-glucan; they observed that the guar gum beverage reduced desire to eat compared to the control beverage, while the beta-glucan beverage increased fullness compared to the control beverage. When evaluating these findings, it must be remembered that fullness and desire to eat measure different facets of subjective appetite and are not merely opposing sensations. In a study by Juvonen et al. [31], it was found that increasing the viscosity of a beverage increased feelings of fullness immediately after consuming it. However, there was no difference in postprandial satiety, and plasma concentrations of hormones related to satiety were higher following the low-viscosity beverage. In addition, the gastric emptying rate was also slower following the low-viscosity beverage. Taken together, these studies suggest that increasing the viscosity of a beverage may increase satiety although this effect may not be sufficiently strong to significantly reduce food intake.

Beverages and Thermogenesis

Macronutrients

It has been proposed that there is hierarchical effect of macronutrients on thermogenesis with protein > CHO > fat [32, 33]. While the consumption of a high-protein diet could theoretically aid weight loss by increasing energy expenditure, this assumes that the rise in energy expenditure would not be accompanied by a compensatory rise in hunger and food intake. In addition, many of these studies have used large amounts of protein, and it may not be feasible under normal dietary intakes to elicit a substantial enough rise in DIT to influence body weight.

There is currently little data available to determine if this hierarchy holds in beverages. In one study using meal replacement beverages, it was found that a high-protein/low-carbohydrate shake elicited a greater DIT than a 100 % protein or low-protein/high-carbohydrate shake [34]. However, the difference was only 31 kcal so the contribution to daily energy expenditure is seemingly minimal. The chapter by McDonald et al. discusses this effect in elderly populations more specifically.

Catechins/Caffeine

Catechins and caffeine contained in beverages may influence energy balance through an effect on thermogenesis. All black teas contain high quantities of catechins such as epicatechin, epicatechin gallate, epigallocatechin, and epigallocatechin-3-gallate (EGCG), although processing decreases the amount of these compounds.

A meta-analysis of six studies found that supplementation with catechin-caffeine or caffeine increased 24-h energy expenditure by about 4.8 % [35]. However, there was no statistically significant effect of these compounds on fat oxidation. However, there may be an interaction between these compounds and exercise with one study finding that acute green tea extract consumption increases fat oxidation during moderate intensity exercise [36].

Potential Mechanisms through Which Beverages May Influence Satiation or Satiety

Cognition

One possibility explaining the poor satiating power of beverages is that people consume beverages to satisfy thirst rather than hunger and this psychological expectation reduces the effect on satiety. Accumulating evidence indicates that humans have expectations about how satiating a food is and this could influence satiation or satiety [37]. In a study with direct relevance to beverages, participants were provided with four different test loads [38]. They were informed that one test load was liquid and remained liquid in the stomach while another was liquid but turned solid in the stomach. It was found that when participants expected the test load to turn to solid, they felt less hungry. Consequently, the effect of beverages on appetite may be influenced by the consumer's expected satiation. That is, if they drink beverages that are expected to satiate (e.g., meal replacement beverages), these may be more satiating than beverages that are consumed primarily to quench thirst.

Oral Processing

Beverages require very little oral processing and can be consumed quickly. This may reduce the effect on satiety for several reasons. First, beverages do not require chewing and recent evidence suggests that mastication contributes to satiation and satiety [39]. Second, meals that can be rapidly ingested may lead to increased energy intake at a meal [40]. Conversely, slowing the rate of consumption of beverages by using a smaller sip size has been shown to reduce consumption of an energy-yielding beverage by ~30 % [41]. Recent developments in fluid delivery systems, such as swirling vortexes, may have an impact on consumer's perceptions of the beverage and influence the amount consumed. Further research is required to understand the effect of fluid delivery systems on energy intake.

Gastric Emptying

Studies have shown that gastric distention contributes to satiation and satiety [42]. When consuming solid foods, there is a significant lag phase between ingestion and gastric emptying while the particle size of the swallowed bolus is reduced [43]. After this lag time, the food empties from the stomach at a linear rate. By comparison, there is no lag phase for beverages and gastric emptying proceeds at a rate directly proportional to the volume in the stomach. Consequently, beverages empty from the stomach faster than solids, likely reducing the duration of gastric distention.

Gastrointestinal Transit

Any differences between the gastrointestinal transit time of beverages and solids could potentially influence satiety through an effect on the pattern of putative satiety hormone response, such as CCK or GLP-1 or ghrelin. It is not clear if liquids have a faster transit time through the small intestine with one study reporting no difference between solids or liquids [44]. Moreover, it is not clear if the transit of liquids through the colon is quicker than solids; studies have reported either a faster transit time [45] or no difference [46]. However, it is not clear if transit time through the large intestine has any appreciable effect on appetite.

Hormonal Response

Several hormones have been linked to feelings of satiation or satiety [47] although their usefulness as a marker of the satiating capacity of foods has been questioned [48]. Beverages may impact the hormonal response in several ways. First, studies have shown a cephalic phase response for several hormones related to satiation and satiety such as CCK and ghrelin [49]. It is pertinent to note that beverages may elicit a small or nonexistent cephalic phase response compared to solid foods [50]. Second, beverages may elicit a different pattern of hormonal response to solid foods due to differences in gastrointestinal transit or nutrient availability. Studies investigating the effect of beverages on the hormonal response are limited in number but suggest the endocrine response is lower following beverages compared to solid food equivalents [51, 52].

Conclusion

Based on the totality of the data, it seems reasonable to conclude that beverages are less satiating than their solid equivalents. However, suggestions based on data from short-term studies (<24 h) that beverages do not elicit any compensatory response appear erroneous as longer-term studies (>4 weeks) suggest that substantial compensation occurs [53]. Currently available data indicate that drinking an energy-yielding beverage with a meal merely increases energy intake and does not elicit a compensatory reduction in the amount of solid food eaten. This effect holds regardless of the macronutrient content of the beverage. However, the macronutrient content of a beverage may influence feelings of satiety. Beverages containing bioactive compounds, such as caffeine or catechins, have the potential to influence energy balance by increasing energy expenditure although the effect may be modest. Due to the increased consumption of beverages, further research is required to fully understand their contribution to the obesity epidemic. In particular, research is required to determine the effect of beverages that differ in their physical or chemical characteristics on energy balance.

References

1. Begg DP, Woods SC. The endocrinology of food intake. Nat Rev Endocrinol. 2013;9(10):584–97.
2. LeBlanc J, Labrie A. A possible role for palatability of the food in diet-induced thermogenesis. Int J Obes (Lond). 1997;21(12):1100–3.
3. Kratz M, Baars T, Guyenet S. The relationship between high-fat dairy consumption and obesity, cardiovascular, and metabolic disease. Eur J Nutr. 2013;52(1):1–24.
4. Stubbs RJ, et al. Breakfasts high in protein, fat or carbohydrate: effect on within-day appetite and energy balance. Eur J Clin Nutr. 1996;50(7):409–17.
5. Raben A, et al. Meals with similar energy densities but rich in protein, fat, carbohydrate, or alcohol have different effects on energy expenditure and substrate metabolism but not on appetite and energy intake. Am J Clin Nutr. 2003;77(1):91–100.
6. Clark MJ, Slavin JL. The effect of fiber on satiety and food intake: a systematic review. J Am Coll Nutr. 2013;32(3):200–11.
7. Rolls BJ, Kim S, Fedoroff IC. Effects of drinks sweetened with sucrose or aspartame on hunger, thirst and food-intake in men. Physiol Behav. 1990;48(1):19–26.
8. DellaValle DM, Roe LS, Rolls BJ. Does the consumption of caloric and non-caloric beverages with a meal affect energy intake? Appetite. 2005;44(2):187–93.
9. Panahi S, et al. Caloric beverages consumed freely at meal-time add calories to an ad libitum meal. Appetite. 2013;65:75–82.
10. Rolls BJ, Bell EA, Thorwart ML. Water incorporated into a food but not served with a food decreases energy intake in lean women. Am J Clin Nutr. 1999;70(4):448–55.
11. Flood JE, Roe LS, Rolls BJ. The effect of increased beverage portion size on energy intake at a meal. J Am Diet Assoc. 2006;106(12):1984–90.
12. Nielson SJ, Popkin BM. Changes in beverage intake between 1977 and 2001. Am J Prev Med. 2005;28(4):413 (2004; 27:205).
13. Elliott SS, et al. Fructose, weight gain, and the insulin resistance syndrome. Am J Clin Nutr. 2002;76(5):911–22.

14. Welsh JA, et al. Consumption of added sugars is decreasing in the United States. Am J Clin Nutr. 2011;94(3):726–34.
15. Malik VS, Schulze MB, Hu FB. Intake of sugar-sweetened beverages and weight gain: a systematic review. Am J Clin Nutr. 2006;84(2):274–88.
16. Pan A, et al. Changes in water and beverage intake and long-term weight changes: results from three prospective cohort studies. Int J Obes (Lond). 2013;37(10):1378–85.
17. Malik VS, et al. Sugar-sweetened beverages and weight gain in children and adults: a systematic review and meta-analysis. Am J Clin Nutr. 2013;98(4):1084–102.
18. Tate DF, et al. Replacing caloric beverages with water or diet beverages for weight loss in adults: main results of the Choose Healthy Options Consciously Everyday (CHOICE) randomized clinical trial. Am J Clin Nutr. 2012;95(3):555–63.
19. de Ruyter JC, et al. A trial of sugar-free or sugar-sweetened beverages and body weight in children. N Engl J Med. 2012;367(15):1397–406.
20. Ortinau LC, et al. The effects of increased dietary protein yogurt snack in the afternoon on appetite control and eating initiation in healthy women. Nutr J. 2013;12:71.
21. Mourao DM, et al. Effects of food form on appetite and energy intake in lean and obese young adults. Int J Obes (Lond). 2007;31(11):1688–95.
22. Poppitt SD, et al. Low-dose whey protein-enriched water beverages alter satiety in a study of overweight women. Appetite. 2011;56(2):456–64.
23. Panahi S, et al. Energy and macronutrient content of familiar beverages interact with pre-meal intervals to determine later food intake, appetite and glycemic response in young adults. Appetite. 2013;60:154–61.
24. Hall WL, et al. Casein and whey exert different effects on plasma amino acid profiles, gastrointestinal hormone secretion and appetite. Br J Nutr. 2003;89(2):239–48.
25. Zafar TA, et al. Whey protein sweetened beverages reduce glycemic and appetite responses and food intake in young females. Nutr Res. 2013;33(4):303–10.
26. Bowen J, Noakes M, Clifton PM. Appetite hormones and energy intake in obese men after consumption of fructose, glucose and whey protein beverages. Int J Obes (Lond). 2007;31(11):1696–703.
27. Monsivais P, et al. Soluble fiber dextrin enhances the satiating power of beverages. Appetite. 2011;56(1):9–14.
28. Carter BE, Drewnowski A. Beverages containing soluble fiber, caffeine, and green tea catechins suppress hunger and lead to less energy consumption at the next meal. Appetite. 2012;59(3):755–61.
29. Mattes RD, Rothacker D. Beverage viscosity is inversely related to postprandial hunger in humans. Physiol Behav. 2001;74(4–5):551–7.
30. Lyly M, et al. Fibre in beverages can enhance perceived satiety. Eur J Nutr. 2009;48(4):251–8.
31. Juvonen KR, et al. Viscosity of oat bran-enriched beverages influences gastrointestinal hormonal responses in healthy humans. J Nutr. 2009;139(3):461–6.
32. Westerterp-Plantenga MS, et al. Satiety related to 24 h diet-induced thermogenesis during high protein carbohydrate vs high fat diets measured in a respiration chamber. Eur J Clin Nutr. 1999;53(6):495–502.
33. Westerterp KR. Diet induced thermogenesis. Nutr Metab. 2004;1:5.
34. Scott CB, Devore R. Diet-induced thermogenesis: variations among three isocaloric meal-replacement shakes. Nutrition. 2005;21(7–8):874–7.
35. Hursel R, et al. The effects of catechin rich teas and caffeine on energy expenditure and fat oxidation: a meta-analysis. Obes Rev. 2011;12(7):E573–81.
36. Venables MC, et al. Green tea extract ingestion, fat oxidation, and glucose tolerance in healthy humans. Am J Clin Nutr. 2008;87(3):778–84.
37. Brunstrom JM, Shakeshaft NG, Scott-Samuel NE. Measuring 'expected satiety' in a range of common foods using a method of constant stimuli. Appetite. 2008;51(3):604–14.
38. Cassady BA, Considine RV, Mattes RD. Beverage consumption, appetite, and energy intake: what did you expect? Am J Clin Nutr. 2012;95(3):587–93.

39. Zhu Y, Hsu WH, Hollis JH. Increasing the number of masticatory cycles is associated with reduced appetite and altered postprandial plasma concentrations of gut hormones, insulin and glucose. Br J Nutr. 2013;110(2):384–90.
40. Viskaal-Van Dongen M, Kok FJ, de Graaf C. Eating rate of commonly consumed foods promotes food and energy intake. Appetite. 2011;56(1):25–31.
41. Weijzen PLG, Smeets PAM, de Graaf C. Sip size of orangeade: effects on intake and sensory-specific satiation. Br J Nutr. 2009;102(7):1091–7.
42. Wang GJ, et al. Gastric distention activates satiety circuitry in the human brain. Neuroimage. 2008;39(4):1824–31.
43. Camilleri M, et al. Relation between antral motility and gastric-emptying of solids and liquids in humans. Am J Physiol. 1985;249(5):G580–5.
44. Bennink R, et al. Evaluation of small-bowel transit for solid and liquid test meal in healthy men and women. Eur J Nucl Med. 1999;26(12):1560–6.
45. Kaufman PN, et al. Effects of liquid versus solid diet on colonic transit in humans – evaluation by standard colonic transit scintigraphy. Gastroenterology. 1990;98(1):73–81.
46. Proano M, et al. Unprepared human colon does not discriminate between solids and liquids. Am J Physiol. 1991;260(1):G13–6.
47. Suzuki K, Jayasena CN, Bloom SR. The gut hormones in appetite regulation. J Obes. 2011;2011, 528401.
48. Mars M, Stafleu A, de Graaf C. Use of satiety peptides in assessing the satiating capacity of foods. Physiol Behav. 2012;105(2):483–8.
49. Smeets PAM, Erkner A, de Graaf C. Cephalic phase responses and appetite. Nutr Rev. 2010;68(11):643–55.
50. Teff KL. Cephalic phase pancreatic polypeptide responses to liquid and solid stimuli in humans. Physiol Behav. 2010;99(3):317–23.
51. Apolzan JW, et al. Effects of food form on food intake and postprandial appetite sensations, glucose and endocrine responses, and energy expenditure in resistance trained v. sedentary older adults. Br J Nutr. 2011;106(7):1107–16.
52. Tieken SM, et al. Effects of solid versus liquid meal-replacement products of similar energy content on hunger, satiety, and appetite-regulating hormones in older adults. Horm Metab Res. 2007;39(5):389–94.
53. Reid M, et al. Effects on obese women of the sugar sucrose added to the diet over 28 d: a quasi-randomised, single-blind, controlled trial. Br J Nutr. 2014;111(3):563–70.

Chapter 13
Beverage Considerations for Persons with Metabolic Syndrome and Diabetes Mellitus

Margaret A. Maher and Lisa Kobs

Keywords Metabolic syndrome • Diabetes • Hyperglycemia • Hypertension • Dyslipidemia • Obesity

Key Points

1. Beverages may provide a rich source of easily consumed nutrients that may reduce metabolic risk factors that contribute to cardiovascular disease when consumed within caloric limits.
2. Protein, vitamins, minerals, and phytochemicals in beverages provide healthful benefits.
3. Easily consumed beverages may also be a source of excess calories with little nutrient value.
4. Beverage intake should be carefully considered when diet planning to reduce metabolic syndrome risk factors and effectively manage diabetes when present.
5. Beverages low in fat and high in protein, while rich in micronutrients and/or phytochemicals, are recommended for calorie control and hunger and thirst satiety.
6. Milks, phytochemical-rich fruit juices, and formulated supplements, along with water, may all be part of a healthy risk-lowering dietary plan.

M.A. Maher, Ph.D., R.D. (✉) • L. Kobs, M.S., R.D.
Biology and Nutrition, University of Wisconsin – La Crosse,
1725 State Street, La Crosse, WI 54601, USA
e-mail: mmaher@uwlax.edu; lkobs@uwlax.edu

© Springer International Publishing Switzerland 2016
T. Wilson, N.J. Temple (eds.), *Beverage Impacts on Health and Nutrition*,
Nutrition and Health, DOI 10.1007/978-3-319-23672-8_13

Introduction: Metabolic Syndrome and Diabetes Mellitus

Diabetes mellitus (DM), whether type 1, type 2, or gestational diabetes, is a condition associated with significant metabolic dysfunction critically impacted by dietary intake. Macronutrient intake is a key concern in successfully managing DM and reducing the likelihood of acute and chronic complications of the disease. Carbohydrate quantity, composition, distribution through the day, and coordination with medication and/or exercise therapies are especially important. Beverages may enable quick overconsumption of concentrated macronutrients. This chapter will address the best use of different beverages for managing diabetes and the symptoms that are related to the metabolic syndrome (MetS).

MetS, often a precursor to diabetes, represents a cluster of four risk factors that occur in combination and pose an increased risk of cardiovascular disease (CVD). The unifying feature of this syndrome is underlying resistance to the actions of the hormone insulin and its interaction with the diet, hence the tendency of persons with MetS to develop type 2 diabetes. Once MetS and/or CVD is present, morbidity and mortality are greatly increased. Conventions for assigning MetS diagnoses vary by organization, but the presence of three of the four accepted risk factors shown in Table 13.1 is a generally acceptable criterion for diagnosis [1].

Obesity has become increasingly prevalent in the United States across genders and ages over the last 30 years [2]. It is associated with genetics but is ultimately a product of dietary caloric overconsumption. It is a key risk factor for MetS. Diet is one modifiable risk parameter that profoundly affects MetS risk factors. Caloric intake and specific food and beverage components affect multiple risk factors of MetS.

Beverages can represent a source of carbohydrates and caloric intake. Other beverage ingredients can also have negative or positive impacts on diabetes and MetS, including sweeteners, dairy components, artificial sweeteners, and alcohol. This chapter describes key considerations of beverage consumption in relation to DM, MetS risk factors, and related clinical outcomes.

Table 13.1 Consensus risk factors and diagnostic cut points for the metabolic syndrome [1]

Risk factor	Cut point
High blood pressure	≥130/85 mmHg (17.3/11.3 kPa) or treatment
Dyslipidemia	≤50 mg/dL (1.29 mmol/L) HDL cholesterol; ≥150 mg/dL (1.69 mmol/L) triglyceride or treatment
Insulin resistance/glucose intolerance	≥100 mg/dL (5.55 mmol/L) fasting glucose or treatment
Central obesity	≥88 cm (0.88 m)

Sweetened Beverages

Few nutrients have been more controversial than sugar, particularly when consumed in beverages, such as soft drinks. In a recent comprehensive meta-analysis, Kelishadi et al. [3] found that consumption of fructose from "industrialized foods" was directly correlated with prime MetS risk factors, namely, elevated blood pressure, raised blood levels of triglyceride and glucose, and a low blood level of HDL cholesterol. Fructose has associations with MetS, obesity, and DM, as well as appetite-regulating effects that favor excess caloric intake [4].

Fructose is present in natural fruit products, in sucrose, and in high-fructose corn syrup. Though excess calories from any source may contribute to obesity and sweetened beverages are easy to consume in excess, there is no consistent difference in the obesogenic potential of different caloric sweetening agents, namely, sucrose and high-fructose corn syrup, in caloric density, sweetness, digestion or absorption, or satiety [5]. This is discussed at greater length in the chapter by White and Nicklas. Despite accepted differences in the way that fructose and glucose are metabolized by the liver, Rippe et al. [5] contend that experiments comparing pure fructose and glucose feeding are not applicable to the human diet since these simple sugars do not appear in pure form in foods or beverages.

The association between sweetened beverages and disease risk has been more extensively studied. Risks of consuming these beverages include an increased risk of obesity [6, 7], type 2 DM [7–9], hypertension, and MetS [7]. It is unclear whether sweetened beverages play a direct role in increased risk or whether these beverages are one component of multiple contributors to increased disease risk.

Diet/Artificially Sweetened Beverage Effects on Risk Factors

Artificially sweetened beverages (ASBs), sometimes described as diet drinks, are an alternative to sugar-sweetened beverages such as sweetened juices, sodas, teas, and energy drinks. They consist of beverages with little or no calorie content and often have little nutritional benefit. The artificial sweeteners used in ASBs are often the same sweeteners used in solid foods. They are used as a substitute to table sugar (sucrose) or high-fructose corn syrup. The US Food and Drug Administration (FDA) has approved eight different artificial sweeteners for human consumption including acesulfame potassium, aspartame, luo han guo extract, neotame, saccharin, stevia, and sucralose. Although the use of artificial sweeteners has been a source of controversy, the FDA has deemed them safe based on animal and human studies [10]. Advantame is the newest sweetener to be deemed safe by the FDA. It has been approved as a general-purpose sweetener for use in a variety of products including nonalcoholic beverages [11].

The consumption of ASB in the USA is less compared to sugar-sweetened beverages, but has increased slightly in the last few decades due to successful marketing campaigns claiming that ASBs are a healthier choice because of their limited calorie content [12]. It is difficult to determine the consumption rates of artificial sweeteners because they are often present in foods in combination with each other or with other nutritive sweeteners. It is estimated that the use of ASB has increased by only 15 % since 1965 [10]. There are demographic differences in consumption of ASB between different groups; for example, adolescents girls consume more than boys [8].

The epidemiological research that has been conducted examining ASBs and disease risk is inconclusive. When investigating ASB and weight gain, it is difficult to determine causation because of the many confounding factors that contribute to observed associations. There may be a protective effect of consuming ASB because they may replace higher-calorie beverages therefore preventing weight gain. The relationships between ASB and type 2 DM and cardiovascular risk factors remain just as unclear, with the possibility of reverse causality (individuals already at high risk of obesity choosing to consume ASB in an attempt to control their weight) contributing to any positive associations [8]. Some observational studies have indicated associations between ASB and central obesity and high blood glucose levels. There have been limited associations between ASB and hypertension, hypertriglyceridemia, or low HDL cholesterol levels. This suggests associations between risk of obesity and type 2 DM, but not for all components of MetS [8, 13].

In randomized trials, the replacement of sugar-sweetened beverages with ASB brings about reduced energy intake and helps prevent weight gain. Many intervention studies have examined artificial sweeteners and metabolic parameters using subjects who have type 2 DM. The interventions often involved administration of the artificial sweetener in pill form. This does not allow for the effect of real-world variables of artificial sweeteners, much less ASB [8].

Another important factor to consider in evaluating the use of ASB in relation to disease risk is their effect on appetite, a topic more fully described in the chapter by Hollis. This is another area where current research can be contradictory. Early research indicated that consumption of artificial sweeteners increases appetite. However, more recent research indicates that consumption of foods containing artificial sweeteners causes no increase in appetite compared with foods containing no artificial sweeteners. This is supported by research conducted using artificial sweetener administration using a nasogastric tube or capsule, which eliminates any oral sensory stimulation influence [12].

Another key question related to artificial sweeteners and increases in appetite is whether additional calories are consumed when consuming artificial sweeteners. Human studies have shown limited results, with some indications that overall calorie intake decreases after multiday periods of consuming artificial sweeteners, whereas overall energy intake increases when consuming sugar-sweetened products [12]. Rodent studies demonstrate more consistent results that consumption of ASB is associated with increased overall calorie consumption and increases in adiposity. If consistent results are similarly found in human studies, these factors could result in increased risk of developing MetS and type 2 DM [14]. However, research conducted in vivo in humans has not shown alterations in appetite or changes in calorie intake with ASB. Glucose levels, insulin levels, and blood pressure have also not been shown to be impacted by artificial sweeteners using in vivo human studies [15].

Several organizations have released scientific statements regarding the consumption of ASB. The Academy of Nutrition and Dietetics recommends that "consumers can safely enjoy a range of nutritive and nonnutritive sweeteners when consumed within an eating plan that is guided by current federal nutrition recommendations, such as the Dietary Guidelines for Americans and the Dietary Reference Intakes, as well as individual health goals and personal preference" [10]. The American Heart Association along with the American Diabetes Association jointly released the recommendations that ASB "when used judiciously, [nonnutritive sweeteners] could facilitate reductions in added sugars intake, thereby resulting in decreased total energy and weight loss/weight control, and promoting beneficial effects on related metabolic parameters. However, these potential benefits will not be fully realized if there is a compensatory increase in energy intake from other sources" [16]. These statements highlight that ASB cannot be addressed in isolation but should be considered along with other dietary factors and that their use should be promoted with caution for persons with DM or MetS.

Fruit and Vegetable Juices

The key nutrient compositions of different fruits and juices are shown in Table 13.2. Fruit and vegetable juices have significant essential nutrient and phytochemical content. They are also known to be concentrated sources of carbohydrates and calories, and consumers may reduce their intake of these healthy diet items in order to prevent weight gain. The fiber content in a standard serving of whole fruit is significantly higher compared to juices; this is also generally true for the antioxidant content [20, 21]. In summary, fruit juices consumed in moderation and with consideration to calorie control as it relates to obesity risk contribute to a healthy metabolic risk-reducing dietary plan.

The USDA fruit and fruit juice per serving equivalency is 1 cup and ½ cup, respectively [21]. One cup is approximately 8 oz or 250 mL.

Vegetable juices have not been studied as extensively as fruit juices but have been shown to be helpful for increasing vegetable intake and promoting weight loss when coupled with a low-calorie diet [22]. Juicing has been touted as a practice to improve health and reduce risk of multiple conditions. However, there are multiple issues associated with home juicing, which should be considered. For example, individuals with kidney disease, such as those with diabetic nephropathy, should be advised to limit fruit and vegetable juices which may be very rich in oxalates to reduce the risk of oxalate toxicity and acute renal failure [23].

Table 13.2 Key nutrient composition of fruits and juices and related comments

Fruit juice	Energy in 1 cup fruit (kcal)	Energy in 1/2 cup unsweetened juice (kcal)	Fiber in 1 cup fruit (g)	Fiber in 1/2 cup unsweetened juice (g)	Key micronutrients and phytonutrients, comments
Apple	57	57	2.6	0.25	There is 47–60 times total polyphenols in fruit versus juice [17]
Orange	81	56	3.6	0.25	The vitamin C content is comparable and vitamin D-fortified juice products are available [18]
Grapefruit	69	48	2.5	0.1	The consumption of grapefruit juice is contraindicated with numerous medications due to gastrointestinal cytochrome P450 competition
Grape	104	76	1.4	0.25	Concord grape juice is third to pomegranate juice and red wine in antioxidant activity [19]
Cranberry	51	58	5.1	0.12	The fruit and juice are rich in polyphenols and vitamin C, but requires sweetening agents to improve palatability
Pineapple	82	66	2.3	0.25	The commercial juice antioxidant activity shown to be higher than fruit [20]
Pomegranate	144	67	7.0	0.10	The juice has superior antioxidant activity compared to other juices and wine [19]

Dairy and Dairy Substitute Beverages

Milk is a rich, potentially low-fat, source of high biological value protein and many micronutrients, such as calcium, phosphorus, and vitamins A, B_1 (thiamin), B_2 (riboflavin), and B_{12} [21]. A more complete review of the nutritional health effect of cow's milk consumption is presented in the chapter by Armas, Frye, and Heaney. Milk is used as the starting material for numerous beverage products that vary in their concentrations of macro- and micronutrients, based on processing methods and/or fortification (such as addition of vitamin D and addition of vitamin A lost in

Table 13.3 Components of natural and artificial milks (approximate amount per 1 fluid oz) [21]

"Milk" type	Energy (kcal)	Protein (g)	Carb (g)	Lipid (g) (SFA-MUFA-PUFA)	Micronutrients: calcium (mg); vitamin D (IU)
Human	22	0.32	2.12	1.35 (0.62-0.51-0.15)	10; 1
Formula 1	19	0.42	2.20	1.07 (0.45-0.41-0.20)	16; 12
Formula 2	20	0.41	2.10	1.08 (0.38-0.40-0.24)	16; 12
Cow whole	19	0.96	1.46	0.99 (0.57-0.25-0.06)	34; 16
Cow skim	11	1.09	1.54	0.08	15; 16
Goat	21	1.09	1.36	1.26 (0.81-0.34-0.05)	41; 16
Soy	14	0.49	1.62	0.69 (0.08-0.15-0.36)	25; 13
Almond	11	0.13	2.00	0.31 (0-0.19-0.06)	56; 13

Data from http://ndb.nal.usda.gov/ndb/foods [21]

processing). Pasteurization destroys most bacteria in milk, but probiotic strains of bacteria are used to ferment milk to produce different beverages and foods. The active cultures consumed therein and their effects on the gut microbiome are a hot area of research. Studies of the effects of gut microbiome status and manipulation on MetS risk factors, especially obesity and insulin resistance, are underway and suggest benefits of certain pre- and probiotics that may be found in beverages and may have health benefits for persons with obesity or MetS [24].

For infants, breast milk is a comprehensive food that meets most nutrient needs [25], though it is low in vitamin D relative to other fortified milks and substitute milks. Breastfed infants have lower growth velocity and leanness compared to formula-fed infants. Hormonal and behavioral factors related to breastfeeding, as well as the nutrient composition and nutrient density of breast milk, have been explored as causative factors for reduced risk of development of obesity, DM, and MetS later in life.

Vegetable beverages, including soy, rice, and nut "milks," are generally inadequate for infants and toddlers, and their exclusive use can lead to severe deficiencies [26]. Table 13.3 details comparisons of different milks in relation to macro- and micronutrient content. Breast milk, which may protect against obesity later in life, is covered in the chapter by Freil and Qasem, while milks made from soy and other plant foods are discussed in the chapter by Woodside.

Vitamin D status has been linked to MetS and DM in recent epidemiological, prospective, and meta-analysis studies [27–30], suggesting an inverse relationship between blood vitamin D indicators and risk of MetS. The major source of vitamin D in the American diet is fortified dairy products and dairy substitutes. Other beverages, including soymilk and orange juice, may also be fortified with vitamin D [21]. This can be advantageous for those who chose not to drink milk, including vegetarians, vegans, and those with lactose intolerance.

Calcium consumption appears to have no effect on type 2 DM specifically [29–31]. However, the consumption of milk and a high dietary intake of calcium appear to have a protective effect against the development of MetS [32, 33]. Diets relatively rich in calcium exert a neutral effect or possibly a lowering action on total cholesterol and LDL cholesterol while having no impact on HDL cholesterol [34]. It is unclear whether it is actually the calcium in dairy foods that has a protective effect against chronic disease or whether the credit belongs to other healthy dietary habits that are associated with dietary calcium [32].

Diets with a generous content of potassium have been associated with many health benefits including with reduced risk of MetS as well as some specific components of MetS such as abdominal obesity and fasting hyperglycemia. This association remains even after adjusting for diet and lifestyle factors [35]. Specifically, low-fat and high-potassium dairy sources, such as milk, have been shown to have a beneficial effect on blood pressure [34, 36] and to have protective effects against insulin resistance and coronary heart disease [37].

Phosphorus in the American diet comes mainly from milk and milk products and other high-protein foods. Kalaitzidis et al. [38] and Park et al. [39] found that individuals with MetS had lower phosphate (and magnesium) levels than healthy controls, and the lower phosphate levels were attributable to lower dietary phosphate consumption. A cross-sectional study was carried out where intake of cheese was studied in combination with consumption of soft drinks (both diet and regular) and their relationship with MetS [40]. An observational study examining total phosphorus consumption in American diets (not just from beverage consumption) found that a high intake of phosphorus (approximately double the US RDA) is associated with increased mortality in healthy adults [41]. These mixed results related to phosphate levels and consumption suggest that adequate, but moderate, phosphate intake from beverages and food is advisable. Diabetics with established kidney disease may have to significantly limit intake of phosphate, sodium, and potassium (from beverages and food) to prevent abnormally high blood levels of the minerals.

In summary, the beneficial impacts of consuming dairy beverages and foods may not be due to any one particular ingredient but from a synergistic combination of all of these components that have been shown to have benefits in terms of disease risk [34, 36]. The health-promoting benefits of these foods were summarized in the 2010 Dietary Guidelines for Americans is the statement: "Moderate evidence also indicates that intake of milk and milk products is associated with a reduced risk of cardiovascular disease and type 2 DM and with lower blood pressure in adults."

Alcohol-Containing Beverages

The relationship between alcohol intake and nutritional health is discussed in the chapter by Temple. Effects of the nonalcoholic components of wine on cardiovascular disease are discussed in the chapter by O'Connor, Halpern, and Walzem. The nonalcoholic content of alcoholic beverages is summarized in Table 13.4. These substances require special attention in terms of their effects on DM and MetS. Clinicians need to remind persons with DM and MetS to remain cautious in this regard.

Table 13.4 Key micronutrient and phytochemical compositions and risk-related comments of different alcohol-containing beverages in usual drink sizes [21]

Alcoholic beverage	Energy (kcal)	Carb/ sugar (g)	Alcohol content (g)	Key micronutrients and phytochemical risk-related comments
Beer (1 12 oz can; 340 g)	153	12.6/0	13.9	Beers contain B vitamins, Ca, and K. Darker, less-filtered, beers contain more flavonoids, but also more calories, and are associated with more accident risk
Wine, white (5 oz; 142 g)	121	3.8/1.4	15.1	White wines contain Ca, K, and variations in phytochemicals. Sweeter versus drier wines contain more sugars and calories. Wine consumption is associated with healthier diets
Wine, red (5 oz; 142 g)	125	3.8/0.9	15.6	Red wines contain calcium, potassium, and niacin. Sweeter versus drier wines contain more sugars and calories. Red wines contain more flavonoids than white wine or beer and specifically contain resveratrol
Distilled spirits (1.5 oz [42 g] of 80 proof)	97–110	0/0	14–16	Distilled spirits contain few micronutrients and phytochemicals. Mixers can add many calories with few nutrients, unless 100 % fruit juice or ASB are used as mixers

Carbonated Beverages and Sodium

Carbonated beverages contain carbon dioxide dissolved under pressure. The term soda is derived from the practice of adding sodium to carbonated beverages as a flavor enhancer and for regulation of acidity. Sodium consumption in individuals who are salt sensitive is known to influence blood pressure, a MetS risk factor. High sodium consumption has also been associated with elevated plasma glucose concentrations and increased central adiposity, both increasing the risk of MetS. These results are from total sodium consumption, including food and beverages [42]. Dietary sodium intake stimulates thirst. This may result in a positive energy balance and overweight in those that consume sugar-sweetened beverages [43]. In comparison, the consumption of a sodium-rich bicarbonated mineral water improved metabolic markers such as lowered total cholesterol and LDL cholesterol, increased HDL cholesterol, and lowered serum glucose, without significant changes in blood pressure in postmenopausal women [44].

Functional Beverage Phytochemicals

The term "functional beverage" does not have a universal definition but often refers to beverages that have a high nutrient content. They may also contain other healthful substances, namely, phytonutrients, some of which act as antioxidants. Some vitamins, such as C and E, also act as antioxidants.

Polyphenols are a class of phytonutrient that are often claimed to have a beneficial health impact. The bioavailability of polyphenols has been found to be lacking due to their metabolism in the digestive tract and liver. Polyphenols may therefore have the most benefit in the upper digestive tract before being metabolized. Beverages that are high in total phenolics, not surprisingly, had higher antioxidant activity [45]. Green tea is one beverage that is rich in polyphenols, but coffee is also high in antioxidants. These beverages are looked at in more detail in the chapter by Suzuki and colleagues that discusses tea and in the chapter by Cavalli and Tavani that discusses coffee.

Manufacturer claims about antioxidant content are not consistent. Juices claiming to be high in antioxidants may have similar values to juices making no such claim [45]. In addition the manufacturing location of different juices can impact polyphenol content, as seen in blackcurrant juice products produced in Europe: higher levels of total polyphenols are found in blackcurrant juices from Germany and Poland than from Finland or the UK [46].

Commercial Beverage Preparations

Home and commercial processing and preparation can alter the nutrient and overall composition of foods and beverages and thereby alter some of their harmful or beneficial effects that impact MetS or DM. This is often due to exposure to heat during processing. Another consideration is storage time and conditions. For instance, lycopene, a carotenoid, is found in tomato juice. The rate of loss when stored for up to 12 months is variable, from below 20 % to as much as 75 % loss. This variability of loss is due to differences in temperature and storage container [47]. Phenolic qualities of a beverage appear to be related to DM and MetS risk, and the quality of these compounds may be degraded during processing.

Commercial fruit juices generally undergo multiple processing steps depending on the variety of juice. These steps include harvesting the fruit, cleaning, squeezing, centrifuging, pasteurization, freezing, and concentrating. In orange juice processing, it has been found that commercial squeezing (industrial squeezing), compared to domestic squeezing (hand squeezing), results in higher phenolic and vitamin C content. Depending on the squeezing method, phenolic absorption in the small intestine and phenolics available for absorption after fermentation using the gut flora may vary. Variations in the pasteurization method used and temperature did not affect phenolic content in orange juice. However, freezing did result in a dramatic decrease in phenolic content, which could have been due to the freezing and thawing processes. The phenolic content of different juices may therefore be highly variable depending on the processing methods used [48].

Conclusion

In summary, nutrient-dense commercial or home-pressed fruit and vegetable juices may provide dietary benefits to persons with metabolic syndrome and diabetes, due to their vitamins, minerals, and phytochemicals, but only when consumed within caloric limits and with careful attention to glycemic control. These juices should not be used to completely replace whole fruits and vegetables, which provide additional benefits, such as more dietary fiber. The benefit of artificially sweetened beverages is mainly for caloric and glycemic control, since many ASBs are not nutrient dense and are used to replace sugar-sweetened beverages like tea and soda. Sugar-sweetened beverages generally contain a high number of calories considering the micronutrients and nutrients provided. When these are regularly consumed or consumed in excess, caloric limits may be easily exceeded and weight gain may occur, adding to cardiometabolic risk. Protein-containing beverages, like milk and supplements, may provide a nutrient-dense source of calories and high biological value protein and contribute to satiety and preservation of lean body mass when weight reduction is underway. Finally, naturally noncaloric beverages, like tea and coffee, can provide needed fluids, sensory satisfaction, and phytochemicals that can complement a cardiometabolic risk-reducing diet, as long as condiments, such as sugar and cream, are added within caloric limits. Addition of spices, such as cinnamon, to these and other beverages may add sensory satisfaction and phytochemicals while not adding calories.

References

1. Alberti KG, Eckel RH, Grundy SM, et al. Harmonizing the metabolic syndrome: a joint interim statement of the International Diabetes Federation Task Force on Epidemiology and Prevention; National Heart, Lung, and Blood Institute; American Heart Association; World Heart Federation; International Atherosclerosis Society; and International Association for the Study of Obesity. Circulation. 2009;120:1640–5.
2. Ogden CL, Carroll MD, Kit BK, Flegal KM. Prevalence of childhood and adult obesity in the United States, 2011–2012. JAMA. 2014;311:806–14.
3. Kelishadi R, Mansourian M, Heidari-Beni M. Association of fructose consumption and components of metabolic syndrome in human studies: a systematic review and meta-analysis. Nutrition. 2014;30:503–10.
4. Johnson RJ, Nakagawa T, Sanchez-Lozada LG, et al. Sugar, uric acid, and the etiology of diabetes and obesity. Diabetes. 2013;62:3307–15.
5. Rippe JM, Angelopoulos TJ. Sucrose, high-fructose corn syrup, and fructose, their metabolism and potential health effects: what do we really know? Adv Nutr. 2013;4:236–45.
6. Malik VS, Schulze MB, Hu FB. Intake of sugar-sweetened beverages and weight gain: a systematic review. Am J Clin Nutr. 2006;84:274–88.
7. Fahgerazzi G, Vilier A, Sartotelli DS, Lajous M, Balkau B, Clavel-Chapelon F. Consumption of artificially and sugar-sweetened beverages and incident type 2 diabetes in the Etude Epide' miologique aupre' s des femmes de la Mutuelle Ge' ne' rale de l'Education Nationale–

European Prospective Investigation into Cancer and Nutrition cohort. Am J Clin Nutr. 2013;97:517–23.

8. Pereira MA. Diet beverages and the risk of obesity, diabetes, and cardiovascular disease: a review of the evidence. Nutr Rev. 2013;71:433–40.

9. Raben A, Richelsen B. Artificial sweeteners: a place in the field of functional foods? Focus on obesity and related metabolic disorders. Curr Opin Clin Nutr Metab Care. 2012;15:597–604.

10. Academy of Nutrition and Dietetics. Position of the Academy of Nutrition and Dietetics: use of nutritive and nonnutritive sweeteners. J Acad Nutr Diet. 2012;112:739–58.

11. Food and Drug Administration. Additional information about high-intensity sweeteners permitted for use in food in the United States. 2014. Retrieved from http://www.fda.gov/food/ingredientspackaginglabeling/foodadditivesingredients/ucm397725.htm#Advantame.

12. Mattes RD, Popkin BM. Nonnutritive sweetener consumption in humans: effects on appetite and food intake and their putative mechanisms. Am J Clin Nutr. 2009;89:1–14.

13. Nettleton JA, Lutsey PL, Wang Y, et al. Diet soda intake and risk of incident metabolic syndrome and type 2 diabetes in the Multi-Ethnic Study of Atherosclerosis (MESA). Diabetes Care. 2009;32:688–94.

14. Nelson G, Hoon MA, Chandrashekar J, Zhang Y, Ryba NJ, Zuker CS. Mammalian sweet taste receptors. Cell. 2001;106:381–90.

15. Renwick AG, Molinary SV. Sweet-taste receptors, low-energy sweeteners, glucose absorption and insulin release. Br J Nutr. 2010;104:1415–20.

16. Gardner C, Wylie-Rosett J, Gidding SS, Steffen LM, Johnson RK, Reader D, Lichtenstein AH. Nonnutritive sweeteners: current use and health perspectives. Circulation. 2012;126:509–19.

17. Hyson DA. A comprehensive review of apples and apple components and their relationship to human health. Adv Nutr. 2011;2:408–20.

18. Tangpricha V, Koutkia P, Rieke SM, Chen TC, Perez AA, Holick MF. Fortification of orange juice with vitamin D: a novel approach for enhancing vitamin D nutritional health. Am J Clin Nutr. 2003;77:1478–83.

19. Seeram NP, Aviram M, Zhang Y, Henning SM, Feng L, Dreher M, Heber D. Comparison of antioxidant potency of commonly consumed polyphenol-rich beverages in the United States. J Agric Food Chem. 2008;56:1415–22.

20. Crowe KM, Murray E. Deconstructing a fruit serving: comparing the antioxidant density of select whole fruit and 100% fruit juices. J Acad Nutr Diet. 2013;113:1354–8.

21. United States Department of Agriculture (USDA) Nutrient Database. http://ndb.nal.usda.gov/.

22. Shenoy SF, Poston WS, Reeves RS, et al. Weight loss in individuals with metabolic syndrome given DASH diet counseling when provided a low sodium vegetable juice: a randomized controlled trial. Nutr J. 2010;9:8.

23. Getting JE, Gregoire JR, Phul A, Kasten MJ. Oxalate nephropathy due to 'juicing': case report and review. Am J Med. 2013;126:768–72.

24. Parekh PJ, Arusi E, Vinik AI, Johnson DA. The role and influence of gut microbiota in pathogenesis and management of obesity and metabolic syndrome. Front Endocrinol (Lausanne). 2014;5:47.

25. Oddy WH. Infant feeding and obesity risk in the child. Breastfeed Rev. 2012;20:7–12.

26. Fourreau D, Peretti N, Hengy B, et al. Pediatric nutrition: severe deficiency complications by using vegetable beverages, four cases report. Presse Med. 2013;42:e37–43.

27. Khan H, Kunutsor S, Franco OH, Chowdhury R. Vitamin D, type 2 diabetes and other metabolic outcomes: a systematic review and meta-analysis of prospective studies. Proc Nutr Soc. 2013;72:89–97.

28. Lim S, Kim MJ, Choi SH, et al. Association of vitamin D deficiency with incidence of type 2 diabetes in high-risk Asian subjects. Am J Clin Nutr. 2013;97:524–30.

29. Elwood PC, Pickering JE, Fehily AM. Milk and dairy consumption, diabetes and the metabolic syndrome: the Caerphilly prospective study. J Epidemiol Community Health. 2007;61:695–8.

30. Gagnon C, Lu ZX, Magliano DJ, et al. Serum 25-hydroxyvitamin D, calcium intake, and risk of type 2 diabetes after 5 years: results from a national, population-based prospective study (the Australian Diabetes, Obesity and Lifestyle study). Diabetes Care. 2011;34:1133–8.

31. Dong JY, Qin LQ. Dietary calcium intake and risk of type 2 diabetes: possible confounding by magnesium. Eur J Clin Nutr. 2012;66:408–10.
32. Azadbakht L, Mirmiran P, Esmailzadeh A, Azizi F. Dairy consumption is inversely associated with the prevalence of the metabolic syndrome in Tehranian adults. Am J Clin Nutr. 2005;82:523–30.
33. Fumeron F, Lamri A, Khalil CA, et al. Dairy consumption and the incidence of hyperglycemia and the metabolic syndrome. Diabetes Care. 2011;32:813–7.
34. Rice BH, Quann EE, Miller GD. Meeting and exceeding dairy recommendations: effects of dairy consumption on nutrient intakes and risk of chronic disease. Nutr Rev. 2013;71:209–23.
35. Shin D, Joh H, Kim KH, Parm SM. Benefits of potassium intake on metabolic syndrome: the fourth Korean National Health and Nutrition Examination Survey (KNHANES IV). Atherosclerosis. 2013;230:80–5.
36. Pfeuffer M, Schrezenmeir J. Milk and the metabolic syndrome. Obes Rev. 2007;8:109–18.
37. Weaver CM. Role of dairy beverages in the diet. Physiol Behav. 2010;100:63–6.
38. Kalaitzidis R, Tsimihodimos V, Bairaktari E, Siamopoulos KC, Elisaf M. Disturbances of phosphate metabolism: another feature of metabolic syndrome. Am J Kidney Dis. 2005;45:851–8.
39. Park W, Kim BS, Lee JE, et al. Serum phosphate levels and the risk of cardiovascular disease and metabolic syndrome: a double-edged sword. Diabetes Res Clin Pract. 2009;83:119–25.
40. Hostmark AT, Haug A. Does cheese intake blunt the association between soft drink intake and risk of the metabolic syndrome? Results from the cross-sectional Oslo Health Study. BMJ. 2012;2:e001476.
41. Chang AR, Lazo M, Appel LJ, Guiterrez OM, Grams ME. High dietary phosphorus intake is associated with all-cause mortality: results from NHANES III. Am J Clin Nutr. 2014;99:320–7.
42. Raisanen JP, Silaste M, Kesanieme YA, Ukkola O. Increased daily sodium intake is an independent dietary indicator of the metabolic syndrome in middle-aged subjects. Ann Med. 2012;44:627–34.
43. Grimes CA, Wright JD, Liu K, Nowson CA, Loria CM. Dietary sodium intake is associated with total fluid and sugar-sweetened beverage consumption in US children and adolescents aged 2–18 y: NHANES 2005–2008. Am J Clin Nutr. 2013;98:189–96.
44. Schoppen S, Perez-Granados AM, Carbajal A, et al. A sodium-rich carbonated mineral water reduces cardiovascular risk in postmenopausal women. J Nutr. 2004;134:1058–63.
45. Costa ASG, Nunes MA, Almeida IMC, Carvalho MR, Barroso MF, Alves RC. Teas, dietary supplements and fruit juices: a comparative study regarding antioxidant activity and bioactive compounds. Food Sci Technol. 2012;49:324–8.
46. Mattila PH, Hellstrom J, McDougall G, et al. Polyphenol and vitamin C contents in European commercial blackcurrant juice products. Food Chem. 2011;127:1216–23.
47. Garcia-Alonso FJ, Bravo S, Casas J, Perez-Conesa D, Jacob K, Periago MJ. Changes in antioxidant compounds during the shelf life of commercial tomato juices in different packaging materials. J Agric Food Chem. 2009;57:6815–22.
48. Gil-Izquierdo A, Gil MI, Ferreres F. Effect of processing techniques at industrial scale on orange juice antioxidant and beneficial health compounds. J Agric Food Chem. 2002;50:5107–14.

Chapter 14
Oral Nutritional Supplementation Using Beverages for Older Adults

Shelley R. McDonald

Keywords Malnutrition • Older adults • Liquid nutritional supplements • Undernutrition • Sip feeds

Key Points

1. Poor nutrition in older adults is associated with many adverse health outcomes, including loss of lean mass, loss of bone mass, poor wound healing, greater risk of infection, longer hospital stays, and increased mortality.
2. Malnutrition and risk of malnutrition need to be identified as early as possible so that a comprehensive assessment and intervention can be implemented.
3. To the extent that oral food intake can be maintained, supplemental beverages should be used primarily to augment a diet of conventional whole foods, not as a replacement for those foods.
4. The evidence shows that dietary supplementation with oral nutritional supplement beverages produces only modest weight gain in older adults.
5. Oral nutritional supplement beverages produce a beneficial effect on mortality but only in those who are undernourished. Thus, they provide little or no health benefit to older adults who are adequately nourished.

S.R. McDonald, D.O., Ph.D. (✉)
Department of Medicine, Duke University Medical Center,
804 Clarion Drive, Durham, NC 27710, USA
e-mail: shelley.mcdonald@duke.edu

© Springer International Publishing Switzerland 2016
T. Wilson, N.J. Temple (eds.), *Beverage Impacts on Health and Nutrition*,
Nutrition and Health, DOI 10.1007/978-3-319-23672-8_14

Introduction

Prevalence of Malnutrition in Older Adults

Older adults, defined as those over 65 years of age, are at high risk for malnutrition or undernutrition due to a number of well-known risk factors including changes in body composition, changes to the GI tract, diminished sensory function, fluid and electrolyte dysregulation, increases in chronic disease, use of medications, institutionalization, financial constraints, social isolation, and frailty [1]. The largest pooled analysis of malnutrition, with more than 6000 adults over 65 years of age worldwide, found that 22.8 % were malnourished with the highest proportions found in those in rehabilitation (50.5 %) and hospital settings (38.7 %). When subjects at risk of being malnourished were included with those who were malnourished, the combined number increased to 69 % for all older adults, 86 % for those hospitalized, and 91.7 % for those in rehabilitation [2].

Consequence of Malnutrition in Older Adults

Poor nutrition in older adults is associated with many negative outcomes including loss of lean body and bone mass, development of pressure sores, slow wound healing, increased risk of infection, longer length of hospitalization, greater likelihood of hospital readmission after discharge, and increased mortality [3–5]. Older adults are more vulnerable to the adverse outcomes from any stressor including malnutrition. The complex interplay between physiological and metabolic changes of aging that alter dietary requirements coupled with social and/or environmental constraints that limit desire to eat and access to food creates this geriatric syndrome of malnutrition that is difficult to treat [6].

Physiological aging, independent of nutritional status, leads to a decline in skeletal muscle mass, increase in abdominal obesity, and reduced intracellular fluid leading to a slowing in basal metabolic rate [1]. But the combination of compromised nutritional intake in addition to age-related changes in physiology, such as blunting of anabolic responses to nutritional substrates, can lead to a significant loss of physical strength and functional status and thus independence [7].

Proliferation of Oral Nutritional Beverage Use in Older Adults

Dietary supplements are enormously popular across the general population. In the light of the above considerations, it is not surprising that older adults are more likely to use supplements than younger people. The market for supplements remains very strong despite the fact that there is no requirement for the FDA to establish either the safety or the effectiveness of supplements before they are marketed [8]. Their use can be expected to increase even faster in future years due to the unprecedented aging of the world's population. Not only are people living longer, but the ratio of older adults to children is projected to be equal for the first time in history by the year 2050 [9]. While this scenario applies to both micronutrient supplements such as multivitamin/mineral and single-nutrient preparations and liquid supplements focusing on protein/calorie repletion, this chapter will focus on the merits of liquid oral nutritional supplements (ONS) and their use by older persons. ONS beverages typically provide calories for energy and are fortified with protein and micronutrients; they are designed as a dietary augmentation in the case of chronic disease, illness, injury, or surgery resulting in an inability for an older adult to meet their nutritional requirements through their usual diet alone and are widely used. Sales of these products are projected to grow worldwide from $9.7 billion in 2010 to $15.6 billion in 2015 [10].

Identifying Malnutrition in Older Adults

Institutionalized Older Adults

The first step to intervention with a treatment plan is the identification of those who are malnourished or at risk of becoming malnourished. One prospective study suggests that undernutrition precedes development of disease and hospitalization in adults older than 70 years [11] and malnutrition is associated with an increased risk of death at 3 months in hospitalized older adults [12, 13]. A widely accepted measure to help identify those who are malnourished or at nutritional risk has been operationalized by the Minimum Data Set (MDS) for use in Medicare-certified nursing homes. It centers on a loss of more than 5 % of body weight over the past month or more than 10 % over the past 6 months [14]. Unplanned weight loss or loss of ten pounds in the preceding 6 months predicts increased mortality in older adults [15].

Older Adults in the Community

In community settings, undernutrition is often unrecognized and thus undertreated. To facilitate the identification of older adults who have malnutrition or are at risk for malnutrition, we need to use standardized screening and assessment tools that have been validated in multiple care settings. An example is the Mini Nutritional Assessment (MNA). It uses multiple domains composed of body mass index (BMI), weight loss, mobility, recent psychological stress or illness, neuropsychological comorbidity, and changes in food intake to identify those with malnutrition, as well as those at risk for malnutrition [2, 16]. Screening is known to significantly increase referrals to a registered dietitian. For example, in one hospital-based study of malnourished patients, the use of the Simplified Nutritional Appetite Questionnaire (SNAQ) screening tool generated referrals in 76 % of those screened vs. 46 % of those not screened [2].

Comprehensive Assessment Is Essential

When malnutrition can be identified (or anticipated as in those at risk), comprehensive assessment to identify and correct the underlying cause should address medical, dental, psychological, social, economic, and nutritional contributors. General medical conditions related to malnutrition include respiratory, cardiac, renal, endocrine, and mood disorders, as well as cancer. These all affect not only nutrient intake but also nutrient utilization. Problems with oral health can make eating uncomfortable or even painful and make food tasteless. Older adults are often isolated and on a fixed income resulting in reductions in both the quantity and quality of food intake. Comorbid medical conditions create multiple dietary restrictions that can often result in limited food choices [6, 14].

If an underlying cause of malnutrition can be identified, then a targeted strategy to increase conventional food intake will likely be more successful. A commonly used approach is to add supplements to the older adult's medical regimen, in the form of either a beverage or a once daily pill. Both types of supplement contain a broad array of vitamins and minerals, but ONS beverages can also provide a sizable amount of energy from the additional combination of carbohydrates, fat, and protein.

Nonpharmacological Treatment Options for Malnourished Older Adults

Support Programs

Many programs and approaches are available to increase the energy content and the quality of the diets that older adults consume, and success may be dictated by the settings in which the programs are implemented. Lower-income older adults living in both rural and urban communities may be able to access more fresh produce through the US Department of Agriculture's Senior Farmers' Market Nutrition Program. Eligible participants are given coupons that can be exchanged for locally grown fruits and vegetables, as well as honey and herbs that are sold in farmers' markets, roadside stands, or community-supported agriculture programs. Home-delivered meals, such as Meals on Wheels, is another example of a senior nutrition program that can increase the access to and quality of food, while congregate meal programs through senior centers can enhance the social aspects of eating in addition to the nutritional value. Older adults living in institutional settings have increased dietary intakes when homelike dining areas, cafeteria-style serving, and snack carts are available [3, 6, 17]. For long-term care facilities, the Code of Federal Regulations requires that the special dietary needs of each resident be met with a nourishing, palatable, attractive, and well-balanced diet. Furthermore, a qualified dietitian must be engaged in the planning and implementation of the dietary programs. Any therapeutic diets provided in long-term care, which would include ONS, must be prescribed by the attending physician.

Use of ONS to Overcome Barriers to Nutritional Support

Despite these many solutions that have been implemented for improving access to nutritious food and for creating environments designed to facilitate optimal nutritional intake for senior adults, older adults still often times have limitations in what they can eat. This may be due to dietary restrictions from medical conditions, underlying disease processes, and/or physical limitations that can result in limited intake or exclusion of many whole foods. When oral intake of conventional foods is insufficient, a supplement is often added to the diet with the goal of preventing adverse outcomes and/or restoring health and function. ONS are primarily protein and calorie products that have differing amounts of energy, fluid, protein, fat, and micronutrients. They are formulated in order to target specific medical conditions, such as weight loss, malnutrition, or loss of muscle. They are available in many forms, such as liquids, powders, puddings, soups, or bars, but the beverage form is the most prevalent, also known as "sip feeds."

ONS beverages are intended to supplement an individual's diet and be integrated into a comprehensive treatment plan. They can be of value for older adults who are unable to have sufficient intake of solid oral foods to meet their metabolic needs. ONS beverages can be especially useful to supplement diets in the event of acute or chronic illness and to maintain some consistency in intake when an older adult transitions across care settings, between home, hospital, post-acute care, or even long-term care. For example, a particular product that is familiar to an older adult and that can be portable across care settings may provide just enough additional nutrition to maintain adequate caloric and macronutrient intake. Thibault's study of hospitalized patients reported that when at least one ONS beverage was consumed daily, the risk of underfeeding decreased and protein intake increased from 80 % of the estimated protein need before supplementation to 115 % after supplementation ($P < 0.001$) [18]. Some of the preparations, such as Nepro and Suplena, are marketed as both supplements and meal replacements. Therefore, they can also be used for those who depend on enteral tube feeding. Table 14.1 lists comparison data for the macronutrient content of some of the more common ONS beverages.

Table 14.1 Composition of selected commercially available adult oral nutritional supplement beverages[a]

Product (manufacturer)	Targeted uses/design features	Energy density (kcal/mL)	Protein (g/100 mL)	Carbohydrate (g/100 mL)	Fat (g/100 mL)
Ensure (Abbott)	"To help get strong on the inside"	0.93	3.8	13.9	2.5
Ensure Complete (Abbott)	Muscle, heart, immune, and bone support	1.5	5.5	21.5	4.6
Ensure High Protein (Abbott)	Recovery from surgery or fractures	1	5.1	13.1	2.5
Ensure Immune Health (Abbott)	Support for the immune system	1.05	3.8	17.7	2.5
Ensure Muscle Health (Abbott)	To help rebuild muscle and strength lost naturally over time	1.05	5.1	13.5	3.4
Ensure Plus (Abbott)	Malnutrition, nutritional risk, or unintentional weight loss	1.5	5.5	21	4.6
Nepro (Abbott)	To help meet the nutritional needs of patients on dialysis	1.8	8.1	16	9.6
ProSure (Abbott)	Cancer cachexia	1.3	20.9 %	57.7 %	18.1 %
Promote (Abbott)	Protein-energy malnutrition or pressure sores	1	6.2	13	2.6
Pulmocare (Abbott)	To help meet the nutritional needs of those with COPD	1.5	6.2	10.5	9.3
Suplena (Abbott)	Stage 3–4 chronic kidney disease (CKD)	1.8	4.5	19.6	9.6
Boost (Nestlé)	Malnutrition, inadequate oral intake, reduced appetite	1	4.2	17.3	1.7
Boost High Protein (Nestlé)	Recovery from illness, injury, surgery, wound, or fracture	1	6.3	13.9	2.5
Boost Plus (Nestlé)	Difficulty maintaining a healthy weight, need for general weight gain, loss of appetite, and unintended weight loss	1.5	5.9	19	5.9
Carnation Breakfast Essentials (Nestlé)		1	4.2	17	1.7

Table 14.1 (continued)

Product (manufacturer)	Targeted uses/design features	Energy density (kcal/mL)	Protein (g/100 mL)	Carbohydrate (g/100 mL)	Fat (g/100 mL)
Oral Impact (Nestlé)	Protection against infection/74 g packets of powder	1	5.6	13.2	2.8
Resource Hepatic 1.5 (Nestlé)	Liver disorders with the need for minimal fluid intake	1.5	4.6	28.5	2.4
Resource High Protein (Nestlé)	Malnutrition, fluid restrictions, burns and trauma, chronic and acute disease, pressure ulcers, and post-surgery/to be added to milk	1.5	11.2 with milk	13.7 with milk	4.4 with milk
Resource Renal 2.0 (Nestlé)	Acute renal failure, chronic renal failure, or those with fluid and/or electrolyte restrictions	2	4	27	8.8
Sustacal (Nestlé)	Loss of appetite, unintentional weight loss, rehab after injury, malnutrition in elderly, perioperative	1	4.25	14.5	2.87
Calogen Extra (Nutricia)	Packaged as 40 mL shots	4	5	4.5	40.3
Cubitan (Nutricia)	To treat chronic wounds	1.25	10	11.7	3.5
FortiFit (Nutricia)	To stimulate muscle synthesis	1.2	>8	NA	NA
Fortimel Compact (available w fiber) (Nutricia)	125 mL unit	2.4	9.6	29.7	9.3
Fortimel Energy (available w fiber) (Nutricia)		1.5	6	18.4	5.8
Fortimel Regular (Nutricia)	200 mL unit	1	10	10.3	2.1
Renilon 7.5 (Nutricia)	Low electrolyte for renal failure requiring dialysis	2	7.5	20	10
Respifor (Nutricia)	Dietary management of COPD	1.5	7.5	22.5	3.3
Souvenaid (Nutricia)	Memory support	1	3	13.2	3.9

www.abbottnutrition.com; www.nutricia.com; www.nestle-nutrition.com; www.nestle.lk/en/brands/nestle-health-science/products; www.carnationbreakfastessentials.com/Products/FAQ.aspx (all accessed July 31, 2014)

[a]All the listed products also contain micronutrients

Evidence for Oral Nutritional Support Beverages

Evidence for Energy Intake

Despite the wide prevalence of usage and the potential importance for maintaining energy balance and protein needs, ONS beverages have not been thoroughly studied. Historically the studies for oral supplementation in older adults have been of poor quality with much heterogeneity. However, the number of trials is increasing so that more specific clinical questions can now be addressed through systematic reviews and meta-analyses. Pooled evidence has repeatedly demonstrated that dietary supplementation with ONS beverages produces a modest weight gain [19]. This can be partly explained by the findings from Hubbard et al. [20] showing that the amount of commercial multi-nutrient beverages consumed as a proportion prescribed is fairly good, with 81 % compliance for those in the community and 67 % for those in hospital. Additionally, ONS in the form of beverages does not appear to compromise intake at meals when given 30–60 min prior [21, 22] or decrease total energy intake throughout the day [23].

Evidence for Clinical Benefits

While ONS beverages can provide additional calories and lead to weight gain, it has not been firmly established that the weight gain translates into improved functional outcomes for cognitive abilities, muscle strength, falls, mobility, or ability to perform activities of daily living (ADLs). A simple gain in fat mass, as has been reported [24], is unlikely to translate into clinically important health improvements. So it is not surprising that most of the systematic reviews and meta-analyses examining the impact of ONS beverages have not identified a mortality benefit with ONS (Table 14.2). However, Milne et al. [19] carried out the largest review and showed a beneficial effect on mortality in those who were undernourished. This underscores that ONS beverages likely have the greatest benefit when used by those with the greatest need.

Nutrient composition may also play a role in the clinical outcomes attributable to ONS beverages. For example, a review by Cawood et al. [26] reported that high-protein ONS may be one particular way to target specific metabolic pathways in order to counteract the catabolic effects of disease; when >20 % of the energy content was provided as protein, study participants had fewer complications, reduced hospital readmissions, and improved grip strength; whether these outcomes are related to the protein content or the overall supplementation cannot be ascertained, because only three trials compared high-protein ONS to standard ONS [26].

Two systematic reviews also suggested that nutritional supplementation can improve particular clinical conditions such as the prevention of pressure ulcers or recovery after hip fracture [29, 30]. However, both of these reviews were excluded

Table 14.2 Health effects of oral nutritional supplement beverages: recent systematic reviews and meta-analyses

Question addressed	Population	Trials/participants	Product	1. Energy intake (kcal/day) 2. Protein intake (g/day)	Duration	Positive outcomes	Neutral or negative outcomes	Reference
Are diet supplements an effective way of improving outcomes for older people at risk from malnutrition?	Range of means for age 65–88; 71 % hospitalized Groups recovering from cancer or in critical care were excluded	62 RCTs and quasi-RCTs/N = 10,187 randomized participants	Usually commercial "sip feeds"	NA	Up to 18 months	• Weight increased by 2.2 % (42 trials) • Mortality change was statistically significant when limited to trials in which participants were defined as undernourished • The risk of complications was reduced (24 trials)	• No evidence of improvement in functional benefit • No reduction in length of hospital stay with supplements • No significant reduction in mortality in the supplemented compared with control groups (42 trials) • No statistically significant effect on length of hospital stay (12 trials)	Milne et al. (2009) [19]

(continued)

Table 14.2 (continued)

Question addressed	Population	Trials/participants	Product	1. Energy intake (kcal/day) 2. Protein intake (g/day)	Duration	Positive outcomes	Neutral or negative outcomes	Reference
What is the effectiveness of oral liquid nutritional supplements (OLNS) for people with dementia in residential facilities?	No ages given, but subjects had dementia and lived in residential facilities	15 studies: RCTs, quasi-experimental studies, cohort studies, case–control studies, and observational studies without control group	NA	NA	NA	• Very slight evidence to suggest that OLNS may increase energy intake	• No evidence that OLNS have an effect on morbidity or mortality • No evidence that OLNS have an effect on functional status	Hines et al. (2010) [25]
Do high-protein ONS counter the catabolic effects of disease and facilitate recovery from illness?	Mean age 74 years; 83 % of trials in patients >65 years	36 RCTs/$N=3790$	High-protein ONS (>20 % energy from protein)	1. 149–995 kcal 2. 10–60 g	2 weeks to 1 year	• Reduced complications • Reduced readmissions to hospital • Improved grip strength • Increased intake of energy and protein with little reduction in normal food intake and improvements in weight	• Inadequate information to compare standard ONS (<20 % energy from protein) with high-protein ONS (>20 % energy from protein)	Cawood et al. (2012) [26]

| What is patients' compliance with ONS across healthcare settings and the influence of patient and ONS-related factors? | Mean age 74 years | 46 studies/N = 4328 | 96 % of ONS used were ready-made, multi-nutrient liquids with energy densities ranging from 1.0 to 4.0 kcal/mL | 1. Overall mean 433 kcal/day (range 144–1045 kcal/day) | 4–365 days | • Overall mean compliance with ONS was 78 % (37–100 %): 67 % hospital and 81 % community | • Compliance across a heterogeneous group of unmatched studies was negatively associated with age and unrelated to amount or duration of ONS prescription | Hubbard et al. (2012) [20] |
| | BMI 22.8 | | | 2. NA | | • Compliance across a heterogeneous group of unmatched studies was positively associated with higher energy-density ONS and greater ONS and total energy intakes | | |

(continued)

Table 14.2 (continued)

Question addressed	Population	Trials/participants	Product	1. Energy intake (kcal/day) 2. Protein intake (g/day)	Duration	Positive outcomes	Neutral or negative outcomes	Reference
What is the effectiveness of ONS compared to placebo or usual care in improving clinical outcomes in older medical and surgical patients after discharge from hospital?	Mean age 81 years	6 trials/$N=716$ randomly assigned participants	Commercial ONS	1. 480–1000 kcal/day 2. 12–30 g	4–16 weeks	• A positive effect on nutritional intake (energy) and/or nutritional status (weight) (in compliant participants) was observed in all trials	• No significant effect on mortality or readmissions	Beck et al. (2013) [27]
Is providing nutritionally complete ONS drinks an effective way of improving clinical outcomes for older people with dementia?	Cognitive impairment with 75 % living in long-term care facilities	12 studies including all research methodologies/$N=$ 1076 in supplement groups and $N=748$ in control groups	ONS drinks	NA	3 weeks to 1 year	• Significant improvement in weight • Significant improvement in BMI • Significant improvement in cognition at 6.5 months follow-up on the MMSE test scores	• No significant effect was found on mortality. • No significant difference was found between the MMSE test scores in the ONS and control groups at 3 months	Allen et al. (2013) [28]

RCT randomized controlled trial, *ONS* oral nutritional supplementation, *BMI* body mass index, *MMSE* Mini Mental State Examination

from Table 14.2 because the supplementation included enteral tube feedings and IV nutrient supplementation. The reviews by Hines et al. [19] and Allen et al. [22] also showed that energy intake can be increased in those with dementia but again with no effect on mortality. A numerical significance was identified on the MMSE with a mean improved score of 1.6 points (SE 0.3) after 6.5 ± 3.9 months of supplementation; however, only four studies evaluated cognition as an outcome, and an increase of 1.6 points is not clinically meaningful [28]. Overall, the evidence that ONS improves the health of older adults is of a small magnitude with respect to weight gain and of uncertain clinical benefit in other domains.

Conclusion

In summary, aging puts the older adult at risk of malnutrition for many of the reasons discussed, and when malnutrition develops, the consequences can be dire. The following question still remains: if we are able to correct the nutritional deficiencies of malnutrition, will this ameliorate the downward spiral associated with malnutrition, aging, and various chronic diseases? Ideally, early identification of unintentional weight loss in older adults or those at risk of malnutrition will trigger an extensive evaluation to help identify the causes and aid in the development of a multifaceted treatment plan to address physical, medical, psychosocial, and economic contributors. The comprehensive strategy to increase the energy intake of older adults should begin with individualized food preferences for conventional whole foods. When this is not enough to increase energy intake, ONS beverages should then be incorporated into the diet as a therapeutic intervention with specific goals for a desired weight target, functional goals, and pleasure surrounding the diet.

More well-designed intervention trials are needed that pay particular attention to comparing a diet with enhanced quality and quantity of whole foods on an isocaloric or isonutrient basis to ONS beverages [3]. Future studies need to be clearly designed with enough sensitivity to identify the relationship of total energy or nutrient composition in a diet to postulated clinical or functional outcomes within specific populations, such as malnourished older adults. It is quite likely that specific ONS beverage formulations will be required for different medical conditions. Until the required research has been carried out, there is only limited evidence to support ONS beverages for producing any desired effects.

References

1. Brownie S. Why are elderly individuals at risk of nutritional deficiency? Int J Nurs Pract. 2006;12(2):110–8.
2. Kaiser MJ, Bauer JM, Ramsch C, Uter W, Guigoz Y, Cederholm T, et al. Frequency of malnutrition in older adults: a multinational perspective using the mini nutritional assessment. J Am Geriatr Soc. 2010;58(9):1734–8.

3. Silver HJ. Oral strategies to supplement older adults' dietary intakes: comparing the evidence. Nutr Rev. 2009;67(1):21–31.

4. Sullivan DH, Morley JE, Johnson LE, Barber A, Olson JS, Stevens MR, et al. The GAIN (Geriatric Anorexia Nutrition) registry: the impact of appetite and weight on mortality in a long-term care population. J Nutr Health Aging. 2002;6(4):275–81.

5. Pichard C, Kyle UG, Morabia A, Perrier A, Vermeulen B, Unger P. Nutritional assessment: lean body mass depletion at hospital admission is associated with an increased length of stay. Am J Clin Nutr. 2004;79(4):613–8.

6. Ross AC, Cabllero B, Cousins RJ, Tucker KL, Zieder TR, editors. Modern nutrition in health and disease. 11th ed. Baltimore: Lippincott Williams and Wilkins; 2012.

7. Evans WJ. Skeletal muscle loss: cachexia, sarcopenia, and inactivity. Am J Clin Nutr. 2010;91(4):1123S–7S.

8. Yetley E. Dietary supplement use in the elderly conference. U.S. Department of Health & Human Services. 2003. [January 4, 2015]. http://ods.od.nih.gov/News/Dietary_Supplement_Use_in_the_Elderly_Conference_(January_14-15_2003)_Overview.aspx.

9. http://www.un.org/esa/population/publications/worldageing19502050/pdf/81chapteriii.pdf. New York: United Nations; 2014 [cited 2014 July 26]. Population Division.

10. Crandall MA. U.S. and global markets for ethical nutrition in healthcare. 2011. Report No.: Contract No.: Report ID: FOD029D.

11. Mowe M, Bøhmer T, Kindt E. Reduced nutritional status in an elderly population (>70 y) is probable before disease and possibly contributes to the development of disease. Am J Clin Nutr. 1994;59(2):317–24.

12. Cerri AP, Bellelli G, Mazzone A, Pittella F, Landi F, Zambon A, et al. Sarcopenia and malnutrition in acutely ill hospitalized elderly: prevalence and outcomes. Clin Nutr. 2014;34:745–51.

13. Heersink JT, Brown CJ, Dimaria-Ghalili RA, Locher JL. Undernutrition in hospitalized older adults: patterns and correlates, outcomes, and opportunities for intervention with a focus on processes of care. J Nutr Elder. 2010;29(1):4–41.

14. Pacala JT, Sullivan GM. Geriatric review syllabus: a core curriculum in geriatric medicine. 7th ed. New York: American Geriatrics Society; 2010.

15. Johnsen C, East JM, Glassman P. Management of malnutrition in the elderly and the appropriate use of commercially manufactured oral nutritional supplements. J Nutr Health Aging. 2000;4(1):42–6.

16. MNA Mini Nutritional Assessment: Nestle Nutrition Institute. 2014 [cited 2014 July 28, 2014]. http://www.mna-elderly.com/default.html.

17. Ruigrok J, Sheridan L. Life enrichment programme; enhanced dining experience, a pilot project. Int J Health Care Qual Assur Inc Leadersh Health Serv. 2006;19(4–5):420–9.

18. Thibault R, Chikhi M, Clerc A, Darmon P, Chopard P, Genton L, et al. Assessment of food intake in hospitalised patients: a 10-year comparative study of a prospective hospital survey. Clin Nutr (Edinburgh). 2011;30(3):289–96.

19. Milne AC, Potter J, Vivanti A, Avenell A. Protein and energy supplementation in elderly people at risk from malnutrition. Cochrane Database Syst Rev. 2009;2:CD003288.

20. Hubbard GP, Elia M, Holdoway A, Stratton RJ. A systematic review of compliance to oral nutritional supplements. Clin Nutr (Edinburgh). 2012;31(3):293–312.

21. Boudville A, Bruce DG. Lack of meal intake compensation following nutritional supplements in hospitalised elderly women. Br J Nutr. 2005;93(6):879–84.

22. Wilson MM, Purushothaman R, Morley JE. Effect of liquid dietary supplements on energy intake in the elderly. Am J Clin Nutr. 2002;75(5):944–7.

23. Ryan M, Salle A, Favreau AM, Simard G, Dumas JF, Malthiery Y, et al. Oral supplements differing in fat and carbohydrate content: effect on the appetite and food intake of undernourished elderly patients. Clin Nutr (Edinburgh). 2004;23(4):683–9.

24. Fiatarone Singh MA, Bernstein MA, Ryan AD, O'Neill EF, Clements KM, Evans WJ. The effect of oral nutritional supplements on habitual dietary quality and quantity in frail elders. J Nutr Health Aging. 2000;4(1):5–12.

25. Hines S, Wilson J, McCrow J, Abbey J, Sacre S. Oral liquid nutritional supplements for people with dementia in residential aged care facilities. Int J Evid Based Healthc. 2010;8(4):248–51.
26. Cawood AL, Elia M, Stratton RJ. Systematic review and meta-analysis of the effects of high protein oral nutritional supplements. Ageing Res Rev. 2012;11(2):278–96.
27. Beck AM, Holst M, Rasmussen HH. Oral nutritional support of older (65 years+) medical and surgical patients after discharge from hospital: systematic review and meta-analysis of randomized controlled trials. Clin Rehabil. 2013;27(1):19–27.
28. Allen VJ, Methven L, Gosney MA. Use of nutritional complete supplements in older adults with dementia: systematic review and meta-analysis of clinical outcomes. Clin Nutr (Edinburgh). 2013;32(6):950–7.
29. Stratton RJ, Ek AC, Engfer M, Moore Z, Rigby P, Wolfe R, et al. Enteral nutritional support in prevention and treatment of pressure ulcers: a systematic review and meta-analysis. Ageing Res Rev. 2005;4(3):422–50.
30. Avenell A, Handoll HH. Nutritional supplementation for hip fracture aftercare in older people. Cochrane Database Syst Rev. 2010;1:CD001880.

Part V
Health Effects of Sports Drinks, Energy Drinks and Water

Chapter 15
Sports Beverages for Optimizing Physical Performance

Ronald J. Maughan and Susan M. Shirreffs

Keywords Dehydration • Hypohydration • Exercise performance • Sports drinks • Sweat loss

Key Points

1. Dehydration, if sufficiently severe, will impair all physiological and cognitive functions. Some impairment of function may be apparent when losses reach 1–3 % of body mass. This applies to both pre-exercise hypohydration and hypohydration accrued during exercise.
2. Ingestion of water may improve exercise performance when exercise lasts longer than about 40–60 min.
3. Addition of carbohydrates, and possibly also sodium, to ingested drinks may further benefit exercise performance.

Introduction

Many different factors combine to produce a successful performance in sporting contests, with genetic endowment playing a large role. Other factors also intervene, but many of these also have a genetic basis, including the ability to adapt to a

R.J. Maughan, Ph.D. (✉)
School of Sport, Exercise and Health Sciences, Loughborough University, Loughborough LE11 3TU, UK
e-mail: r.maughan@lboro.ac.uk

S.M. Shirreffs, Ph.D.
Research and Development, GSK, AS1, Brentford, Middlesex, UK

© Springer International Publishing Switzerland 2016
T. Wilson, N.J. Temple (eds.), *Beverage Impacts on Health and Nutrition*,
Nutrition and Health, DOI 10.1007/978-3-319-23672-8_15

training program and probably also the psychological factors that encompass motivation, competitiveness, and tactical awareness. Consistent intensive training is a major factor in the success of most elite performers, but there is a limit to the training load that can be sustained without illness or injury. Of those factors that can be altered by conscious effort, nutrition, which is perhaps only a very small part of the overall picture, is of considerable importance because it is arguably the factor that athletes can most tightly control.

In competition, there is scope for modification of the diet in the pre-event period, and, in some sports, for ingestion of food and/or fluids during the event itself. In some events, this means taking drinks (and solid foods in some cases) without interrupting the exercise. In games such as tennis, there are regular breaks in play that allow opportunities for food and drink to be consumed. In most team games, there are no scheduled breaks, except for the half-time interval, but brief breaks in play do allow players to take drinks.

There is a substantial amount of evidence to support the use of water and of commercial sports drinks to enhance performance, but there is also considerable controversy in this area. Some loud voices argue that the evidence base is insufficient for any conclusions to be reached [1], that dehydration at the levels normally encountered has little effect on performance [2], and even that the sports drinks industry is responsible for the deaths of some runners by encouraging excessive drinking [3]. Many factors have contributed to these controversies, including poor methodology in many studies and misinterpretation or misrepresentation of others.

Limitations to Endurance Performance

The major causes of fatigue in prolonged exercise are generally thought to be depletion of the body's limited carbohydrate (CHO) store and the twin problem of dehydration and hyperthermia [4]. There is, however, no single clearly defined cause of fatigue in most exercise situations, and many different factors probably contribute to the subjective sensation of fatigue and reduced exercise capacity that occurs in the later stages of any intense exercise. The decision to slow down or to let the leaders go in a race situation is a conscious one based on a subjective assessment of one's current physiological status and the distance remaining. The brain, consciously or otherwise, is therefore of paramount importance, and it may be that the cause of fatigue lies within the central nervous system rather than in the periphery, as was generally recognized a century ago.

Most laboratory studies into the efficacy of fluid ingestion have used simple models of cycling or running at constant speed to the point of fatigue. The limitations of this approach have been recognized, and various other experimental models are now commonly used, including simulated time-trial performance, multiple sprint shuttle running, and an assessment of the ability to maintain skill throughout exercise. For most serious athletes in a race, however, the challenge is more like a time to fatigue task rather than a time trial: the aim is to win and that means staying with the leaders for as long as possible. The point at which a decision is made by the performance athlete to drop off the pace in a race is very similar to the decision to stop exercising in a laboratory test where simply slowing is not an option.

It is also important to recognize that sports drinks are more often consumed by recreational exercisers for whom enjoyment and the prospect of health benefits are more important than performance. Anything that can make the exercise feel easier is potentially of much value for these individuals. In these respects the needs of recreational exercisers are quite distinct from those of elite athletes.

Hydration and Performance

Dehydration is the process of reducing the body's water content, while hypohydration is a state of water deficit. The methods used to induce hypohydration in laboratory settings usually involve exercise, heat exposure, fluid restriction, or a combination of these, and it is often hard to separate the process from the end result. It is well established that hypohydration will, if sufficiently severe, adversely affect all body functions. This applies both to pre-existing hypohydration present at the onset of exercise and to the hypohydration that develops if body water losses are not replaced during exercise. This includes both mental and physical performance, though various functions will be affected to different degrees, with cognitive performance perhaps better preserved than physical performance. However, at the relatively modest levels of hypohydration incurred in most sports or occupational tasks, performance effects may be too small to measure. Most [5, 6] but not all [2] reviews of the literature have concluded that a body water deficit of about 2 % of the starting body mass will result in a meaningful impairment of performance, with greater effects in warm environments and in exercise of longer duration.

It is often asserted that results generated in the laboratory environment have no relevance to the athlete in the field because the exercise test lacks ecological validity, and the absence of forced air flow over the body surface confounds the results [7]. These arguments ignore the facts: as noted above, the time to fatigue test may be more relevant to the competitive athlete than the simulated time trial. Many laboratory studies do indeed use forced convection, but for the recreational exerciser who pedals a cycle ergometer or runs on a treadmill in an overheated health club, there is usually no air movement.

Some of the studies used as evidence that drinking does not benefit performance have used inappropriate models, and reviews or meta-analyses based on these studies will inevitably reach erroneous conclusions. Goulet [2], for example, performed a meta-analysis based on five studies and concluded that: "Compared with euhydration, EID (up to 4 % weight loss) does not alter cycling performance during out-of-doors exercise conditions." In one of the studies included in this meta-analysis, however, subjects were required to cycle as far as possible in 60 min while receiving either no fluid or attempting to ingest sufficient fluid to replace the volume that had been lost in a familiarization trial (approximately 1.7 L) [8]. During the trial where fluid was given, the cyclists were able to drink a mean volume of 1.49 L, but this resulted in mean ratings of abdominal fullness in excess of 4 on a scale that went from 1 (no discomfort) to 5 (extreme discomfort) and was, unsurprisingly, accompanied by a reduced mean distance covered in 1 h (from 43.1 to 42.3 km). This should not be taken as evidence that drinking per se is harmful: rather, this study shows that drinking in amounts that cause discomfort impair performance. Other studies included in this meta-analysis are also flawed, so the conclusions have little value.

Aims of Fluid Ingestion

In their 1984 Position Stand on the prevention of thermal injuries in distance running, the American College of Sports Medicine (ACSM) said that cool water is the optimum fluid for ingestion during endurance exercise [9]. However, there is a substantial body of evidence to support the benefits of consuming drinks containing added sugars, electrolytes, and flavoring ingredients. This updated message was a key part of the 2007 ACSM Position Stand on exercise and fluid replacement [10]. Commercially formulated sports drinks are intended to serve a variety of purposes when consumed during exercise. These include:

- Supply of substrate
- Prevention of dehydration
- Electrolyte replacement

In addition, these drinks may be used for pre-exercise hydration and for postexercise recovery. To meet these various needs, the formulation of ingested beverages is likely to differ in some respects. In addition, because of the biological variability between individuals, no single formulation will be optimal for all athletes in all situations. Issues of taste preference further complicate the formulation of the ideal product. Although manipulation of the composition to suit individual circumstances is not practical for commercial manufacturers, an understanding of the issues involved will allow consumers to make the best choice from the options available. The major components of sports drinks that can be manipulated to alter their functional properties are shown in Table 15.1. To some extent these factors can be manipulated independently, although addition of increasing amounts of CHO or electrolyte will generally be accompanied by an increase in osmolality, and alterations in the solute content will have an impact on taste characteristics, mouth feel, and palatability.

The recommendation for cool water was based largely on the taste preferences of individuals during exercise in a warm environment, where chilled beverages are certainly preferred and are consumed in greater quantities [11]. There is an additional reason for taking cool beverages: it helps cool the body and thereby enhances performance [12].

Table 15.1 Characteristics of carbohydrate–electrolyte sports drinks

CHO type
CHO concentration
Osmolality
Electrolyte content—sodium and potassium
Anion content
pH and buffer capacity
Carbonation level
Flavoring ingredients
Vitamin content
Other ingredients (amino acids, herbal extracts, etc.)

Carbohydrate Content: Concentration and Type

The Advantages of Adding Carbohydrates to Sports Drinks

CHO ingested during exercise enters the blood glucose pool, provided that it is absorbed. If performance is limited by the size of the body's limited endogenous liver or muscle glycogen stores, then exercise capacity should be improved when CHO is consumed. Several studies have shown that the ingestion of glucose during prolonged intense exercise prevents the development of hypoglycemia by maintaining or raising the circulating glucose concentration; consequently, beneficial effects of CHO ingestion are seen during both cycling [13] and running [14]. As well as prolonging the time for which a fixed power output can be sustained, improvements are seen in time-trial performance, in multiple sprint performance, and in the performance of skilled tasks, as well as in a reduced subjective perception of effort [10]. This ergogenic effect may be related to a sparing of the body's limited muscle glycogen stores by the oxidation of the ingested CHO, but increasing CHO availability can improve performance even when glycogen availability is not limiting [15]. The primary benefit of ingested CHO is probably its role in supplementing the endogenous stores in the later stages of exercise to allow a relatively high rate of CHO oxidation to be maintained. This may stem from the fact that the amount of oxygen required to perform a given task is about 10 % less when CHO is used as a fuel than when fat is used [16].

As well as providing an energy substrate for the working muscles, the addition of CHO to ingested drinks promotes water absorption in the small intestine, provided the concentration is not too high. Because of the role of sugars and sodium in promoting water uptake in the small intestine, it is sometimes difficult to separate the effects of water replacement from those of substrate and electrolyte replacement when CHO–electrolyte solutions are ingested. Below et al. [17] have shown that ingestion of CHO and water have separate and additive effects on performance capacity and concluded that ingestion of dilute CHO solutions optimizes performance. Most subsequent literature reviews have come to the same conclusion.

Types of Carbohydrate

In most of the early studies, the ingested CHO was in the form of glucose. However, sucrose and oligosaccharides have also been shown to be effective in maintaining the blood glucose concentration when ingested during prolonged exercise; as a result they also improve endurance capacity [17]. There are theoretical advantages in the use of sugars other than glucose. Substitution of glucose polymers for glucose allows an increased CHO content without an increased osmolality and may also have taste advantages, but the available evidence suggests that the use of glucose polymers or sucrose rather than free glucose does not alter the blood glucose response or the effect on exercise performance.

Ingested fructose is generally less readily oxidized than glucose or glucose polymers, but a mixture of glucose and fructose in equal amounts may have some advantages. There may be benefits in including different kinds of CHO in a sports drink, including free glucose, sucrose, fructose, and maltodextrin. This has taste implications which may influence the amount consumed. Providing a number of transportable solutes may maximize the rate of sugar and water absorption in the small intestine [18], and this can increase total exogenous CHO oxidation [19].

Concentration of Carbohydrate

The optimum concentration of sugar to be added to drinks depends on individual circumstances. A high CHO concentration delays gastric emptying, thus reducing the amount of fluid that is available for absorption, but also increases the rate of CHO delivery. If the CHO concentration is high enough to result in a markedly hypertonic solution, a transient net secretion of water into the intestine will result, and this will actually increase the risk of dehydration [20]. This may explain why high sugar concentrations (>10 %) often result in gastrointestinal disturbances [21]. Where the primary need is to supply an energy source during exercise, increasing the sugar content of drinks increases the delivery of CHO to the site of absorption in the small intestine. Beyond a certain limit, however, simply increasing CHO intake no longer increases the rate of oxidation of exogenous CHO [22]. Dilute glucose–electrolyte solutions may be as effective, or even more effective, in improving performance as more concentrated solutions [23–25]; adding as little as 90 mmol/L glucose may improve endurance performance [24].

Osmolality

It has become common to refer to CHO–electrolyte sports drinks as isotonic drinks, as though tonicity is their most important characteristic. While the osmolality of sports drinks is certainly important, the composition of the drinks and the nature of the solutes are of greater importance.

Although osmolality is often identified as an important factor influencing the rate of gastric emptying of liquid meals, there seems to be rather little effect of variations in the concentration of sodium or potassium on the emptying rate, even when this substantially changes the osmolality of ingested drinks. The effect of increasing osmolality is most consistently observed when nutrient-containing solutions are studied, and the most significant factor influencing the rate of gastric emptying is the energy density [26, 27]. There is an acceleration of emptying when glucose polymer solutions are substituted for free glucose solutions with the same energy density: at low (about 40 g/L) concentrations, this effect is small, but it becomes appreciable at higher (180 g/L) concentrations. Where the osmolality is the same (as in the 40 g/L glucose solution and 180 g/L polymer solution), the increasing energy density is of far greater significance in slowing the rate of gastric emptying [27]. This effect may therefore be important when large amounts of energy must be replaced after exercise, but is unlikely to be a major factor during exercise where more dilute drinks are taken.

Water absorption occurs largely in the proximal segment of the small intestine, and although water movement is itself a passive process driven by local osmotic gradients, it is closely linked to the active transport of solutes. Osmolality therefore plays a key role in the flux of water across the upper part of the small intestine. Net flux is determined largely by the osmotic gradient between the luminal contents and intracellular fluid of the cells lining the intestine. Absorption of glucose is an active, energy-consuming process linked to the transport of sodium. The rate of glucose uptake is dependent on the luminal concentrations of glucose and sodium, and dilute glucose–electrolyte solutions with an osmolality which is slightly hypotonic with respect to plasma will maximize the rate of water uptake [28]. Solutions with a very high glucose concentration will not necessarily promote an increased glucose uptake relative to more dilute solutions but, because of their high osmolality, will cause a net movement of fluid into the intestinal lumen, resulting in a transient loss of body water; this will exacerbate any pre-existing dehydration [20]. The absorption of fructose is not an active process in man: it is absorbed more slowly than glucose and promotes less water uptake, but combinations of sugars that are absorbed by different mechanisms can promote increased CHO and water uptake and increase the contribution of exogenous CHO to substrate oxidation during exercise [18, 19].

Most of the popular sports drinks are formulated to have as osmolality close to that of body fluids and are promoted as isotonic drinks, but based on evidence that was discussed earlier, hypotonic solutions are more effective when rapid rehydration is desired [29]. A higher osmolality is inevitable when large amounts of CHO are included in sports drinks, but the optimum amount of CHO necessary to improve exercise performance may be less than previously thought [23–25].

Electrolyte Composition and Concentration

Sound evidence indicates that the only electrolyte that should be added to drinks consumed during exercise is sodium, which is usually added in the form of sodium chloride [20]. Sodium stimulates sugar and water uptake in the small intestine and helps maintain extracellular fluid volume. Most soft drinks of the cola or lemonade variety contain virtually no sodium (1–2 mmol/L); sports drinks commonly contain about 10–30 mmol/L; oral rehydration solutions intended for use in the treatment of diarrhea-induced dehydration, which may be fatal, have higher sodium concentrations, in the range 30–90 mmol/L. A high sodium content, although it may stimulate jejunal absorption of glucose and water, tends to make drinks unpalatable. This is a problem as in order to stimulate consumption it is important that drinks intended for ingestion during or after exercise should have a pleasant taste. The choice of anion that accompanies sodium in functional beverages has implications for osmolality, taste, pH, stability, and other factors.

When the exercise duration is likely to exceed 3–4 h, there may be advantages in adding sodium to drinks to avoid the danger of hyponatremia. This problem has been reported to occur in such events when excessively large volumes of low-sodium drinks are taken. Physicians dealing with individuals in distress at the end of long-distance races often deal with hyperthermia and hypernatremia associated with dehydration, but it has become clear that a small number of individuals at the end of very prolonged events may be suffering from hyponatremia in conjunction with either hyperhydration [30, 31] or hypohydration [32]. All the reported cases have been in slower participants in marathon, ultramarathon, or triathlon events, and there are few reports of cases where the exercise duration is less than 4 h. The factors associated with this hyponatremia have been extensively discussed by Noakes [3]. Some important points are generally ignored, however. Most studies have not assessed pre-exercise sodium status, so there is no way of knowing whether hyponatremia was present in affected individuals prior to exercise. We should also recognize that the standard reference range embraces 95 % of the normal population, so we would expect 2.5 % of any sample to be either above or below the reference range. Whether the standard reference range of 135–145 mmol/L that is usually derived from hospital patients is also applicable to participants in endurance events is not known.

These reports indicate that some supplementation with sodium salts may be required in extremely prolonged events where large sweat losses can be expected and where it is possible to consume large volumes of fluid. Most CHO–electrolyte sports drinks intended for consumption during prolonged exercise contain a sodium concentration of about 10–30 mmol/L, which is rather lower than the normal sweat sodium concentration (Table 15.2). The formulation of these drinks might represent a reasonable strategy for providing substrates and water (although it can be argued that a higher sodium concentration would enhance water uptake and that a higher CHO content would increase substrate provision), but these recommendations may not be appropriate in all circumstances.

Table 15.2 Approximate concentration (mmol/L) of the major electrolytes present in sweat, plasma, and intracellular (muscle) water in humans (values collated from a variety of sources; see Maughan [4] for further details)

	Plasma	Sweat	Intracellular
Sodium	137–144	40–80	10
Potassium	3.5–4.9	4–8	148
Calcium	4.4–5.2	3–4	0–2
Magnesium	1.5–2.1	1–4	30–40
Chloride	100–108	30–70	2

Flavoring Components

Taste is an important factor influencing the consumption of fluids, a topic also discussed by Spence in Chap. 21 of this book. The thirst mechanism is rather insensitive and will not stimulate drinking behavior until some degree of dehydration has occurred [33]. This absence of a drive to drink is reflected in the rather small volumes of fluid that are typically consumed during exercise: in endurance running events, voluntary intake seldom exceeds about 0.5 L/h [34]. Sweat losses normally exceed this, even in cool conditions, and a fluid deficit is therefore almost inevitable. Several factors influence palatability, and the addition of a variety of flavors has been shown to increase fluid intake relative to that ingested when only plain water is available. Hubbard et al. [35] and Szlyk et al. [36] found that the addition of flavorings resulted in an increased consumption (by about 50 %) of fluid during prolonged exercise. More recently, Bar-Or and Wilk [37] reported that the fluid intake of children during exercise is much influenced by taste preference. The children were presented with a variety of flavored drinks, but the only one that resulted in sufficient fluid being ingested to offset sweat losses was a grape-flavored beverage. In many of these studies, added CHOs and/or electrolytes accompanied the flavoring agent, and the results must therefore be interpreted with some caution.

Given the need to add electrolytes to fluids intended to maximize the effectiveness of rehydration, there are clearly palatability issues that influence the formulation. Effective postexercise rehydration requires replacement of electrolyte losses as well as the ingestion of a volume of fluid in excess of the volume of sweat loss [38]. When sweat electrolyte losses are high, replacement with drinks with a high sodium content can result in an unpalatable product. This can be alleviated to a large degree by substituting other sodium salts, such as sodium citrate, to replace some of the sodium chloride. The addition of CHO has a major impact on taste and mouth feel, and a variety of different sugars with different taste characteristics can be added.

Other Active Ingredients

There is a growing trend for sports drinks to include other components that might affect the functional characteristics of the drink. Many of the drinks aimed at the active individual include a range of vitamins and minerals, but it is widely agreed that these are not generally necessary. There is also little convincing evidence for beneficial effects of the addition of purported ergogenic compounds such as taurine, ginseng, aspartate, or glutamine [39]. There is rather more experimental evidence to support the use of caffeine [40], and some commercially available products now contain small amounts of this substance.

Promoting Postexercise Recovery

Key Challenges in Postexercise Recovery

An effective strategy to promote recovery from exercise is vital for all athletes during periods of heavy training and competition. The nature of the recovery process depends on the nature of the sport, the training and nutritional status of the athlete, the time in the training/competition cycle, and the time available before the next exercise bout. In some sports, where competition is infrequent and highly demanding, recovery relates to recovery between training sessions which may be carried out two or even more times per day for prolonged periods. Good examples of such sports are marathon running and professional boxing. In other sports, such as professional basketball and baseball, or in professional road cycling, the greater part of the competition season, which lasts for several months, is occupied with almost daily competition, and recovery means preparing for the next day's competition.

Key issues in the recovery process for the athlete in training are:

- Restoration of fluid and electrolyte balance
- Replenishment of fuel stores
- Stimulation of the anabolic and catabolic pathways involved in the process of adaptation
- Avoidance of illness, infection, and injury
- Psychological recovery

When recovery is discussed, the focus is usually on the first two of these processes, but the third and fourth are vital if performance capacity is to be enhanced in response to the training regimen and if overload and injury are to be avoided. Remodeling of the tissues is a vital part of the adaptation to training. For strength and power athletes, this means increasing the actin and myosin content of muscle in order to increase its force-generating capacity. For the endurance athlete, important goals of training are to increase the muscle's content of mitochondrial enzymes, to promote the growth of new capillaries, and to bring about other local changes that increase the capacity for aerobic metabolism. Overtraining, illness, and chronic fatigue are problems for some athletes, and there may be nutritional strategies to reduce the hazards that inevitably accompany the sustained intensive training that is necessary to optimize performance. Psychological recovery in preparation for the next training session is also crucial if an intensive training program is to be sustained. Numerous other homeostatic mechanisms may also be involved, including restoration of acid–base status and restoration of thermal balance.

Restoration of Fluid and Electrolyte Balance

The extent of fluid and electrolyte losses during exercise depends on the volume of sweat lost and on the composition of the sweat. This, in turn, depends on the size and surface area of the individual, the intensity and duration of the exercise, the training and acclimation status of the individual, and the environmental conditions. Sweat rates may range from 0 to about 3 L/h, with the main electrolytes lost being sodium (20–80 mmol/L), chloride (20–60 mmol/L), and potassium (4–8 mmol/L). Sweat losses vary greatly between individuals even when the other factors are similar. It is therefore difficult to predict loss and the need for replacement. Formulating general guidelines for replacement strategies is therefore almost impossible, and individualization of rehydration strategies is essential [41].

The important aspects of volume replenishment are the ingestion of an adequate quantity of fluid and replacement of electrolyte losses. The need for ingestion of fluid is obvious, and it remains common to recommend that athletes drink 1 L of fluid for each kilogram of mass lost during training. The volume of fluid consumed, however, must exceed that lost in sweat—perhaps by as much as 50 %—if effective rehydration is to be achieved [38]. This stems from the need to allow for ongoing urine and other losses during the recovery period. Restoration of euhydration (a state of fluid balance) after exercise-induced sweat losses will not be achieved without replacement of the electrolytes lost in sweat [42]. These electrolytes (especially sodium) prevent the drop in plasma sodium concentration and plasma osmolality that occurs with the ingestion of large volumes of plain water. If plasma osmolality and sodium concentration fall, a diuresis is initiated, leading to the prompt loss of a significant fraction of the ingested fluid. The thirst mechanism is also inhibited by these changes, leading to the termination of drinking before a volume sufficient to meet the body's needs has been ingested. This poses an obvious risk of dehydration.

The addition of salt to drinks can prevent these changes in plasma composition, thereby reducing the urinary loss of water and maintaining the drive to drink. If food is eaten together with water, the electrolytes present in the food eaten may achieve this, but there are many situations, especially when the recovery time is short, when athletes may not be willing or able to tolerate solid food, or where the amount and type of food eaten may not supply an adequate amount of sodium [43]. In this situation, the drinks consumed during the recovery period must provide sufficient electrolytes to replace the sweat losses. Because the electrolyte concentration of sweat varies so greatly between individuals, it is not possible to produce general recommendations that will meet the needs of all athletes in all situations. Nonetheless, the average sweat sodium concentration is about 50 mmol/L, and it is recognized that this amount of sodium must be replaced to maintain volume homeostasis. The ingestion of salt tablets is seldom necessary, but may be contemplated when sweat losses are exceptionally high or if the intake of food is limited.

Muscle Glycogen Resynthesis

CHO is the major fuel used by the muscles during high-intensity exercise, but the body's CHO stores are rather small. The glycogen store in the liver amounts to only about 80–100 g, and the total muscle glycogen content is only about 300–500 g. This is sufficient for about one to three hours of continuous exercise at moderately high intensity. However, brief high-intensity sprints cause rapid depletion of muscle glycogen. These losses must be replaced in the recovery period after training, and replenishment of the glycogen stores should be essentially complete between training sessions if an intensive training or competition program is to be sustained [44]. Although strategies to promote fat oxidation and thus spare the limited CHO stores have been extensively investigated, there are compelling reasons to use CHO as a fuel during hard exercise. About 10 % less oxygen is required when using CHO as an oxidative substrate than when using fat, so where oxygen supply is limiting, this may make a crucial difference to performance capacity.

Several factors determine the extent and time course of the replenishment of the glycogen stores after training. The body has a limited capacity for the conversion of non-CHO substrates to glucose, the precursor of glycogen. The key factor in glycogen resynthesis is therefore the amount of CHO supplied by the diet [45]. Other factors include the timing of CHO intake, the type of CHO ingested, and the type and amount of other macronutrients present in the food consumed.

For the athlete training at least once per day, and perhaps two or three times, and who also has to work or study, practical difficulties arise in meeting the demand for energy and CHO. Most athletes find it difficult to train hard in the first hour or two after a meal, and the appetite is also suppressed for a time after hard exercise. In this situation, it is particularly important to focus on ensuring a rapid recovery of the glycogen stores between training sessions. This is best achieved by consuming CHO as soon as possible after training as the rate of glycogen synthesis is most rapid at that time. At least 50–100 g (1–2 g/kg body weight) should be consumed in the first hour, and a high CHO intake continued thereafter. There is clearly a maximum rate at which muscle glycogen resynthesis can occur, and there appears to be no benefit in increasing the CHO intake to levels in excess of 100 g every 2 h [44].

The type of CHO is less crucial than the amount consumed. However, there may be some benefit from ingesting foods with a high glycemic index (i.e., those foods that produce a substantial elevation of the blood glucose concentration) at this time to ensure a rapid elevation of the blood glucose level. There is limited evidence to suggest that foods with a high glycemic index promote a more rapid rate of glycogen synthesis in the postexercise period. The addition of small amounts of protein to CHO ingested at this time can also increase the rate of glycogen synthesis [44]. This effect has been attributed to an enhanced insulin secretion, but further experimental data are needed to confirm this.

Protein Synthesis and Tissue Remodeling

It is clear that a prolonged period of training causes substantial changes in the structural and functional characteristics of skeletal muscle and other tissues. These changes take place between training sessions. There is good evidence of adaptive changes in muscle structure and function in response to only a few exercise sessions [46]. These changes are different from those that are commonly observed after a single exercise bout, when the observed responses are largely catabolic in nature and manifest themselves as muscle damage and soreness. Nonetheless, there must be adaptive changes involving synthesis of new proteins in response to each training stimulus. It is likely that the methods currently available are simply inadequate to measure these changes with any degree of reliability.

Muscle glycogen synthesis is often a priority in the recovery period, but synthesis of new proteins should perhaps be seen as being of equal or even greater importance. Because little attention has been paid to this area, it is not as yet known what factors may be manipulated to influence these processes. The hormonal environment is one obvious factor that may be important, and nutritional status can influence the circulating concentration of a number of hormones that have anabolic properties, the most obvious example being insulin. Cell volume appears to be another important regulator of metabolic processes, including the synthesis of both glycogen and protein [47]; there may be ways to manipulate cell volume in order to promote tissue synthesis. During and after exercise there may be large changes in cell volume, secondary to osmotic pressure changes caused by metabolic activity, hydrostatic pressure changes, or by sweat loss. The full significance of these findings for the postexercise recovery process and the roles they play in adaptation to a training program remain to be established. Manipulation of fluid and electrolyte balance and the ingestion of a variety of osmotically active substances or their precursors offer potential for optimizing the effectiveness of a training regimen. In an attempt to meet these multiple objectives after training, the use of milk-based drinks that provide carbohydrate, protein, and electrolytes has become popular with athletes.

Fatigue, the Brain, and Effects on Skilled Performance

It is well recognized that the brain relies on a regular supply of glucose from the blood as its primary fuel source, so anything that compromises this supply is likely to have adverse effects on its functional capacity. A fall in blood glucose has long been recognized as a possible cause of fatigue in prolonged exercise. More recent evidence does not entirely support the idea that hypoglycemia is a major factor in fatigue, but has reaffirmed that hyperthermia, dehydration, and reduced CHO availability can precipitate early onset of fatigue [48].

Dehydration is associated with impairment of some aspects of cognitive function and with unwelcome subjective symptoms such as headache, nausea, inability to concentrate, and tiredness [49]. Providing fluids before and during exercise can limit the severity of these symptoms and can help maintain performance of skilled tasks that involve judgement, hand–eye coordination, and fine motor skills. It is not entirely clear from these studies whether the primary effect is by the prevention of dehydration or as a result of the supply of CHO.

It has more recently been recognized that other aspects of central nervous system function may be affected by the metabolic, cardiovascular, and thermal changes taking place during prolonged exercise. There is some experimental evidence to support the hypothesis that changes in the activity of central serotonergic and/or dopaminergic neurons can modulate fatigue signals arising in the periphery [50]. This hypothesis proposes that an increased concentration of serotonin (5-hydroxytryptamine, 5HT) in the brain is associated with the onset of fatigue: increases in brain 5HT can result from an increase in the transport of the precursor tryptophan (*Trp*) from the plasma across the blood–brain barrier. Increasing the plasma concentration of the branched chain amino acids (BCAA), which are competitive inhibitors of Trp uptake, can reduce 5HT accumulation in the brain, and these observations have led to suggestions that BCAA should be added to drinks intended for consumption during prolonged exercise.

Although the evidence supporting a role of 5HT in the fatigue process seems strong, attempts to improve performance by the administration of BCAA during exercise have not generally been successful. In spite of these rather unpromising findings, sports drinks containing BCAA and other neurotransmitter precursor amino acids have been marketed.

Promoting Hyperhydration

It has been suggested that if dehydration is one of the major factors contributing to fatigue in prolonged exercise, then increasing body water content prior to exercise should, by analogy with glycogen loading, improve performance. Drinking large volumes of plain water provokes a diuretic response, but some degree of temporary hyperhydration appears to result when drinks with high (100 mmol/L) sodium concentrations are ingested. An alternative strategy that has been attempted with the aim of inducing an expansion of the blood volume prior to exercise is to add glycerol to ingested fluids. Glycerol exerts an osmotic action. Although its distribution in the body water compartments is variable, glycerol expands the extracellular space and some of the water ingested with the glycerol is retained [51]. However, the elevated osmolality of the extracellular space results in some degree of intracellular dehydration, the implications of which are unknown. It might be expected that the raised plasma osmolality will have negative consequences for thermoregulatory capacity. The evidence for improved thermoregulatory function and exercise performance after administration of glycerol and water prior to prolonged exercise is far from convincing [52].

Future Developments

It seems unlikely that there will be major changes to the basic formulation of the mainstream sports drinks in the foreseeable future. Commonly used formulations are based on a solid foundation of research that shows beneficial effects of ingestion of CHOs and water during exercise. There has been a move in the clinical oral rehydration field towards the use of hypotonic rather than isotonic drinks, but it is not clear that this will be adopted by the sports drink manufacturers as they favor isotonic formulations. There may be benefits of an increased level of sodium for postexercise rehydration, but this may not have any benefit during exercise for most athletes. A separate postexercise drink may be attractive, and there is scope for the addition of protein (or protein hydrolysates) to such a drink to promote protein synthesis after training. Many drinks currently contain a range of other ingredients, and it is easy to make claims for those that are attractive to the consumer. It seems likely that the mainstream sports drinks, with a simple and well-proven sugar, salt, and water combination, will continue to dominate the sports drink market.

Conclusion

Dehydration, if sufficiently severe, will impair all physiological functions, including exercise performance. Forced abstention from drinking will also have adverse effects in addition to the purely physiological actions. The level of hypohydration that affects performance will depend on the intensity, duration, and complexity of the exercise task, the ambient environmental conditions, and the experience and physiology of the individual. In addition to providing water, drinks can provide other nutrients, especially carbohydrate and electrolytes. The optimum composition of ingested drinks will depend on the circumstances, as outlined above.

References

1. Heneghan C, Perera R, Nunan D, Mahtani K, Gill P. Forty years of sports performance research and little insight gained. BMJ. 2012;345:e4797.
2. Goulet EDB. Effect of exercise-induced dehydration on endurance performance: evaluating the impact of exercise protocols on outcomes using a meta-analytic procedure. Br J Sports Med. 2013;47:679–86.
3. Noakes TD. Waterlogged. Champaign: Human Kinetics; 2012.
4. Maughan RJ. Fluid and electrolyte loss and replacement in exercise. J Sports Sci. 1991; 9(Suppl 1):117–42
5. Judelson DA, Maresh CM, Anderson JM, et al. Hydration and muscular performance—does fluid balance affect strength, power and high-intensity endurance? Sports Med. 2007;37:907–21.
6. Cheuvront SN, Kenefick R. Dehydration: physiology, assessment, and performance effects. Compr Physiol. 2013;4:257–85.
7. Goulet EDB, Dion T, Savoie FA. Does mild hypohydration really reduce cycling endurance performance in the heat? Medi Sci Sports Exerc. 2014;46:207.
8. Robinson TA, Hawley JA, Palmer GS, et al. Water ingestion does not improve 1-h cycling performance in moderate ambient-temperatures. Eur J Appl Physiol. 1996;71:153–60.
9. American College of Sports Medicine. Position stand on prevention of thermal injuries during distance running. Med Sci Sports Exerc. 1984;16:ix–xiv.
10. Sawka MN, Burke LM, Eichner ER, Maughan RJ, Montain SJ, Stachenfeld NS. Exercise and fluid replacement. Med Sci Sports Exerc. 2007;39:377–90.
11. Mundel T, King J, Collacott E, Jones DA. Drink temperature influences fluid intake and endurance capacity during exercise in a hot, dry environment. Exp Physiol. 2006;91:925–33.
12. Lee JKW, Shirreffs SM, Maughan RJ. Cold drink ingestion improves exercise endurance capacity in the heat. Med Sci Sports Exerc. 2008;40:1637–44.
13. Coggan AR, Coyle EF. Carbohydrate ingestion during prolonged exercise: effects on metabolism and performance. Ex Sport Sci Rev. 1991;19:1–40.
14. Tsintzsas OK, Liu R, Williams C, Campbell I, Gaitanos G. The effect of carbohydrate ingestion on performance during a 30-km race. Int J Sport Nutr. 1993;3:127–39.
15. Pitsiladis Y, Maughan RJ. The effects of exercise and diet manipulation on the capacity to perform prolonged exercise in the heat and cold in trained humans. J Physiol. 1999;517:919–30.
16. Krogh A, Lindhard JL. The relative values of fat and carbohydrate as sources of muscular energy. Biochem J. 1920;14:290–363.
17. Below P, Mora-Rodriguez R, Gonzalez-Alonso J, Coyle EF. Fluid and carbohydrate ingestion independently improve performance during 1 h of intense cycling. Med Sci Sports Exerc. 1995;27:200–10.
18. Shi X, Summers RW, Schedl HP. Effect of carbohydrate type and concentration and solution osmolality on water absorption. J Appl Physiol. 1995;27:1607–15.
19. Jentjens RLPG, Moseley L, Waring RH, Harding LK, Jeukendrup AE. Oxidation of combined ingestion of glucose and fructose during exercise. J Appl Physiol. 2004;96:1277–84.
20. Evans GH, Shirreffs SM, Maughan RJ. Acute effects of ingesting glucose solutions on blood and plasma volume. Br J Nutr. 2009;101:1503–8.
21. Davis JM, Burgess WA, Slentz CA, Bartoli WP, Pate RR. Effects of ingesting 6% and 12% glucose/electrolyte beverages during prolonged intermittent cycling in the heat. Eur J Appl Physiol. 1988;57:563–9.
22. Jeukendrup AE, McLaughlin J. Carbohydrate ingestion during exercise: effects on performance, training adaptations and trainability of the gut. In: Maughan RJ, Burke LM, editors. Sports nutrition: more than just calories—triggers for adaptation. Nestle Nutrition Institute Workshop Series, Vol. 69. Basel: Karger AG; 2011. p. 1–17.
23. Smith JW, Pascoe DD, Passe DH, et al. Curvilinear dose—response relationship of carbohydrate (0–120 g· h^{-1}) and performance. Med Sci Sports Exerc. 2013;45:336–41.

24. Maughan RJ, Bethell L, Leiper JB. Effects of ingested fluids on homeostasis and exercise performance in man. Exp Physiol. 1996;81:847–59.
25. Watson P, Shirreffs SM, Maughan RJ. Effect of dilute CHO beverages on performance in cool and warm environments. Med Sci Sports Exerc. 2012;44:336–43.
26. Vist GE, Maughan RJ. The effect of increasing glucose concentration on the rate of gastric emptying in man. Med Sci Sports Exerc. 1994;26:1269–73.
27. Vist GE, Maughan RJ. The effect of osmolality and carbohydrate content on the rate of gastric emptying of liquids in man. J Physiol. 1995;486:523–31.
28. Wapnir RA, Lifshitz F. Osmolality and solute concentration—their relationship with oral rehydration solution effectiveness: an experimental assessment. Pediatr Res. 1985;19:894–8.
29. Schedl HP, Maughan RJ, Gisolfi CV. Intestinal absorption during rest and exercise: implications for formulating oral rehydration beverages. Med Sci Sports Exerc. 1994;26:267–80.
30. Noakes TD, Goodwin N, Rayner BL, Branken T, Taylor RKN. Water intoxication: a possible complication during endurance exercise. Med Sci Sports Exerc. 1985;17:370–5.
31. Noakes TD, Norman RJ, Buck RH, Godlonton J, Stevenson K, Pittaway D. The incidence of hyponatremia during prolonged ultraendurance exercise. Med Sci Sports Exerc. 1990;22: 165–70.
32. Hiller WDB. Dehydration and hyponatraemia during triathlons. Med Sci Sports Exerc. 1989;21:S219–21.
33. Hubbard RW, Sandick BL, Matthew WT, et al. Influence of thirst and fluid palatability on fluid ingestion during exercise. In: Gisolfi CV, Lamb DR, editors. Perspectives in exercise science and sports medicine, vol. 3. Carmel: Benchmark; 1990. p. 39–95.
34. Noakes TD. Fluid replacement during exercise. Exerc Sports Sci Rev. 1993;21:297–330.
35. Hubbard RW, Sandick BL, Matthew WT. Voluntary dehydration and alliesthesia for water. J Appl Physiol. 1984;57:868–75.
36. Szlyk PC, Sils IV, Francesconi RP, Hubbard RW, Armstrong LE. Effects of water temperature and flavoring on voluntary dehydration in men. Physiol Behav. 1989;45:639–47.
37. Bar-Or O, Wilk B. Water and electrolyte replenishment in the exercising child. Int J Sports Nutr. 1996;6:93–9.
38. Shirreffs SM, Taylor AJ, Leiper JB, Maughan RJ. Post-exercise rehydration in man: effects of volume consumed and sodium content of ingested fluids. Med Sci Sports Exerc. 1996;28: 1260–71.
39. Maughan RJ. Risks and rewards of dietary supplement use by athletes. In: Maughan RJ, editor. Sports nutrition. Oxford: Wiley-Blackwell; 2014. p. 291–300.
40. Burke L, Desbrow B, Spriet L. Caffeine for sports performance. Champaign: Human Kinetics; 2013.
41. Maughan RJ, Shirreffs SM. Development of individual hydration strategies for athletes. Int J Sport Nutr Exerc Metab. 2008;18:457–72.
42. Maughan RJ, Owen JH, Shirreffs SM, Leiper JB. Post-exercise rehydration in man: effects of electrolyte addition to ingested fluids. Eur J Appl Physiol. 1994;69:209–15.
43. Maughan RJ, Leiper JB, Shirreffs SM. Restoration of fluid balance after exercise-induced dehydration: effects of food and fluid intake. Eur J Appl Physiol. 1996;73:317–25.
44. Maughan RJ, Burke LM. Practical nutritional recommendations for the athlete. In: Maughan RJ, Burke LM, editors. Sports nutrition: more than just calories—triggers for adaptation. Nestle Nutrition Institute Workshop Series, Vol. 69. Basel: Karger AG; 2011. p. 131–49.
45. Ivy JL, Katz AL, Cutler CL, Coyle EF. Muscle glycogen synthesis after exercise: effects of time of carbohydrate ingestion. J Appl Physiol. 1988;64:1480–5.
46. Green HJ, Jones S, Ball-Burnett ME, et al. Early muscular and metabolic adaptations to prolonged exercise training in man. J Appl Physiol. 1991;70:2032–8.
47. Lang F. Effect of cell hydration on metabolism. In: Maughan RJ, Burke LM, editors. Sports nutrition: more than just calories—triggers for adaptation. Nestle Nutrition Institute Workshop Series, Vol. 69. Basel: Karger AG; 2011. p. 131–49.
48. Maughan RJ, Shirreffs SM, Watson P. Exercise, heat, hydration and the brain. J Am Coll Nutr. 2007;26:604S–12.

49. Shirreffs SM, Merson SJ, Fraser SM, Archer DT. The effects of fluid restriction on hydration status and subjective feelings in man. Br J Nutr. 2004;91:951–8.
50. Meeusen R. Exercise, nutrition and the brain. Sports Med. 2014;44:47–56.
51. Riedesel ML, Allen DL, Peake GT, Al-Qattan K. Hyperhydration with glycerol solutions. J Appl Physiol. 1987;63:2262–8.
52. van Rosendal SP, Strobel NA, Osborne MA, Fassett RG, Coombes JS. Performance benefits of rehydration with intravenous fluid and oral glycerol. Med Sci Sports Exerc. 2012;44:1780–90.

Chapter 16
Energy Drinks: The Elixirs of Our Time

Frances R. Ragsdale

Keywords Energy drinks • Caffeine • Taurine • Ginseng • Ginkgo • Red Bull • Monster • Government oversight

Key Points

1. Energy drinks have become very popular in spite of or because of their ability to maintain a nebulous ingredient content and identity.
2. Market value ($27.5 billion 2013) and sales of energy drinks (4.8 billion L/year 2011) continue to grow. Sales are expected to reach $37.1 billion by 2017.
3. Caffeine is the primary active ingredient of energy drinks.
4. Adverse effects appear to be related to caffeine toxicity, although it has been difficult to document adverse effects in controlled study conditions.
5. Government oversight focuses on adolescents and youth and is widely variable across different nations and regulatory bodies.

Introduction

Drinkable nutritional tonics and elixirs date back to the proprietary medicines of the eighteenth, ninetieth, and twentieth centuries in Western civilization, but have been present in the international market since the beginning of time. These proprietary tonics promoted physical enhancement, mental well-being, or treatment for almost any malady and were sold not only at medicine shows and from street vendors but

F.R. Ragsdale, Ph.D. (✉)
Department of Biology, Winona State University, 226 Pasteur Hall, Winona, MN 55987, USA
e-mail: fragsdale@winona.edu

© Springer International Publishing Switzerland 2016
T. Wilson, N.J. Temple (eds.), *Beverage Impacts on Health and Nutrition*,
Nutrition and Health, DOI 10.1007/978-3-319-23672-8_16

also at retail stores with enormous popularity. With the introduction of US government oversight into food safety at the start of the twentieth century, most of these street remedies/tonics disappeared. Red Bull emerged in the early 1990s from South Asia and entered the global market creating a new consumable category—"energy drink" (ED). Today, there are hundreds of brands of these drinks, and they have become the new elixir for much of the younger population. They have a nebulous ingredient list, although most brands contain sugars, caffeine, vitamins, and herbal extracts. The marketing of EDs offer consumers "a lifestyle in a can"; their use is associated with high-intensity lifestyles as lived (in the popular imagination) by pro-athletes and musicians. Users are promised more energy, improved mood, better cognition, faster reaction times, and enhanced athletic prowess. Research that supports these claims is nearly as difficult to find as is identifying a common ingredient list. This chapter discusses the past, present, and future of EDs as a commonly consumed and sometimes controversial type of beverage.

Defining Energy Drinks Is Intended to Be Difficult

Historical Perspective

During the eighteenth and nineteenth centuries in the United States and Europe, proprietary tonics promised physical enhancement, mood improvement, or the treatment of almost any ailment. These concoctions were sold not only at medicine shows and from street vendors but also at retail stores. The popularity of these "medicine show" syrups was enormous. The appearance of Glucozade (i.e., Lucozade), manufactured in 1927, might be considered to be one of the first EDs of the twentieth century [1]. Glucozade was formulated to provide a boost of energy to patients suffering from the flu or other common illnesses. In 1929 the manufacturers removed the G from the brand to create Lucozade. This drink contained under 50 mg of caffeine and distribution of this product was quite restrictive, promoting the use of this beverage to patients in hospital and clinical settings, and the general public was aware of the brand because of advertising that "Lucozade aids recovery."

By the 1930s and with the advent of chemical patents, the Wiley Law and US FDA governmental regulations through the Bureau of Chemistry, elixirs and tonics disappeared from mainstream markets. However, outside of the United States and Europe, manufacturers throughout Asia continued their alchemy with elixirs. In the 1960s the Japanese drink Livonian D, an energy brew manufactured and distributed by Taisho Pharmaceutical, gained popularity among factory workers and club-goers for that added energy kick [2]. But distribution of this product, with its medicinal taste and distribution in a nondescript brown bottle, did not expand to the world market. Lucozade continued to be manufactured and in 1985 shifted its campaign emphasis away from the treatment of the sick to "replace lost energy." But it wasn't until the release of Red Bull in Austria and the world market in 1987 that the modern caffeinated ED was born [3]. This ED is a carbonated modification of an elixir from Asia, which was then released in Thailand and then Australia, Europe, and the United States. Red Bull became synonymous with the term "energy drink" and today holds the top sales position worldwide. Due in part to the success of Red Bull, other manufacturers followed suit and released EDs into the global market; in fact, by the mid-2000s there were over 500 brands being sold [4]. These products include Monster, Rockstar, and a plethora of other drinks, each with its own proprietary mix of ingredients.

Today, most EDs, especially those manufactured for the Western market, are highly sweetened beverages with "proprietary" ingredients such as carbonation, stimulants, taurine, vitamin B complex, ginkgo, and ginseng. Some use artificial sweeteners, while others have purposefully migrated away from synthetics to alternative sugar substitutes such as honey, agave nectar, or high-fructose corn syrup. Most, if not all, of the ingredients of EDs have purported health benefits, although none of these benefits have been directly tied to ED consumption; documentation of physiological changes following consumption of a single serving of an ED such as Red Bull or Monster remains very difficult to quantify [5–7].

Manufacturers' Market Strategy and Audience

EDs were initially marketed as energy supplements to young adult males who perceived themselves as playing and partying hard. Manufacturers were marketing an image of a macho, virile athlete where an average man could escape the conformity of his nine-to-five job and follow his dreams. Miller [8] argues this media campaign was all about selling the "jock identity." ED brand names like Full Throttle, No Fear, or Bawls screamed to this audience, but even Red Bull and Monster appealed to this population. The manufacturers of Monster even stated that their brand name needed to speak to the macho adult image—their lifestyle [9]. In the first 5 years, young men constituted 85 % of the consumer market suggesting the product designs portrayed a macho, virile, thrill-seeking lifestyle [8]. ED manufacturers promoted this jock identity by sponsoring professional sports events in BMX racing, snowboarding, skateboarding, and car racing (NASCAR, Formula One, and stock cars). This marketing strategy creates brand recognition and establishes a pool of celebrities ready to endorse ED products. Red Bull may have gone to unusual ends with this campaign by devoting about one-third of its marketing budget to it. These investments include ownership of a US soccer franchise (Red Bull New York), several Austrian soccer teams, and a hockey team as well as several racecar sponsorships. This strategy proved profitable as over this time frame ED sales experienced double-digit growth.

Thus, the original public image of EDs revolved around a male-dominated, very masculine lifestyle. In order to attract females to this market, brand names like Vixen, Go Girl, and Enviga appeared with campaign slogans that suggested the ED consumer should strive to be "all that she can." The manufacturers again targeted athletic young women. Collectively, this group of young adult ED consumers became the "young transitionals," young adults who appeared to have spending money in their pockets and time to party [10].

EDs have always appealed to the physically active adult populations even when they are not extreme competitors but just athletes looking to boost their performance or fuel their workout. Part of this marketing strategy focused on the health-conscious consumer and exercise enthusiast. This group includes people with a preference for organic and fair-trade products and who had shifted away from artificial sweeteners and synthetics to natural sugar substitutes. Monster, manufactured under the Hansen beverage company, with its appeal of all natural ingredients, fell into this category. Many weight-conscious consumers also fell into this category. Advertising dollars were also spent to target individuals interested in non-mainstream sports, including rock climbing, parasailing, and BASE jumping [11]. Caffeine is one of the best-tested ergogenic supplements to enhance performance. And moderate caffeine consumption by an athlete through the ingestion of an ED just seemed to make sense as a way of supplying nutrients and a short boost of energy for that exercise workout.

Soon the market strategy evolved to exploit other populations who might be interested in quick energy, including college students. Campaigns to recruit "Collegiate Ambassadors Teams" and "Active Brand Partners" were developed to appeal to college students who might need additional energy to study for that "all-nighter" or as a coffee alternative to get ready for the 8 o'clock class. At least one manufacturer marketed "Finals" gift boxes of their beverages. These types of marketing campaigns are very inexpensive and highly successful.

One of the latest market niches appears to be advertising to target the growing population of aging baby boomers. With celebrity endorsements like John Ratzenberger (i.e., Cliff Clavin character from Cheers), to advertisements appearing in senior-specific publications (AARP magazine), the ED industry has focused its attention on senior citizens [12].

Sales of all EDs were up between 14–21 % in 2012 [13] and 6.7 % in 2013, which contrasts with a relatively stagnant soda market [14]. Taking into account the size of a single serving (8.4–12 oz), EDs cost about four times more than carbonated soda. Despite the high price and the potential health risks of EDs, customers are still ingesting these drinks in large quantities. Red Bull continues to be the most popular ED; the company grossed $10.9 billion worldwide in 2012. Red Bull and Monster are the top selling EDs in the United States; they sold $3.4 billion (43 % of market sales) and $3.1 billion dollars (39 % of market sales), respectively, in the first half of 2013 [14]. Rockstar is the third most popular brand in the United States with 10 % of the market share. This ED company moved away from the athlete-exercise market to appeal to individuals attracted to the "Hollywood"/celebrity high energy, sex appeal lifestyle [15]. Overall, the per capita consumption of EDs in the United States grew to 22 eight-ounce (approx. 5 L) servings in 2012 [16]. This equates to the consumption of one ED drink every 3 days for every person in the United States.

US and European markets remain the primary audience for EDs, but some companies worry that these markets may have approached saturation. The new growth arenas may be in markets such as the Far East and South America. Brazil was the site for recent market growth by Red Bull, and with the 2014 World Cup and the 2016 Olympics in Rio de Janeiro, the country is poised to become a central distribution site. Furthermore, China, with the growth of the middle/upper class, exposure of the populous to the Western lifestyle, and an increase in disposable personal income, is an enticing future market for ED manufacturers. The ED market continues to exploit new niches and attract/convert alternate caffeine users to their beverages while striving to maintain the initial consumer base as they mature and age.

Part of this market strategy, to reach all audiences, was to avoid labeling EDs as beverages and to instead market them as functional supplements. The vague nature of the definition of "energy drink" is a marketing tactic where the term loosely coined by the beverage industry refers to any caffeinated beverage with other ingredients that are purported to provide the consumer with a boost of energy [17]. Labeling requirements for products distributed as supplements must comply with the Dietary Supplement Health and Education Act of 1994, although these guidelines are quite lax and do not require specific caffeine content labeling. Other definitions for EDs minimize the use of the term "caffeinated" and substitute the more generic term "stimulant" into the proprietary mix. Adding to the ambiguity of the initial definition, a stimulant can now include caffeine, guarana, theobromine, theophylline, or even sugar. This marketing strategy has allowed manufacturers to explore alternate ingredient markets and different consumer bases. Lax FDA oversight for these supplements has allowed ED manufacturers great latitude in the labeling of their products.

Recently, some companies in the beverage industry have begun to strategically market EDs as a broader category of "beverage" by providing precise caffeine information as mandated by the Nutrition Labeling and Education Act of 1990 [18]. Rockstar and Monster EDs began this practice in 2013. Prior to this market push, some labels listed both caffeine and guarana extracts separately even though guarana is a plant-based product naturally rich in caffeine [19]. Theophylline and theobromine are purine alkaloids and also minor metabolites of caffeine metabolism commonly found in teas and chocolate. These methyl xanthines are currently making their way to EDs due to their stimulatory effect.

General Content of Nebulous Energy Drinks

In general, EDs contain sugar and caffeine as well as a mixture of herbs (e.g., ginseng and ginkgo biloba), amino acids, electrolytes, and vitamins designed to be palatable to the "Western" diet and taste buds. Most EDs have a slight medicinal taste, and most manufacturers suggest consuming the beverages cold for optimal flavor. Most are consumed like soft drinks. While the chapter in this book by Nelson, Rush, and Wilson discusses general properties of beverage ingredients, a more detailed description of some of ED ingredients is helpful.

Caffeine

Chemically, caffeine is a methyl xanthine that is quickly absorbed by the gut within about 20 min of ingestion. Once in the blood, the half-life of caffeine is highly variable from 2 to 10 h, depending on individual metabolism, life events, and habits [20, 21].

Systematically, caffeine is known to cause the release of catecholamines (e.g., epinephrine), alter glycogen/free fatty acid metabolism, and promote CNS/muscle attenuation. It may also be associated with an increase in ambulatory blood pressure. Intracellularly caffeine stimulates the $\beta1$ and $\beta2$ adenosine receptors, blocks the actions of adenosine (specifically the A1 and A2 adenosine receptors), and inhibits the actions of phosphodiesterase, thereby increasing intracellular calcium and cAMP concentrations [22]. Both cellular mechanisms increase cAMP and elevate intracellular calcium levels that can lead to enhanced excitability in cells. Most research supports caffeine's effect on performance via this competition for the adenosine receptor (for reviews, see [22–24]).

The average consumption of caffeine by the adult public is between 200 and 400 mg/day (3.5–5.3 mg/kg/day), making the developed world a major potential market for EDs [25]. This amount of caffeine will produce a mild stimulatory effect in most people. At this level, caffeine has also been shown to improve athletic performance by postponing fatigue, increasing muscle efficiency, and improving oxygen utilization (e.g., [26, 27]). Caffeine has been shown to enhance psychomotor function [28, 29].

The caffeine levels in EDs are highly variable (6–242 mg/serving) [30]. Based on the serving sizes of many of these beverages (8.4–12 oz), the caffeine content falls well within the range of ordinary coffee, tea, or carbonated soda (134–245 mg/serving, 48–175 mg/serving, 65 mg/350 mL, respectively). Most ED manufacturers designate an 8–12 oz serving size, similar to the original Red Bull and Monster packaging. Then Monster heralded the 16 oz, pop-top can containing two servings, but in reality this volume is intended to be fully consumed immediately upon opening due to the fact that the container cannot be resealed. Even so, the amount of caffeine in this volume is still similar to that contained in two large espresso coffee drinks. Now EDs come in all sizes, including 24 oz cans with resealable tops (Fig. 16.1).

Excess caffeine may cause irritability of the body's excitable tissues (e.g., nerves and muscles), creating feelings of irritability, nausea, anxiety, restlessness, and gastrointestinal disturbances to name a few. Furthermore, caffeine intoxication is medically defined as consumption over 400 mg. A lethal dose is estimated to be 10 g [31], a level that exceeds the caffeine content of a single serving of Red Bull or Monster by a factor of at least 20. Caffeine may be chemically addictive, although the literature is not consistent in this regard. The lack of an absolute understanding of how caffeine functions in the human body is surprising given the global popularity of caffeine.

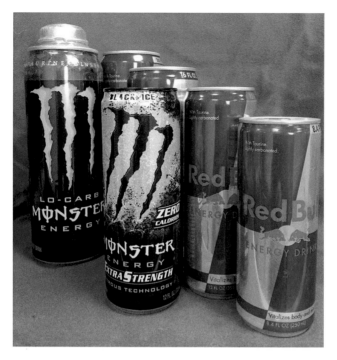

Fig. 16.1 Can sizes of Red Bull and Monster available in convenience stores across the United States. The 8.4 oz (250 mL) Red Bull is the smallest container on the market. The 12 oz (355 mL) containers are the most common and are labeled as a single serving. Beyond this size companies tend to categorize a serving as 8 oz (240 mL). The 20 oz (591 mL) Red Bull is labeled as 2.5 servings, but has a pop-top. The 24 oz (710 mL) Monster is the size that comes in a resealable container and is labeled as containing 3 servings

Sugar

In addition to the caffeine, many EDs contain considerable amounts of sugar (21–34 g/8 oz serving) [32], although some brands can also be found in a "diet" form where nonnutritive synthetic sweeteners are used. At least part of the energy "kick" associated with this type of beverage has been attributed to ingestion of carbohydrates [33] (also see chapters by White and Nicklas and by Maughan and Shirreffs in this book). Again, some manufacturers have shifted away from high-fructose corn syrup and maltodextrin to honey and agave nectar. So far it has been hard to tease apart the influence of caffeine and sugar in combination with the other ED additives, such as the herbs and amino acids. Some EDs do come in an artificially sweetened version (e.g., Red Bull, Monster, Rockstar). Currently, only one study has compared the influence of Red Bull and low-calorie Red Bull [5]. In this study there was a significant glycemic response by the high-calorie version compared to the low-calorie drink, but there were no cardiovascular or renal differences between the two groups.

Taurine

Taurine is a naturally occurring organic acid. Aside from being synthesized by the body, taurine can also be ingested from dietary sources including meat and dairy products. Supplements of up to 3000 mg/day are considered safe [34]. The approximate dose of taurine in an ED is about 1000 mg/8 oz serving. The addition of this amino acid is not specified for any one physiological action, but may be added for its purported neurological or neuromuscular effects. Taurine is known to play a role in neuroprotection and neurotransmitter actions and cardiovascular function. Its cellular actions occur by modulating intracellular calcium via several mechanisms. Taurine may be beneficial in skeletal muscle training, or with diabetic care, heart disease, or anxiety due to its purported antioxidant activity [35–39], but not at the levels delivered in an ED. Other investigators have suggested that taurine in conjunction with caffeine can enhance cognitive performance, although mental improvements that are specific to this combination have not been demonstrated [35, 40, 41]. The influence of taurine in EDs is not well understood, but its use may be an attempt to offset the stimulatory/adverse effects of caffeine and carbohydrates on body systems.

Vitamins

The B vitamin complex is a group of eight vitamin compounds and is another prototypical ingredient found in many EDs. For example, the concentration of B vitamins in Red Bull is over the recommended daily intakes set by the Institute of Medicine of the National Academy of Sciences. According to the manufacturers, this amount of B vitamins will allow the consumer to "sail through his day" [10]. A single serving of a typical ED contains about 350–500 % of the recommended daily allowance of vitamin B6 and 100–200 % of both B12 and B3 [42].

In general, these vitamins maintain muscle tone and skin development and enhance immune and nervous system function, which adds to a feeling of alertness and may increase the body's metabolism. Vitamin B12 is involved in blood cell production and nerve development at the systemic level and DNA synthesis at the cellular level. There is no reliable information concerning the tolerable upper limits (TUL) for vitamin B12 for adults or youth [43]. Vitamin B6 is involved in basic cellular metabolism and heme synthesis and with nerve development. The TUL for vit. B6 is 100 mg/day for adults and then is scaled down in a weight-dependent fashion for youth so that ingestion of one 16 oz (0.47 L) with 10 mg of B6 is about one-third the limit. Niacin is associated with cell metabolism and has been used in the treatment of lipidemia. The TUL for niacin is 35 mg/day for adults and drops to 20 mg/day for adolescents. This means that one 16 oz (0.47 L) serving of an ED exceeds the consumption limit that is likely to pose no risk. A single case of hepatotoxicity has been reported in a young adult after the consumption of 10 EDs and is the smallest reported dose for niacin toxicity [44].

Because B vitamins are involved in metabolism and stress management, this gives manufacturers of EDs an additional way by which they can target their energetically active consumer base. Apart from vitamin B12, most B vitamins are not stored in the body when consumed in excess, but rather overdoses are eliminated in the urine following discontinued use. This generality that B vitamins cannot be overdosed due to their water solubility suggests to the public that EDs are safe for consumption. However, acute physiologic responses may occur with overindulgence even in terms of 3 or more cans per day, and this might be especially important to consider when discussing consumption by adolescents.

Herbal Ingredients

Ginseng is an extract from the *Panax ginseng* plant that has long been used as folk medicine designed to boost immune actions, improve mood, and increase energy levels [45, 46]. The plant extract is typically processed prior to its marketable form. Ginseng has been used by some Asian cultures as a remedy for various diseases and to promote longevity [47]. Physiologically, ginseng is known to interfere with blood clotting, enhance cellular glucose absorption, and act as a stimulant [48]. Ginseng and some of its metabolites may enhance cognition. The amount of ginseng varies widely in EDs (2–200 mg in 8 oz) [49], and the actual influence ginseng has when ingested in an ED has yet to be determined (see [50]).

Ginkgo, a plant extract from the *Ginkgo biloba* tree, is thought to have nootropic effects and cerebral and cardiovascular benefits related to antiplatelet activation and improve blood circulation, many of which are related to the extract's antioxidant properties [51]. The incidence of hemorrhage or excessive bleeding associated with ginkgo seems to be associated with dosages that exceed 240 mg/day, an amount that greatly exceeds that in EDs (15–20 mg/8 oz) [30]. In fact, this level of ginkgo extract is well below that associated with any cardiovascular or neurologic benefit or risk.

Guarana is a supplement derived from the berries of the *Paullinia cupana* plant. These berries contain about twice as much caffeine as the comparable amount of coffee beans. The extract also contains other xanthine alkaloids, including theobromine and theophylline. The amount of guarana added to EDs is highly variable ranging from 1.4 to 300 mg/12 oz serving [49]. Most functions of guarana mirror, and are commonly thought to be from, the effects of caffeine, including antioxidant activities, improved mental cognition, and enhanced lipid metabolism. However, Scholey and Haskell [52] conclude that the slower metabolism and absorption of guarana compared to caffeine may allow more sustained effects.

Other minor herbal ingredients usually present in trace amounts in EDs include L-carnitine, glucuronolactone, creatine, L-theanine, and extracts of the acai berry.

Promises and Performance

ED slogans, such as "Giving Wings to People and Ideas," "Unleash the Beast," "… made to help hard working people," and "Designed for those who lead active lifestyles," all make strong promises [11, 15, 53]. Some studies do suggest improved athletic performance, improved alertness (psychomotor performance) and cognitive abilities, as well as elevation of mood [5, 26, 40, 54, 73]. Yet, overall, there is little evidence that the combined ingredients in EDs, aside from caffeine, contribute to any of these abilities (see review by [55]).

Caffeine ingestion below the 400 mg/day threshold, and well within the limits of many EDs, has been associated with improved performance in swimming and cycling and has been attributed to nutrient mobilization and/or CNS and muscular system attenuation. An increase in reaction times and an increase in pain tolerance have also been attributed to a single serving of Red Bull [5]. The levels of caffeine in a single serving of ED have also been associated with enhanced mood and cognitive abilities [40].

Adverse Effects

As with all caffeine-containing beverages, EDs are not suitable for all consumers and deaths have been reported worldwide [56]. ED manufacturers have issued warnings against excessive consumption of their products. Most of these drinks have additional warning labels on their cans against consumption by children, by women who are pregnant or breast-feeding, and by caffeine-sensitive individuals. The actual wording of these warnings varies from paragraph-length warnings of potential side effects to simple recommendations that these beverages are inappropriate for children and pregnant women. All of these warnings are predominantly based on the caffeine consumption guidelines. Recommendations regarding caffeine consumption for pregnant women suggest an upper limit of 200 mg/day. A dosage of less than 100 mg/day of caffeine for children and 2.5 mg/kg/day for adolescents has also been suggested [57]. Yet over half of ED sales continue to be to adolescents and persons under the age of 26 [58].

According to the FDA, there were a total of 276 adverse events and 34 fatalities associated with ED consumption between 2004 and early 2014. Furthermore, data from poison control centers indicate that most ED-related calls are related to children under the age of 6 [59]. Most of the adverse effects attributed to EDs have been suggested to be due to an excessive intake of caffeine no matter the age of the consumer [60, 61]. These adverse effects may include insomnia, anxiety, restlessness, nausea, vomiting, seizure, and tachycardia that can result in cardiac arrest. Lethal caffeine toxicity has been suggested to occur at 10 g of caffeine. Caffeine toxicity may include nausea, anxiety, headaches, seizures, and restlessness and cardiovascular incidences including hypokalemia and cardiac arrest [31]. The curious fact concerning most of the documented fatalities is that medical crisis occurred below the lethal threshold. An overdose of caffeine from EDs would mean ingesting between 10 and 30 servings (5–15 cans), depending on the specific ED consumed. With adolescents and young adult populations, there is concern that these individuals lack the knowledge to avoid an excessive intake of caffeine. In particular, children and adolescents may be vulnerable to the effects of caffeine, especially effects involving critical thinking and impulse control concerning discrimination of risks associated with reckless behaviors [62].

Further concerns about young ED consumers come when EDs are mixed with alcohol. Although not the first cocktails to mix caffeine with alcohol, these sweetened beverages fit right into the party scene associated with the ED lifestyle. These caffeine-loaded cocktails are thought to diminish an individual's perception of drunkenness and facilitate excess consumption. Discussion of these concerns and review of the literature for EDs mixed with alcohol is outside the scope of this chapter.

A literature search using PubMed with the key words of "energy drink" yielded 204 citations. Of these, only 19 reports were found dealing with EDs alone and deleterious or fatal psychiatric, cardiovascular, or neurologic conditions. Among young adults, the incidence of sudden cardiac death following the consumption of EDs is very low. Even with EDs alone, naïve drinkers may experience traumatic consequences with excess consumption due to caffeine sensitivity. Of the 19 deleterious cases reported in the primary literature, of which there were nine fatalities, extenuating circumstances including excessive exercise and ED consumption or alcohol-ED ingestion triggered fatal cardiovascular events. The cardiovascular conditions included atrial fibrillation, reverse takotsubo cardiomyopathy, supraventricular tachycardia, spontaneous coronary artery dissection, and hypertension [63].

All nine fatalities were attributed to acute ED abuse with or without alcohol or other additives. Of the psychiatric conditions, all appeared to be exacerbations of sleeplessness, medication withdrawal, or blatant ED abuse. Most of the cases passed the 400 mg/day threshold for excessive caffeine consumption, but none of these cases of adverse effects came anywhere close to the 10 g lethal dosage for caffeine. No reports were found in the literature where a single serving of an ED caused adverse effects.

Seifert and others [59] reviewed the information from the US National Poison Data System and found that only 0.2 % of all calls (over 2.3 million in total) were related to EDs including the effects of EDs plus additional additives (alcohol); of these inquiries, only a very small portion were for EDs alone. Most of the reports were for abuse of EDs by male children and were nonfatal [61]. To put this in perspective statistically, if the same number of promiscuous individuals in the target market group engaged in unprotected sexual activities, more will be infected with chlamydia than overdose on EDs.

Governmental Oversight

Over 166 countries permit the sales of EDs, making the global market worth $27.5 billion in 2013 [64]. Since the introduction of EDs into the market, at least six countries have banned the products outright, and numerous others have created legislation in an attempt to keep them out of the hands of children and "at-risk" populations. One country, France, banned EDs, but 12 years later repealed that action in favor of legislation governing the distribution of the products. In November of 2014,

Lithuania adopted a law that made the sale of EDs to minors punishable by a fine up to 400 litas (116 euros, $146). Earlier in 2014 Saudi Arabia banned the sale of EDs in educational and sports facilities as well as from government buildings [64, 65].

Today, many of the ED manufacturers in the United States have accepted the American Beverage Association guidelines for responsible labeling that include caffeine content disclosure, warnings for vulnerable groups, discourage marketing of EDs as a mixer for alcoholic beverages, and avoidance of marketing to children. Most of the litigation against ED manufacturers is for wrongful death suits, but governmental oversight and legislation focus on the marketing campaigns that appear to target the young and vulnerable. Red Bull and Monster have been scrutinized for their marketing campaigns.

Most of the regulatory actions/oversight include requirement of warning labeling on the packaging and restricting/preventing sales to youth or young adults in nightclubs, bars, and taverns. The sale of EDs to children and adolescents is restricted in many countries throughout the world. In 2011, Canada moved to define EDs as foods rather than a "natural health product," thereby placing these beverages under tougher governmental regulation effective [66]. In the United States, FDA actions included issuing warning letters to companies marketing malt beverages with caffeine [67] and the FDA vowing to continue to investigate the addition of caffeine to numerous products [68].

The FDA's investigation into caffeine appears to be, at least in part, due to an open letter from a group of pediatricians and researchers concerned for the welfare of children [69]. Several states, including Maryland, Kentucky, and Tennessee, have all proposed legislation to ban EDs from minors, although no state has proceeded to an outright ban [70]. The Center for Science in the Public Interest, a consumer advocacy group, has asked the FDA to lower the caffeine limits of beverages to that of cola-styled sodas (71 mg/12 oz). Canadian physicians have also joined in this campaign to restrict energy drink usage by juveniles [71]. However, the European Food Safety Authority (EFSA) recently released its draft assessment on caffeine consumption and concluded that 400 mg of caffeine a day from all sources is not a safety concern [72, 74].

Conclusion

From 2006 to 2012, ED consumption almost doubled from just over 600 million gallons to just under 1200 million gallons sold worldwide. EDs continue to be sold front and center in most convenience stores throughout the United States. Colorful marketing campaigns and sport sponsorships continue to attract young and now older, energy-desiring consumers. Brands with catchy names (e.g., Rockstar, Jolt, Full Throttle, Lightning Bolt) continue to provide suggestions of that caffeine "punch" for the weary potential consumer. Worries by the general public over excessive caffeine consumption will continue to arise as modern societies are driven to compete harder in work, social, and athletic settings. Concerns over excess consumption of caffeine-laced alcoholic cocktails by the public, but especially our youth and young adult populations, will keep ED products in the news and will have concerned citizens appealing for legislative intervention in order to protect our vulnerable populations (i.e., young people) around the world. Even the news of litigation surrounding wrongful deaths due to overconsumption of EDs seems to fuel the market for these beverages and has catapulted the ED market to new annual highs for capital earnings for the manufacturers. Continual maneuvering by manufacturers of EDs to tweak the proprietary ingredients of their products and reach new markets ensures that these energy elixirs are here to stay.

References

1. Ward L. The history of Lucozade. 2014. http://www.thefactsite.com/2009/03/history-of-lucozade.html. Accessed Nov 2014.
2. Japanese Energy Drinks. 2014. Lipovitan D. http://japaneseenergydrinks.blogspot.com/. Accessed July 2014.
3. Red Bull Website. http://www.redbull.com/us/en. Accessed Mar 2015.
4. Breda JJ, Whiting SH, Encamacao R, Norberg S, Jones R, Reinap M, Jewell J. Energy drink consumption in Europe: a review of the risks, adverse health effects, and policy options to respond. Front Public Health. 2014;2:134.
5. Ragsdale FR, Gronli TD, Batool N, et al. Effect of Red Bull energy drink on cardiovascular and renal function. Amino Acids. 2010;38:1193–200.
6. Denzer DL, Ragsdale FR, Wilson T. Effects of Monster energy drink on cardiovascular and renal function. FASEB J. 2009;23:901.1.
7. Wilson T, Gronli TD, Batool SN, et al. Effect of Red Bull energy drink on cardiovascular and renal function. FASEB J. 2008;22:888.3.
8. Miller K. Wired: energy drinks, jock identity, masculine norms, and risk taking. J Am Coll Health. 2008;56:481–90.
9. Zegler J. Creating a monster. 2007. http://www.bevindustry.com/articles/84551-creating-a-monster-1. Accessed Mar 2015.
10. Clemency K. Moms are consuming more energy drinks than you might think. 2013. http://www.nielsen.com/us/en/insights/news/2013/moms-are-consuming-more-energy-drinks-than-you-might-think.html. Accessed Jan 2014.
11. Red Bull.com. 2010. http://energydrink-us.redbull.com/red-bull-editions?medium=tsa&gclid=CLiyyePs88MCFYRAaQodzwcARQ&gclsrc=aw.ds. Accessed June 2010.
12. Daily News. Energy Drink market to target senior citizens in 2012 as way to experience more active lifestyle. 2012. http://www.nydailynews.com/life-style/health/energy-drink-market-target-senior-citizens-2012-experience-active-lifestyle-article-1.999786. Accessed July 2013.
13. Munarriz R. Soda sales are slipping, but energy drinks are still buzzing. 2014. Daily Finance Investor Center. http://www.dailyfinance.com/on/energy-drink-sales-rising-soda-sales-slipping/. Accessed July 2014.
14. Caffeine Informer. Top selling energy drink brands. 2014. http://www.caffeineinformer.com/the-15-top-energy-drink-brands. Accessed July 2014.
15. Rockstarenergy.com. 2012. http://rockstarenergy.com/. Accessed Aug 2014.
16. Wong V. Overcaffeination concerns haven't dented energy drink on mood, memory and information processing in healthy volunteers without caffeine abstinence. Psychopharmacology (Berl). 2013;158:322–8.
17. Woodruff C. What's really behind the jolt in your energy drink? 2013. http://www.huffingtonpost.com/2013/08/15/energy-drinks-health-danger-caffeine-ingredients-n-3750826.html. Accessed Jan 2014.

18. Engber D. Who made that energy drink? 2013. The New York Times Magazine. www.nytimes. com/2013/12/08/magazine/who-made-that-energy-drink.html?module=Search&mabReward =relbias%3Ar. Accessed June 2014.
19. Schimpl FC, daSilva JF, Goncalves JF, Mazzafera P. Guarana: revisiting a highly caffeinated plant from the Amazon. J Ethnopharmacol. 2012;150:14–31.
20. Debry G. Coffee and health. New Barnet: Johy Libbey; 1994.
21. Nehlig A, Debry G. Caffeine and sports activity: a review. Int J Sport Med. 1994;15:215–23.
22. Fredholm BB, Battig K, Holmen J, Nehlig A, Zvartau EE. Actions of caffeine in the brain with special reference to factors that contribute to its widespread use. Pharmacol Rev. 1999;51:83–133.
23. Sokmen B, Armstrong LE, Kraemer WJ, Casa DJ, Dias JC, Judelson DA, Maresh CM. Caffeine use in sports: considerations for the athlete. J Strength Cond Res. 2008;22:978–86.
24. Spriet LL, Gibala MJ. Nutritional strategies to influence adaptations to training. J Sports Sci. 2004;22:127–41.
25. Schreiber GB, Maffeo CE, Robins M, Masters MN, Bond AP. Measurement of coffee and caffeine intake: implications for epidemiologic research. Prev Med. 1988;17:280–94.
26. Forbes SC, Candow DG, Little JP, Magnus C, Chilibeck PD. Effect of Red Bull energy drink on repeated Wingate cycle performance and bench-press muscle endurance. Int J Sport Nutr Exerc Metab. 2007;17:433–44.
27. Sinclair CJ, Geiger JD. Caffeine use in sports. A pharmacological review. J Sports Med Phys Fitness. 2000;40:71–9.
28. Stuart GR, Hopkins WG, Cook C, Cairns SP. Multiple effects of caffeine on simulated high-intensity team-sport performance. Med Sci Sports Exerc. 2005;37:1998–2005.
29. Foskett A, Ali A, Gant N. Caffeine enhances cognitive function and skill performance during simulated soccer activity. Int J Sport Nutr Exerc Metab. 2009;19:410–23.
30. Consumer Reports.org. The buzz on energy-drink caffeine. 2012. http://www.consumerreports.org/cro/magazine/2012/12/the-buzz-on-energy-drink-caffeine/index.htm. Accessed Jan 2013.
31. Nawrot P, Eastwood JS, Rotstein J, Hugenholt A, Feeley M. Effects of caffeine on human health. Food Addit Contam. 2003;20:1–30.
32. Sifferlin A. "What's in your energy drink?". 2013. CNN. http://www.cnn.com/2013/02/06/health/time-energy-drink/. Accessed 7 July 2014.
33. Adan A, Serra-Grabulosa J. Effects of caffeine and glucose, alone and combined, on cognitive performance. Hum Psychopharmacol. 2010;25:310–7.
34. Zeratsky K. Taurine is listed as an ingredient in many energy drinks. What is taurine? Is it safe?. 2005. http://www.mayoclinic.org/healthy-living/nutrition-and-healthy-eating/expert-answers/taurine/faq-20058177. Accessed June 2014.
35. Seidl R, Peyri A, Nicham R, Hauser E. A taurine and caffeine-containing drink stimulates cognitive performance and well-being. Amino Acids. 2000;19:635–42.
36. Kang YS, Ohtsuki S, Takanaga H, Tomi M, Hosoya K, Terasaki T. Regulation of taurine at the blood–brain barrier by tumor necrosis factor-alpha, taurine and hypertonicity. J Neurochem. 2002;83:1188–95.
37. Franconi F, Loizzo A, Ghirlanda G, Seghieri G. Taurine supplementation and diabetes mellitus. Curr Opin Clin Nutr Metab Care. 2006;9:32–6.
38. Kong WX, Chen SW, Li YL, Zhang YJ, Wang R, Min L, Mi X. Effects of taurine on rat behaviors in three anxiety models. Pharmacol Biochem Behav. 2006;83:271–6.
39. Xu YJ, Arneja AS, Tappia PS, Dhalla NS. The potential health benefits of taurine in cardiovascular disease. Exp Clin Cardiol. 2008;13:57–65.
40. Alford C, Cox H, Wescott R. The effects of Red Bull energy drink on human performance and mood. Amino Acids. 2001;21:139–50.
41. Warburton DM, Bersellini E, Sweeney E. An evaluation of a caffeinated taurine drink on mood, memory and information processing in healthy volunteers without caffeine abstinence. Psychopharmacology (Berl). 2001;158:322–8.
42. Higgins JP, Tuttle TD, Higgins CL. Energy beverages: content and safety. Mayo Clin Proc. 2010;85:1033–41.

43. Dietary Reference Intakes. 2012. http://iom.edu/Activities/Nutrition/SummaryDRIs/~/media/Files/Activity%20Files/Nutrition/DRIs/ULs%20for%20Vitamins%20and%20Elements.pdf. Accessed 15 Mar 2015.
44. Vivekanandarajah A, Ni S, Waked A. Acute hepatitis in a woman following excessive ingestion of an energy drink: a case report. J Med Case Rep. 2001;5:227.
45. Kennedy DO, Scholey AB, Wesnes KA. Dose dependent changes in cognitive performance and mood following acute administration of Ginseng to healthy young volunteers. Nutr Neurosci. 2001;4:295–310.
46. Kennedy DO, Scholey AB, Wesnes KA. Modulation of cognition and mood following administration of single doses of Ginkgo biloba, ginseng, and a ginkgo/ginseng combination to healthy young adults. Physiol Behav. 2002;75:739–51.
47. Nam MH, Kim SI, Liu RJ, et al. Proteomic analysis of Korean ginseng (*Panax ginseng* C. A. Meyer). J Chromatogr B Analyt Technol Biomed Life Sci. 2005;815:147–55.
48. Chung KF, Dent G, McCusker M, Guinot P, Page CP, Barnes PJ. Effect of a ginkgolide mixture (BN52063) in antagonizing skin and platelet responses to platelet activating factor in man. Lancet. 1987;1:248–50.
49. Loeb H. Do the ingredients in energy drinks work? 2010. MensHealth.com. http://www.menshealth.com/mhlists/effectiveness_of_energy_drinks/printer.php. Accessed Jan 2014.
50. Smith I, Williamson EM, Putnam S, Farrimond J, Whalley BJ. Effects and mechanisms of ginseng and ginsenosides on cognition. Nutr Rev. 2014;72:319–33.
51. Ramassamy C. Emerging role of polyphenolic compounds in the treatment of neurodegenerative diseases: a review of their intracellular targets. Eur J Pharmacol. 2006;545:51–64.
52. Scholey A, Haskell C. Neurocognitive effects of guarana plant extract. Drugs Fut. 2008;33:869.
53. Monster Energy.com. http://www.monsterenergy.com/. Accessed June 2014.
54. Gendle MH, Smucker DM, Stafstrom JA, Helterbran MC, Glazer KS. Attention and reaction time in university students following consumption of Red Bull. Open Nutr J. 2009;3:8–10.
55. McLellan TM, Liberman HR. Do energy drinks contain active components other than caffeine. Nutr Rev. 2012;70:730–44.
56. Kapner AD. Ephedra and energy drinks on college campuses. 2011. The Higher Education Center for Alcohol and Other Drug Abuse and Violence. http://www.higheredcenter.org/files/product/energy-drinks.pdf. Accessed Nov 2011.
57. Seifert SM, Seifert JL, Hershorin ER, Lipshultz SE. Health effects of energy drinks on children, adolescents, and young adults. Pediatrics. 2011;127:511–28.
58. Arria AM, O'Brien MC, Griffiths RR, Crawford PB. Physicians open letter to FDA. 2013. http://graphics8.nytimes.com/packages/pdf/business/BestofScienceLetter_v22.pdf. Accessed June 2014.
59. Seifert SM, Seifert SA, Schaechter JL, et al. An analysis of energy-drink toxicity in the National Poison data system. Clin Toxicol. 2013;51:565–74.
60. Stallings VA, Yaktine AL, editors. Committee on nutrition standards for foods in schools. Nutrition standards for foods in schools: leading the way toward healthier youth. Washington, DC: National Academies Press. http://www.nap.edu/catalog/11899.html.
61. Burrows T, Pursey K, Neve M, Stanwell P. What are the health implications associated with the consumption of energy drinks? A systematic review. Nutr Rev. 2013;71:135–48.
62. Temple JL. Caffeine use in children: what we know, what we have to learn, and why we should worry. Neurosci Biobehav Rev. 2009;33:793–806.
63. Goldfarb M, Tellier C, Thanassoulis G. Review of published cases of adverse cardiovascular events after ingestion of energy drinks. Am J Cardiol. 2014;113:168–72.
64. Yahoo News. AFP. Lithuania enacts ban on energy drinks for minors, in global first. 2014. http://news.yahoo.com/lithuania-enacts-ban-energy-drinks-minors-global-first-131726749.html;_ylt=A0LEVoDDPLBUWEoAdQoPxQt.;_ylu=X3oDMTByMG04Z2o2BHNlYwNzcgRwb3MDMQRjb2xvA2FjMmQ2dGlkAw. Accessed Nov 2014.
65. Yahoo News. AFP. Saudi Arabia bans adverts for energy drinks. 2014. https://uk.news.yahoo.com/saudi-arabia-bans-adverts-energy-drinks-121839209.html#COiRHv6. Accessed Nov 2014.

66. Health Canada. Caffeinated energy drinks. 2012. http://www.hc-sc.gc.ca/fn-an/prodnatur/caf-drink-boissons-eng.php. Accessed 7 July 2014.

67. US Dept. of Health and Human Services. Questions and answers: caffeinated alcoholic beverages. 2010. http://www.fda.gov/Food/IngredientsPackagingLabeling/FoodAdditivesIngredients/ucm233726.htm. Accessed Dec 2010.

68. Hamburg M. Caffeine in food and dietary supplements: examining safety. 2013. US Dept. of Health and Human Services. http://www.fda.gov/newsevents/speeches/ucm363925.htm. Accessed Dec 2014.

69. Meier B. Doctors urge FDA to restrict caffeine in energy drinks. 2013. New York Times. http://www.nytimes.com/2013/03/20/business/doctors-urge-fda-to-restrict-caffeine-in-energy-drinks.html?_r=0. Accessed Dec 2014.

70. Stoll JD, Esterl M, Robinson F. Lithuania bans energy drinks sales to minors: country hopes other EU nations will follow its lead. 2014. Wall Street Journal. http://www.wsj.com/news/articles/SB10001424052702304908304579563690934380648. Accessed June 2014.

71. Doctor's Nova Scotia. CBC news. 2012. http://www.cbc.ca/news/canada/nova-scotia/story/2012/11/15/ns-energy-shot-death.html. Accessed Dec 2014.

72. Harrison-Dunn A. EFSA: 400mg of caffeine a day is safe. 2015. http://www.nutraingredients.com/Regulation-Policy/EFSA-400mg-of-caffeine-a-day-is-safe?utm_source=newsletter_special_edition&utm_medium=email&utm_campaign=16-Jan-2015. Accessed Jan 2015.

73. Ivy JL, Kamer L, Ding Z, Wang C, Bernard JR, Liao YH, Hwang J. Improved cycling time-trial performance after ingesting a caffeine energy drink. Int J Sport Nutr Exerc Metab. 2009;19:61–78.

74. Ferdman R. The American energy drink craze in two highly caffeinated charts. 2014. Accessed June 2014. http://qz.com/192038/the-american-energy-drink-craze-in-two-highly-caffeinated-charts/#/h/56821,2/. Accessed Mar 2015.

Chapter 17
The Nutritional Value of Bottled Water

Norman J. Temple and Kathryn Alp

Keywords Bottled water • Mineral water • Tap water

Key Points

1. In 2011 estimated sales of bottled water in the USA were 9.2 billion gallons (34.8 billion liters), generating 11.1 billion dollars in revenue.
2. Bottled water typically costs several thousand times more than tap water.
3. Bottled water is heavily marketed with advertising often suggesting superiority to tap water but the supporting evidence is weak.
4. There are several compelling reasons to choose tap water rather than bottled water (except in specific circumstances).

Introduction

The human body is approximately 60 % water by weight; around 75 % of lean tissue is made up of water, and less than 25 % of adipose tissue consists of water. Water performs many essential functions including the transport of nutrients and waste products around the body, acting as a medium for metabolic reactions, maintaining the structure of large molecules, and acting as coolant by way of sweat. Water is essential to survival, and 2–3 L of water a day is recommended for the average person representing a minimum of 1 mL/kcal. This amount, contrary to popular belief, comes not only from beverages but also from water found in food.

N.J. Temple (✉) • K. Alp
Centre for Science, Athabasca University, Athabasca, AB, Canada, T9S 3A3
e-mail: normant@athabascau.ca

© Springer International Publishing Switzerland 2016
T. Wilson, N.J. Temple (eds.), *Beverage Impacts on Health and Nutrition*,
Nutrition and Health, DOI 10.1007/978-3-319-23672-8_17

Approximately 800 million people do not have access to clean water, and up to eight million people die annually as a result of water-related diseases [1]. Waterborne illness was first scientifically demonstrated by John Snow in London in 1854 when he showed that drinking water was the source of an epidemic of cholera. Many similar discoveries since then are a major reason why bottled water has been viewed favorably, especially in regions of developing countries where drinking water poses a risk of infection. However, in developed countries with safe tap water, bottled water is consumed for a many reasons, including preference in taste, perceived risks from tap water, and convenience [2, 3].

Evian was the first company to commercially produce bottled water, which was done in France in 1829. Since then the bottled water industry has grown to behemoth proportions. Bottled water sales in the USA have grown at an impressive pace since 2000 and now represent one of the largest beverage categories by volume, second only to soft drinks. In 2011, global consumption of bottled water was estimated at 61.4 billion US gallons (232 billion liters). In 2011 estimated sales in the USA were 9.2 billion gallons (34.8 billion liters), generating revenue of 11.1 billion dollars [4]. Only 1.3 % of the bottled water was imported. The average annual consumption in the USA is estimated at approximately 111 L/person [4], equivalent to 304 mL per person per day. However, this may be an underestimate as data from NHANES based on surveys between 2005 and 2010 indicates that the average American adult consumed 502 mL/day of bottled water, a quantity that is approaching the volume of tap water consumed (644 mL/day) [5]. The global leader in per capita consumption per year is Mexico, averaging 248 L. Six of the ten top consumers are European countries [4].

Bottled water is heavily marketed and is sold at every corner store and grocery store with a seemingly ubiquitous availability. The reason for this heavy marketing stems from its price which is several thousand times that of tap water [6]. A price comparison with gasoline is informative: gasoline in Canada costs between $1.20 and $1.40 per liter, whereas bottled water costs 50c or 60c per liter for cheaper brands and up to $2 or $3 per liter for some imported brands. Four companies dominate the global bottled water market: Nestlé and Danone are the giants, but Coca-Cola and PepsiCo have also entered the arena, focussing primarily on the US market [4].

Labeling Laws and Regulation of Bottled Water

Bottled water falls under different labeling laws than other food products, and laws are further detailed regarding different types of bottled water. According to the regulations of the Food and Drug Administration (FDA), bottled water includes products with the following labels: bottled water, drinking water, artesian water, mineral water, sparkling bottled water, spring water, and purified water [7].

"Purified water" may be purified by distillation, deionization, or reverse osmosis and may be labeled as such. Artesian water is collected from a well that taps an aquifer (a layer of porous rock, sand, and earth that contains water) [8]. Mineral water is extracted from an underground water source. It must contain at least 250 ppm total dissolved solids. Minerals and trace elements may not be added to the water [8]. Spring water is derived from an underground formation from which water flows naturally to the surface. It must be collected only at the spring or through a borehole that taps the underground formation feeding the spring. Its composition cannot be altered [8]. If the water contains a sufficient amount of dissolved gases, such as carbon dioxide, it will be effervescent (i.e., "sparkling"). Sparkling bottled water may not contain a larger concentration of gases than it had when it emerged from its source. Water products with added carbonation, such as soda water (or club soda) and tonic water, are regulated by the FDA as soft drinks [7].

Additionally, flavored water and nutrient-added beverages are becoming increasingly popular—these are just bottled water with added flavoring or nutrients such as vitamins or electrolytes [7].

Bottled water sold in Canada must adhere to similar regulations as those in the USA. The federal responsibility for the regulation of bottled water sold in Canada is shared by Health Canada and the Canadian Food Inspection Agency [9].

When a brand of bottled water sold in the USA or Canada contains significant amounts of a particular mineral, this is usually indicated on the label. If a mineral appears in the nutrition facts label, but not the ingredients label, then the mineral was added artificially. However, sometimes a mineral is present in the water when collected in addition to being added as a supplement for reasons to taste, health claim, or appearance.

While the names of the various types of bottled water are regulated, and bottling companies must adhere to safety regulations [8], they do not need to disclose whether the purified water being sold is merely tap water. Indeed, much of the bottled water sold in North America is, in actuality, municipal tap water that has gone through an additional purification step, such as distillation, reverse osmosis, filtration, or ozonation.

The following three categories are used in the European Union (EU): (1) natural mineral water originating from a ground water reservoir; (2) spring water, namely, groundwater in a natural state but bottled at the source; and (3) other types of bottled drinking water, including bottled tap water [10]. North American and European standards are similar as far as health claims on bottled water with the exception that the USA permits a health claim regarding fluoride and dental caries.

Nutrient Content

Mineral Content

Bottled water can be a significant source of a wide variety of minerals, including calcium, magnesium, and sodium [10]. Surveys carried out in North America in the 1990s reported that the mean concentrations of calcium in bottled spring water and bottled mineral water are 18 and 100 mg/L, respectively; for magnesium the values are 8 and 24 mg/L; while for sodium they are 4 and 371 mg/L [11]. It must be stressed that the actual values vary widely depending on the actual source of the water. The DRI values for adults (as mg/day) are 1000–1200 for calcium, 310–420 for magnesium, and 1300–1500 for sodium. This indicates that bottled spring water is a very minor source of these minerals. But if an adult drinks one liter per day of bottled mineral water, then this may make a significant contribution to the intake of all three of these minerals. The potential nutritional benefit of this source of calcium and magnesium is counterbalanced by the sodium.

Bottled waters, especially those originating in Europe, are highly variable in their content of calcium, magnesium, and sodium [11]. As with mineral water from North America, mineral water bottled in Europe can make a significant contribution to the intake of all three minerals: around 4 % to 20 % of the DRI for both calcium and magnesium and as much as 75 % to 85 % of the DRI for sodium.

A survey was carried out in 2010 on bottled water purchased in Ottawa, Canada [12]. Concentrations of calcium and magnesium in bottled spring water and bottled mineral water were somewhat higher than the values indicated above. What was most noteworthy was that the sodium content of bottled mineral water was low compared to the above values (mean of 103 vs 371 mg/L). These findings indicate that consumption of one liter per day of bottled mineral water can contribute approximately 11 %, 14 %, and 7 % of the DRI for adults for calcium, magnesium, and sodium, respectively. It must again be stressed that the actual values vary widely depending on the actual source of the water. This survey also revealed that the potassium content of bottled water is low.

How does the mineral content of bottled water compare with tap water? North American tap water is generally a modest source of calcium and magnesium [11]. Consumption of one liter per day of tap water could contribute 3 % to 5 % of the DRI for these minerals. A positive feature of tap water is that it rarely has a high concentration of sodium (very few sources exceed 150 mg/L, whereas many brands of bottled mineral water contain >200 mg/L) [11].

The mineral content of bottled mineral water may be sufficiently high that it has a potential impact on health and is eligible for health claim approval. As intake of calcium and magnesium is often well below the DRI [13], the contribution from bottled mineral water is potentially beneficial. This may be of most clinical relevance with regard to magnesium as low intakes are associated with type 2 diabetes, metabolic syndrome, hypertension, atherosclerotic disease, sudden cardiac death, osteoporosis, migraine headache, asthma, and colon cancer [14].

Conversely, the high sodium content of some types of bottled mineral water is potentially harmful. An estimated 91 % of American adults consume in excess of the Tolerable Upper Limit for sodium (2300 mg/day) [15]. The excessive salt content found in the diets of almost everyone has been firmly established as causing an elevation in blood pressure. Conversely, a decrease in salt intake significantly lowers blood pressure, especially in persons with hypertension [16, 17]. Cohort studies have reported a positive association between salt intake and risk of both coronary heart disease and stroke [16]. Clearly, bottled mineral water is a two-edged sword.

Flouride

Flouride is a potentially contentious trace element frequently added to tap water. It attaches to dental enamel and thereby makes it stronger and more resistant to decay, especially in children [18, 19]. For that reason it is especially important that children consume an adequate amount of fluoride. Fluoridated tap water is a major source of fluoride in the USA, Canada, and many other countries. A notable disadvantage of bottled water is that the large majority of brands have low levels of fluoride [20, 21].

Safety of Drinking Water

A common reason for selecting bottled water is that many people lack confidence in the safety of tap water. There is much truth to this belief in developing countries where hundreds of millions of people lack access to safe, clean water. However, even in highly developed countries instances of contamination of tap water have occurred in recent years [22, 23]. The most common cause is microbial agents. Water can become contaminated with microbial agents from different sources that include human sewage and septic tanks, animal waste, and storm water. Discharge of wastewater can also serve as a source of contamination for municipal drinking water systems downstream from wastewater outfalls. These sources are reservoirs for various types of microbial agents including bacteria, viruses, and protozoa. Pharmaceutical contamination is also of concern. Wastewater treatment fails to completely remove all pharmaceuticals. As a result tap water contains low levels of pharmaceuticals but very little is known about the possible effects of this on human health [24].

Despite these safety concerns it would be a mistake to conclude that bottled water is therefore safer: some studies have found bacteriological contamination in bottled water [20]. Levels of inorganic substances above the recommended maximum have been reported in some surveys [10]. Arsenic is the most problematic substance in that regard. Another concern is that plastic bottles are a source of estrogen-like compounds at concentrations high enough to have a biological effect [25]. Despite these potentially important issues, those engaged in the marketing of bottled water often suggest in their advertising that their products are somehow superior to tap water.

Conclusion

The safety issues identified above have contributed to the sometimes negative view many people have of tap water. But it is vital to objectively weigh the risks and benefits of tap water and of bottled water. On balance, there are several compelling reasons to choose tap water rather than bottled water (except in specific circumstances):

- A liter of bottled water typically costs several thousand times more than tap water.
- Much of the bottled water sold in North America is merely municipal tap water that has passed through an additional purification step.
- There is no good evidence that bottled water is any safer than tap water and may, in fact, pose a greater risk from microbial agents and hazardous chemicals.
- Bottled water is damaging to the environment as it requires energy to produce the plastic bottles which often end up in landfills. It also requires far more energy to transport bottled water than tap water.

In conclusion, greater education and better public policy surrounding tap water are necessary to inform the public so that, at the very least, the decision to choose bottled water over tap water is an informed one. A good first step would be to impose a tax on bottled water.

References

1. UNESCO. World Water Day 2013. 2013. http://www.unwater.org/water-cooperation-2013/en. Accessed 18 Aug 2014.
2. Doria MF. Bottled water versus tap water: understanding consumers' preferences. J Water Health. 2006;4:271–6.
3. Saylor A, Prokopy LS, Amberg S. What's wrong with the tap? Examining perceptions of tap water and bottled water at Purdue University. Environ Manage. 2011;48:588–601.
4. Rodwan JG. Bottled Water 2011: the recovery continues. U.S. and international developments and statistics. BWR. 2012; p. 13–21. http://www.Bottledwater.org. Accessed 18 Aug 2014.
5. Drewnowski A, Rehm CD, Constant F. Water and beverage consumption among adults in the United States: cross-sectional study using data from NHANES 2005–2010. BMC Public Health. 2013;12:1068.
6. Al-Awqati Q. Thirst, and (bottled) water everywhere. Kidney Int. 2007;71:1191–2.
7. FDA. Food facts from the U.S. Food and Drug Administration. FDA regulates the safety of bottled water beverages including flavored water and nutrient-added water beverages. 2014. http://www.fda.gov/food/resourcesforyou/consumers/ucm046894. Accessed 24 Aug 2014.
8. FDA. Bottled water everywhere: keeping it safe. 2010. http://www.fda.gov/forconsumers/consumerupdates/ucm203620.htmpdf. Accessed 24 Aug 2014.
9. Canada Food Inspection Agency. Labelling requirements for water. 2014. http://www.inspection.gc.ca/food/labelling/food-labelling-for-industry/water/eng/1392050209634/1392050277168?chap=1#s3c1. Accessed 24 Aug 2014.
10. Marcussen H, Holm PE, Hansen HCB. Composition, flavor, chemical foodsafety, and consumer preferences of bottled water. CRFSFS. 2013;12:333–52.
11. Azoulay A, Garzon P, Eisenberg M. Comparison of the mineral content of tap water and bottled waters. J Gen Intern Med. 2001;16:168–75.
12. Bertinato J, Taylor J. Mineral concentrations in bottled water products, Implications for Canadians' mineral intakes. Can J Diet Pract Res. 2013;74:46–50.
13. Moshfegh A, Goldman JD, Ahuja J, et al. What we eat in America, NHANES 2005–2006: usual nutrient intakes from food and water compared to 1997 dietary reference intakes for

vitamin D, calcium, phosphorus, and magnesium. 2009. http://www.ars.usda.gov/SP2UserFiles/Place/12355000/pdf/0506/usual_nutrient_intake_vitD_ca_phos_mg_2005-06.pdf. Accessed 26 Aug 2014.

14. Rosanoff A, Weaver CM, Rude RK. Suboptimal magnesium status in the United States: are the health consequences underestimated? Nutr Rev. 2012;70:153–64.

15. Cogswell ME, Zhang Z, Carriquiry AL, Gunn JP, Kuklina EV, Saydah SH, Yang Q, Moshfegh AJ. Sodium and potassium intakes among US adults: NHANES 2003–2008. Am J Clin Nutr. 2012;96:647–57.

16. Aburto NJ, Ziolkovska A, Hooper L, et al. Effect of lower sodium intake on health: systematic review and meta-analyses. BMJ. 2013;346:f1326.

17. He FJ, Li J, Macgregor GA. Effect of longer term modest salt reduction on blood pressure: cochrane systematic review and meta-analysis of randomised trials. BMJ. 2013;346:f1325.

18. American Dietetic Association. Position of the American Dietetic Association: The impact of fluoride on dental health. J Am Diet Assoc. 1994;94:1428–31.

19. Centers for Disease Control and Prevention. Water Fluoridation Facts. 2013. http://www.cdc.gov/fluoridation/faqs/. Accessed 26 Aug 2014.

20. Lalumandier JA, Ayers LW. Fluoride and bacterial content of bottled water vs tap water. Arch Fam Med. 2000;9:246–50.

21. Quock RL, Chan JT. Fluoride content of bottled water and its implications for the general dentist. Gen Dent. 2009;57:29–33.

22. Chauret C. Tap water and the risk of microbial infection. In: Wilson T, Temple N, editors. Beverages in nutrition and health. Totowa: Humana; 2004. p. 335–48.

23. Centers for Disease Control and Prevention. Surveillance for waterborne disease outbreaks associated with drinking water and other nonrecreational water—United States, 2009–2010. MMWR. 2013;62:714–20. http://www.cdc.gov/mmwr/preview/mmwrhtml/mm6235a3.htm?s_cid=mm6235a3_w. Accessed 26 Aug 2014.

24. Strauch K. Invisible pollution. AAOHN J. 2011;59:525–32.

25. Wagner M, Oehlmann J. Endocrine disruptors in bottled mineral water: estrogenic activity in the E-Screen. J Steroid Biochem Mol Biol. 2011;127:128–35.

Part VI
Marketing of Soft Drinks and Effects of Beverage Sweeteners

Chapter 18
Marketing of Soft Drinks to Children and Adolescents: Why We Need Government Policies

Norman J. Temple and Kathryn Alp

Keywords Advertising • Marketing • In-school marketing • Food and beverage industry • Sugar-sweetened beverages • Self-regulation • Government regulation

Key Points

1. Carbonated beverage companies in the USA spent an estimated $395 million on youth-directed marketing in 2009.
2. The largest marketing expenditures are for advertising on television, in-school marketing, and supporting events.
3. Since 2006, the food and beverage industry has launched self-regulation initiatives in the USA and other countries. The industry has committed to reducing the amount of advertising for unhealthy foods that is directed to children. This also applies to in-school marketing.
4. This self-regulation has had little impact on the amount of advertising for unhealthy foods that is directed to children.
5. Government regulation remains the most effective way to control the marketing of sugar-rich, carbonated beverages, and of other unhealthy foods, to children and adolescents.

N.J. Temple (✉) • K. Alp
Centre for Science, Athabasca University, Athabasca, AB, Canada, T9S 3A3
e-mail: normant@athabascau.ca

© Springer International Publishing Switzerland 2016   269
T. Wilson, N.J. Temple (eds.), *Beverage Impacts on Health and Nutrition*,
Nutrition and Health, DOI 10.1007/978-3-319-23672-8_18

Introduction

Chapter 19 reviews the evidence that consumption of sugar-sweetened beverages (SSBs) is harmful to health. Based on an impressive body of evidence, it is now clear that these beverages play a role in obesity and in several chronic diseases of lifestyle including type 2 diabetes and coronary heart disease. A consensus has developed among those with expertise in nutrition that consumption of SSBs, as well as of other sources of added sugar, should be reduced. Alas, there are major barriers blocking the achievement of that goal. One barrier is that SSBs are heavily marketed.

This chapter surveys the marketing of SSBs with a focus on children and adolescents. This marketing is closely tied in with the marketing of other unhealthy food products. For that reason, much of the discussion is fairly general about the marketing of unhealthy food products.

Types of Marketing and Expenditure

Large corporations, including food and beverage companies, spend billions of dollars on the marketing of their products. The bulk of this money is spent on conventional advertising such as on television. However, marketing in today's world is now highly sophisticated and embraces a wide range of novel techniques. Prominent ones include using the internet, joint promotions with movies and television programs, and product packaging that targets children [1, 2].

A report published in 2012 by the Federal Trade Commission (FTC) reported expenditure on advertising by the food industry in the USA for 2009 [3]. The figures cited below are extracted from that report. These figures are an underestimate as, first, they reflect information collected in 2009, and, second, they are based on the 48 companies that provided information for the report.

Total food advertising was $9.65 billion of which $2.47 billion was for carbonated beverages and $1.03 billion for juice and noncarbonated beverages. The food industry spent approximately $1.8 billion on advertising to children and adolescents [3]. After adjusting for inflation, there was a decrease of 19.5 % from 2006, most likely caused by the recession. It seems probable that spending has rebounded since 2009. Spending was divided equally between age groups 2 to 11 and 12 to 17. Carbonated beverage companies reported $395 million in youth-directed expenditures, of which about 97 % was aimed at teenagers.

Television was used as the vehicle for a major part of food advertising directed to youth. In total the food industry spent $740 million on advertising directed to youth. Of this $62 million was for the advertising of carbonated beverages to those aged 12 to 17 but less than a million dollars for advertising of these products to those aged 2 to 11. The food industry also spent $23 million on advertising of carbonated beverages on the radio and a further $2.2 million advertising these products in the print media. A fast-growing trend is marketing using the new media such as the Internet and mobile devices. This includes using Facebook and Twitter. Here $23 million was spent advertising carbonated beverages [3], almost entirely to those aged 12 to 17.

An estimated $82 million, or 21 %, of carbonated beverage youth marketing was spent in schools. This takes the form of partnerships between beverage companies and schools (see below). However, this category of marketing decreased after 2006.

Food companies have spent increasing amounts on event marketing. The majority of this money—$79 million—has been used for the promotion of carbonated beverages to teens.

This type of marketing now accounts for almost 20 % of all marketing of carbonated beverages to youth.

Another form of promotion is athletic sponsorship. Roughly $25 million was spent by companies producing carbonated beverages in this form of marketing. These companies also spent $24 million on celebrity endorsements directed to teens.

There are yet more marketing tools used by the food industry in order to promote their products. One that is in widespread use is giving away toys and assorted other merchandise. Another marketing tool is product placement in television shows and movies. The product may be integrated into the storylines of movies or television programs appealing to children or teens.

The above numbers refer to the USA. But this is a global problem. Many sporting events around the world are sponsored by food companies. For example, Brazil staged the World Cup in 2014. This event received large sponsorship payments from McDonald's and Coca-Cola. This will be repeated in 2016 when Brazil hosts the Olympics. This inextricably links the foods sold by these companies with sport and physical fitness. The impact of this is likely to be very large as hundreds of millions of people around the world watch these events on television.

There is abundant evidence that the large majority of food advertising directed to children is for unhealthy foods. Most research in this area has focused on television advertising. A study conducted in the USA in 2009 reported that children aged 2 to 11 years watched an average of 10.9 to 12.7 food-related television advertisements per day, with 86 % of them being for products high in saturated fat, sugar, or sodium [4]. Similarly, a study carried out in 2008 in North and South America, Western Europe, Australia, and Asia evaluated television advertisements shown during children's viewing times. This global study found that between 53 % and 87 % of the food advertisements were for unhealthy foods [5].

Evidence shows that advertising to children is effective at generating a desire to consume the advertised foods [1, 6]. Studies have clearly shown that young children, especially those under the age of eight years, do not comprehend the persuasive intent of advertising [1, 6]. One result of this is that children develop a distorted understanding of which foods are part of a normal diet.

Beverage Marketing in Schools

In the 2009–2010 school year, 16,700 schools or districts in the USA had contracts with beverage companies [7]. Beverage contracts are advantageous to schools as they can provide revenue and other noncash benefits [8]. With funding to education and schools continuously being inadequate, it is no wonder schools opt for exclusive beverage contracts. However, in recent years, many jurisdictions have imposed regulations to curtail this form of marketing. Since about 2006, advertising and marketing to children in schools has also been affected by self-regulation by industry (see below).

Self-Regulation by the Food Industry

Evidence has been steadily building for many years that our diets are playing a major role in the epidemic of chronic diseases of lifestyle. There is a widespread realization that the marketing activities of the food industry are aggravating the problem. In particular, the global epidemic of obesity, both in the USA and around the world, has led to increased pressure for action. The food industry has been facing a public relations crisis, especially with regard to its heavy marketing of unhealthy food products to children. In response to this, the food industry launched self-regulation initiatives. Sometimes these have been carried out as joint actions where the food industry works together with advocates of public health in the formulation of new policies.

In 2006 the Alliance for a Healthier Generation (a joint initiative of the William J. Clinton Foundation and the American Heart Association) worked with representatives of The Coca-Cola Company, Dr Pepper Snapple Group, PepsiCo, and the American Beverage Association [7] to establish the Alliance School Beverage Guidelines [7, 9]. The industry committed to changing the type of beverages available in schools across the USA. The guidelines limit beverage sales in elementary and middle school to water, fat-free or low-fat milk, and 100 % juice. The limit on energy content means that diet soda and lower-calorie sports drinks may be sold in high schools but not regular cola drinks.

Another major initiative was launched in 2006. The Council of Better Business Bureaus partnered with 16 major food and beverage companies and launched the Children's Food and Beverage Advertising Initiative (CFBAI). The stated goal is to improve food-marketing practices [10, 11]. The companies that signed up to CFBAI pledged to market only "healthier dietary choices" or "better-for-you" foods in child-targeted media. The companies also agreed not to advertise food or beverage products in elementary schools. In addition, they agreed not to pay for or actively seek placement of their products in entertainment directed at children.

A similar policy action was launched in Canada in 2007: the Canadian Children's Food and Beverage Advertising Initiative [12]. An international version of this was launched in 2008 by the International Food & Beverage Alliance [13]. There is a great deal of overlap of the companies involved in the US, the Canadian, and the international policy actions.

Self-Regulation versus Government Regulation: Which Is the Way Forward?

At first glance, the food industry deserves to be congratulated for its initiatives. It does appear that the Alliance School Beverage Guidelines has succeeded in bringing about a major cut in the sale of regular cola drinks in schools across the USA. However, the CFBAI action is another story as the policy has many weaknesses [14]. For example, it excludes advertising on prime-time television shows popular with children but also viewed by a broader audience. The policy appears to be based on the assumption that teenagers do not watch television after 9 pm. A study published in 2009, 3 years after the policy had been implemented, analyzed the effectiveness of the CFBAI and found that there was scant evidence of any real shift in food advertising for children toward healthier products. The study concluded that advertisements for healthy products accounted for a very small fraction of all advertising by participating companies and that most advertising still promoted foods of low nutritional value [15].

So why did the food industry go to all the trouble to develop the CFBAI? Why did they not formulate polices that would have a real impact on the marketing of unhealthy foods? An examination of the practices of the food industry reveals compelling evidence that the primary goal of the industry is to stop government regulations. The industry saw a real danger that if they did nothing, then the government would step in and implement effective regulations. CFBAI appears to have been, first and foremost, a public relations exercise so that the food industry can tell the government: "There is no need for government regulations. We are taking action."

In 2011 Harris and Graff [14] from the Rudd Center for Food Policy and Obesity at Yale University wrote:

> Public health professionals have suggested that industry self-regulatory efforts (e.g., CFBAI) provide more public relations benefit to the food industry than real health benefits for children and that overreliance on such efforts could exacerbate the childhood obesity crisis.

A survey of food advertising on Canadian television revealed a similar story [16]. Between 2006 (the year before the new policy was implemented) and 2011, advertising viewed by children aged 2 to 11 years showed no indication of overall improvement. While there was some decrease in the advertising of soft drinks, there was an even greater decrease in the advertising of diet soft drinks and juices. Meanwhile, advertising of fast food probably went up.

The following cases reveal that the food industry will go to great lengths to prevent the government from implementing regulations that may curtail the sale of unhealthy foods and thence reduce profits. In 2010 the European parliament debated the adoption of traffic light food labels. This policy is opposed by the food industry as it makes it easy for consumers to determine which foods are unhealthy. The last thing the food companies that produce and sell soft drinks want is red lights on their products. Such labels deliver a clear message "Junk food. Do not consume." To stop this from happening, the food industry carried out massive lobbying. They spent an estimated one billion euros (US$1.3 billion) in a successful attempt to defeat the proposed law [17, 18]. Australia provides a similar example. A few years ago the government of that country was planning to implement a new system for front-of-package food labels. As in Europe this posed a serious danger of making it easy for consumers to identify unhealthy food products.

Not surprisingly, the food industry strongly opposed the government proposals [19]. In 2006, the food industry introduced a voluntary system. The apparent motive for self-regulation had less to do with making food labels easier to understand and more to do with giving ammunition to their lobbyists who could then say to the government: "We have fixed the problem. There is no longer a need for your scheme." Self-regulation by the food industry in Australia has proven to be a badly flawed policy. A survey conducted in 2012 revealed that the food industry was routinely ignoring key parts of its own code of practice, namely, by not stating the quantity of saturated fat and sugar in energy-dense, nutrient-poor snacks (i.e., the foods where these labels are most needed) [20].

The food industry in Australia also carried out a self-regulation action in the area of food marketing to children (the Responsible Marketing to Children Initiative) [21]. A 2010 study concluded that "until one reads the fine print, the self-regulatory commitments of companies signed to the [policy] may appear to be responsible. However, this study shows that the commitments are permissive and allow companies to circumvent the stated intent of the Initiative." [21]

Not surprisingly, public health advocates have become increasingly cynical of the value of self-regulation by the food industry [22]. Instead, the demand is for government regulation. Examples of such policies include adding an extra sales tax to unhealthy foods or by curtailing its marketing. This argument was made in 2013 by an international group of experts in a discussion of policy options to prevent chronic diseases of lifestyle by reducing sales of tobacco, alcohol, and highly processed foods [23]. They argue as follows:

> Because growth in sales, turnover, and profit are the main goals of transnational corporations, supporters of public regulation believe that self-regulation and working from within are ineffective and counter-productive. Most advocate statutory regulations, analogous to those used to control firearms, road traffic, drugs and tobacco....

This expert group also argues that "Regulation, or the threat of government regulation, is the only way to change transnational corporations; therefore the audience for public health is government and not industry."

The World Health Organization (WHO) has also urged governments to take action. In 2011 they published recommendations on the marketing of food and non-alcoholic beverages to children [24]. One of the recommendations is "the reduction of the impact on children of marketing of foods high in saturated fats, trans-fatty acids, free sugars or salt by reducing both children's exposure to it and its power."

There is little doubt that any serious attempts by governments to take action would be met by fierce opposition from those food corporations that owe their huge profits to the sale of unhealthy foods.

Conclusion

Marketing, including advertising, to children and adolescents is highly prevalent worldwide. The largest marketing expenditures are for advertising on television, for in-school marketing, and for giving support to events. Most of this marketing is for sugar-rich, carbonated beverages and for other unhealthy food products. Advertising and marketing to children influences their food choices, health, and nutrition-related knowledge.

In response to the overwhelming body of evidence of harm caused by unhealthy food products, there have been growing demands for regulations that will limit the marketing of these foods to children. The food and beverage industry has responded by launching self-regulation initiatives in the USA and in other countries. However, this self-regulation has had little impact on the amount of advertising for unhealthy foods that is directed to children.

Advocates of public health are increasingly demanding that governments impose regulations as this is the most effective way to control the marketing of unhealthy foods, including sugar-rich, carbonated beverages, to children and adolescents.

References

1. Story M, French S. Food advertising and marketing directed at children and adolescents in the US. Int J Behav Nutr Phys Act. 2004;1:3.
2. Hawkes C. Marketing food to children: the global regulatory environment. Geneva: WHO; 2004. http://whqlibdoc.who.int/publications/2004/9241591579.pdf. Accessed 11 Sept 2014.
3. Federal Trade Commission. A review of food marketing to children and adolescents, follow-up report. 2012. http://www.ftc.gov/sites/default/files/documents/reports/review-food-marketing-children-and-adolescents-follow-report/121221foodmarketingreport.pdf. Accessed 8 Sept 2014.
4. Powell LM, Szczypka G, Chaloupka FJ. Trends in exposure to television food advertisements among children and adolescents in the United States. Arch Pediatr Adolesc Med. 2010;164:794–802.
5. Kelly B, Halford JC, Boyland EJ, et al. Television food advertising to children: a global perspective. Am J Public Health. 2010;100:1730–6.
6. Institute of Medicine, Committee on Food Marketing and the Diets of Children and Youth, McGinnis JM, Appleton Gootman J, Kraak VI, editors. Food marketing to children and youth: threat or opportunity? Washington (DC): National Academies Press; 2006. http://www.nap.edu/openbook.php?record_id=11514. Accessed 11 Sept 2014.

7. American Beverage Association. Alliance school beverage guidelines. Final progress report. 2010. http://www.ameribev.org/files/240_School%20Beverage%20Guidelines%20Final%20 Progress%20Report.pdf. Accessed 11 Sept 2014.
8. GAO (United States Government Accountability Office). School meal programs: competitive foods are widely available and generate substantial revenues for schools. 2005. http://www. gao.gov/products/GAO-05-563. Accessed 11 Sept 2014.
9. American Beverage Association. The guidelines. 2014. http://www.ameribev.org/nutrition-science/school-beverage-guidelines/the-guidelines/. Accessed 11 Sept 2014.
10. Kolish ED, Peeler CD, Council of Better Business Bureaus. Changing the landscape of food & beverage advertising: the children's food & beverage advertising initiative in action. A progress report on the first six months of implementation: July–December 2007. 2008. http://oyc. yale.edu/sites/default/files/Changing-the-Landscape.pdf. Accessed 11 Sept 2014.
11. Kolish ED, Hernandez M, Council of Better Business Bureaus. Changing the landscape of food & beverage advertising: the children's food and beverage advertising initiative: a report on compliance and progress during 2011. 2012. http://www.bbb.org/storage/16/documents/ cfbai/CFBAI%20Report%20on%20Compliance%20and%20Progress%20During%202011. pdf. Accessed 11 Sept 2014.
12. Canadian Children's Food and Beverage Advertising Initiative. 2010. http://www.adstandards.com/en/childrensinitiative/CCFBAI_EN.pdf. Accessed 11 Sept 2014.
13. International Food and Beverage Association. Responsible marketing and advertising to children. 2014. https://ifballiance.org/our-commitments/responsible-marketing-advertising-to-children/. Accessed 11 Sept 2014.
14. Harris JL, Graff SK. Protecting children from harmful food marketing: options for local government to make a difference. Prev Chronic Dis. 2011;8:A92–8.
15. Kunkel D, McKinley C, Wright P. The impact of industry self-regulation on the nutritional quality of foods advertised on television to children. 2009. http://www.childrennow.org/ uploads/documents/adstudy_2009.pdf. Accessed 11 Sept 2014.
16. Potvin Kent M, Wanless A. The influence of the Children's Food and Beverage Advertising Initiative: change in children's exposure to food advertising on television in Canada between 2006-2009. Int J Obes. 2014;38:558–62.
17. Hickman M. Laid bare, the lobbying campaign that won the food labelling battle. The Independent. 2010. http://www.independent.co.uk/life-style/food-and-drink/news/laid-bare-the-lobbying-campaign-thatwon-the-food-labelling-battle-2003686.html. Accessed 15 Dec 2013.
18. Anon. Food industry wins battle on "traffic light" labels. EurActiv. 2010. http://www.euractiv. com/food-industry-wins-battle-traffic-light-labels-news-495324. Accessed 15 Dec 2013.
19. Magnusson RS. Obesity prevention and personal responsibility: the case of front-of-pack food labelling in Australia. BMC Public Health. 2010;10:662.
20. Carter OB, Mills BW, Lloyd E, et al. An independent audit of the Australian food industry's voluntary front-of-pack nutrition labelling scheme for energy-dense nutrition-poor foods. Eur J Clin Nutr. 2013;67:31–5.
21. Hebden L, King L, Kelly B, Chapman K, Innes-Hughes C. Advertising of fast food to children on Australian television: the impact of industry self-regulation. Health Promot J Austr. 2011;21:229–35.
22. Stuckler D, Nestle M. Big food, food systems, and global health. PLoS Med. 2012;9, e1001242.
23. Moodie R, Stuckler D, Monteiro C, et al. Profits and pandemics: prevention of harmful effects of tobacco, alcohol, and ultra-processed food and drink industries. Lancet. 2013;381:670–9.
24. WHO. Reducing food-marketing pressure on children. 2011. http://www.euro.who.int/en/ health-topics/disease-prevention/nutrition/news/news/2011/01/reducing-food-marketing-pressure-on-children. Accessed 11 Sept 2014.

Chapter 19
Sugar in Beverages: Effects on Human Health

Norman J. Temple and Kathryn Alp

Keywords Sugar-sweetened beverages (SSBs) • Sucrose • Sugar • Obesity • Metabolic syndrome • Type 2 diabetes • Coronary heart disease • Dental caries

Key Points

1. Sugar-sweetened beverages (SSBs) include soda and cola drinks, sports and energy drinks, fruit drinks with added sugar, and sweetened coffee and tea.
2. Beverages such as fruit juice or milk, that contain naturally occurring sugars but have no added sugar, are not considered SSBs.
3. Sucrose is a disaccharide sugar in which glucose and fructose are covalently linked. However, the type of sugar added to most SSBs is high-fructose corn syrup. This typically contains 55 % fructose and 45 % glucose.
4. Strong evidence shows that consumption of SSB is positively associated with overweight/obesity, the metabolic syndrome, type 2 diabetes, coronary heart disease, and dental caries.
5. The American Heart Association proposed an upper limit for added sugar in the diet: 100 kcal (25 g) per day for women or 150 kcal (37.5 g) for men. This is equivalent to about 5–6 % of dietary energy. Draft guidelines published by the World Health Organization recommend limiting added sugars to no more than 10 % of total energy intake per day. It further recommends a reduction to no more than 5 % of energy or about 25 g of sugar per day.
6. A 355-mL can of SSB contains approximately 40 g of sugar (150 kcal). Drinking one can per day translates to about 6–7 % of energy intake. Ideally, therefore, both adults and children should limit consumption of SSBs to one can per day or the equivalent amount of added sugar from other foods.

N.J. Temple (✉) • K. Alp
Centre for Science, Athabasca University, Athabasca, AB, Canada, T9S 3A3
e-mail: normant@athabascau.ca

© Springer International Publishing Switzerland 2016
T. Wilson, N.J. Temple (eds.), *Beverage Impacts on Health and Nutrition*,
Nutrition and Health, DOI 10.1007/978-3-319-23672-8_19

Introduction

In the late 1960s and through the 1970s, John Yudkin argued that sugar (i.e., added sugar) was implicated in several diseases, including coronary heart disease (CHD) [1–3]. However, the supporting evidence was rather weak and the hypothesis never gained widespread acceptance. Recent evidence has added much weight to this belief that that sugar plays an important role in the etiology of several diseases.

The major focus here is sugar-sweetened beverages (SSBs). These include all non-diet, nonalcoholic beverages containing added sugars. They supply roughly half of the added sugar consumed by American adults [4]. Soda and cola drinks make up about two-thirds of the total intake of SSBs, while the remainder includes such beverages as sports and energy drinks, fruit drinks with added sugar, and sweetened coffee and tea. Beverages such as fruit juice or milk, that contain naturally occurring sugars but have no added sugar, are not considered SSBs.

Sucrose is a disaccharide sugar in which glucose and fructose are covalently linked through a glycosidic bond. During digestion, sucrose breaks down to equal amounts of glucose and fructose, which are monosaccharide sugars. Since the mid-1980s, the type of sugar added to most SSBs has been high-fructose corn syrup (HFCS). This typically contains 55 % fructose and 45 % glucose present in the free or unbonded state. The use of the words "high-fructose" in the name of HFCS is rather misleading given the 55/45 % ratio of fructose to glucose. The evidence presented in the chapter by White and Nicklas strongly indicates that the health effects of HFCS are no different to those of sucrose.

Consumption of SSBs increased dramatically in the USA after 1965. The proportion of Americans consuming soda or cola drinks increased from 20.8 % in 1965 to 43.5 % in 2002 [5]. Similarly, during the same time period, the energy supplied by these drinks rose from 35 to 143 kcal/day. However, a downward trend in SSB consumption has been observed after its peak in 2000. Between 2000 and 2010, total energy intake supplied by SSBs decreased from 196 to 151 kcal/day in adults and from 223 to 153 kcal/day among young people (age 2 to 19 years) [6]. An intake of around 150 kcal/day is equivalent to about one can (355 mL) of cola. The proportion of total energy intake in 2010 contributed by SSBs was 6.3 %, 10.4 %, and 6.9 % at ages 6–11, 12–19, and >20 years, respectively [6]. Consumption of SSBs is very uneven across the population. For example, among young people (age 2 to 19 years), more than one-third reported that on a given day they consumed no SSB, while 31.2 % reported consumption of two or more servings.

The Effect of Sugar-Sweetened Beverages on Human Health

Research Methods

Establishing the clear connection between intake of SSBs and risk of the disorders discussed in this chapter is supported by several prospective cohort studies. At the time of recruitment, the subjects in such studies are free of the diseases being investigated. Follow-up periods may be as short as a year or as long as 20 years. During that time, the subjects are monitored and all changes in health of relevance to the study are recorded. Methodological advances over the last 30 years have been of immense importance in the design of cohort studies that generate accurate findings. It is no coincidence that this has occurred simultaneously with the widespread adoption of computers. Much research has been carried out in the area of how to carry out accurate diet assessments. In order to increase accuracy, these are often repeated several times over a number of years. Cohort studies today employ large and accurate databases that give the composition of hundreds of foods. A crucial part of cohort studies is the analysis of findings. It is well recognized that many diet and lifestyle factors are strongly associated with each other. As a result, there is the ever-present danger of error due to confounding. Multivariate analysis is carried out in order to minimize this problem. So, for example, a study that aims to show whether SSBs are associated with change in body weight will make adjustments for such factors as age, education, smoking, physical activity, and various components of the diet.

Randomized controlled trials (RCTs) are another important research tool in this area. Whereas cohort studies have follow-up periods of many years, RCTs seldom have a duration beyond a few weeks or months. RCTs are therefore mainly of value for investigating short-term dietary changes on body functioning rather than on actual risk of a disease. RCTs can be carried out to investigate the impact of SSBs on body responses to an increased or decreased intake of these beverages. For example, RCTs can be used to determine whether SSBs affect energy balance and cause changes in body weight. They can also be used to study the metabolic consequences of ingesting SSBs.

Weight Gain and Obesity

The high sugar content of SSBs and the resultant caloric content can potentially result in an excess energy intake and therefore lead to weight gain. The absence of dietary fiber is of particular importance as it causes SSBs to have weak satiating ability. There is only limited compensation for the energy consumed in SSBs (i.e., the reduction in the energy consumption from other foods is less than the energy supplied by SSBs) [7].

A recent meta-analysis and systematic review by Malik et al. [8] examined the relationship between consumption of SSBs and weight. The analysis included cohort studies and RCTs (at least two weeks in length). It included 15 cohort studies in children and adolescents and 7 in adults. Most cohort studies observed a positive association between intake of SSBs and weight gain in both children and adults. The findings indicate that in children and adolescents an additional one serving per day of SSB (equivalent to one can of cola) is associated with an increase in BMI of 0.06 per year. Similarly, the findings indicate that in adults an additional one serving per day of SSB is associated with 0.22 kg of extra weight gain per year. Malik et al. also described an additional 11 cohort studies in children and 6 in adults but which were not included in the meta-analysis. Most of these studies also reported a positive association between consumption of SSBs and weight gain.

The RCTs in children and adolescents reported a decrease in BMI when the intake of SSBs was reduced. In some studies, this was done by substituting noncaloric beverages (e.g., diet cola). Consistent with this, studies in adults observed an increase in body weight of 0.85 kg when SSBs were added to the diet [8].

The Metabolic Syndrome, Diabetes, Cardiometabolic Risk Factors, and Coronary Heart Disease

The exact definition of the metabolic syndrome is still being debated. It is characterized by the presence of the following features: a high waist circumference (i.e., fat accumulation around the waist), insulin resistance, high blood pressure, an elevated blood level of triglycerides, and a low blood level of HDL cholesterol. Obesity is a major risk factor for both the metabolic syndrome and type 2 diabetes (T2D). As SSBs appear to be causally related to risk of obesity, this therefore also implicates SSBs as a risk factor for both metabolic syndrome and T2D. That this is indeed the case was clearly shown in a meta-analysis and systematic review that included three cohort studies of the metabolic syndrome and eight of T2D [9]. The findings revealed that persons who drink 1–2 servings of SSBs per day (compared with those who drink little or none) have a 20 % higher risk of developing the metabolic syndrome and a 26 % higher risk for T2D.

Consumption of SSBs is also associated with disturbances in a cluster of various risk factors for T2D and coronary heart disease (CHD). Some of these risk factors are also components of the metabolic syndrome. SSBs are associated with the blood levels of several inflammatory markers including C-reactive proteins (CRP), interleukin-6, and tumor necrosis factors [10, 11]. The beverages are also associated with a higher blood pressure, a higher blood level of triglycerides, and a lower blood level of HDL cholesterol [10, 12, 13]. Another important factor is that SSBs have a high dietary glycemic load [7].

The above evidence reveals that consumption of SSBs is associated with cardiometabolic risk factors, the metabolic syndrome, and T2D. Based on this solid body of evidence, it can be predicted that SSBs also increase the risk of CHD. Supporting evidence has come from a meta-analysis of four cohort studies [14]. The findings indicate that an increase in intake of SSBs of one serving per day is associated with a 16 % increased risk of developing CHD.

Dental Caries

Dental caries are a serious public health problem. The US government has identified reducing the prevalence of dental caries as one of their goals for *Healthy People 2020* [15].

A diet containing excessive amounts of sugar can facilitate the growth of oral bacteria, including streptococci and lactobacilli which are the primary bacteria involved in the etiology of dental caries [16]. Many studies have demonstrated that consumption of SSBs is associated with an increased risk of dental caries [16, 17]. A dose-response relationship between SSBs and dental caries was reported in a recent four-year cohort study [18]. This association was clearly seen even after adjusting for possible confounding factors including the use of fluoride toothpaste.

There are several aspects of SSBs that may increase the risk of dental caries. SSBs contain sugar that feeds the bacteria that contribute to dental caries. SSBs also contain acids, such as phosphoric acid, that cause erosion of tooth enamel. Furthermore, consumption of SSBs often displaces other beverages such as milk and water which pose no harm to the teeth [17].

Diet Quality

SSBs are empty calories; their consumption tends to displace nutritious foods from the diet. Methodological issues create a problem with respect to documenting this correlation [19]. In particular, people who have a relatively high intake of SSBs often differ from the rest of the population in other aspects of their diet quite apart from beverages. However, studies strongly suggest that people who frequently drink SSBs tend to have a lower intake of milk and fruit juice as well as of calcium and of various other nutrients [4, 20, 21]. Not surprisingly, this was also shown to be the case for the total intake of added sugar [22].

Dietary Recommendations

SSBs are implicated in several chronic diseases of lifestyle and their consumption should be limited. In response to this strong body of evidence, the American Heart Association proposed an upper limit for added sugar in the diet: 100 kcal (25 g) per day for women or 150 kcal (37.5 g) for men [23]. This is equivalent to about 5–6 % of dietary energy. Similarly, the World Health Organization (WHO) published draft guidelines in 2014 that proposed that added sugar intake should be limited to no more than 10 % of energy intake and recommended a further reduction to no more than 5 % of energy or about 25 g of sugar per day [24].

A 355-mL can of SSB contains approximately 40 g of sugar. Ideally, therefore, both adults and children should limit consumption of SSBs to one can per day or the equivalent amount of added sugars from other foods. A lower intake is preferable, though compliance is likely to be difficult to achieve given our current dietary patterns and beverage options. Indeed, as was discussed earlier in this chapter, a large section of the American population consumes the equivalent of two or more cans per day.

Fruit juices are far more nutritious than SSBs. In stark contrast to SSBs, fruit juices have a rich content of micronutrients and phytochemicals. Although fruit juices are similar to SSBs in terms of carbohydrate concentration, they have a slightly lower glycemic index (GI) (apple juice, orange juice, and Coca-Cola have GI values of 40, 50, and 58, respectively) [25]. Fruit juices are therefore preferable to SSBs, but their ease of consumption and low satiety mean they can contribute to excessive energy intake. Vegetable juices are preferable as they have a lower carbohydrate content than fruit juice and, in general, a lower GI [25]. Whole fruit or vegetables are of superior nutritional value than fruit and vegetable juices as they provide fiber and have greater satiety.

Sugar-Sweetened Beverages as a Public Health Challenge

There is strong evidence that SSBs are a public health challenge. What is an appropriate countermeasure? Better public policy, improved education, and access to healthier options are all steps required to make the above guidelines more achievable. However, while dietary guidelines are useful, they seldom achieve a major impact on the dietary behavior of the general population, especially young people. In Chap. 18, we argued that government regulation is the most effective way to control the marketing of SSBs (and of other unhealthy foods) to children and adolescents. This includes many policy approaches that have been proposed in order to reduce consumption of SSBs, including restrictions on advertising, restrictions on sale (especially to children), and improved food labeling. One approach that may be especially effective is to impose a tax on SSBs [26].

Conclusion

For many years, there was debate over the role of sugar in health. Research studies, mostly published over the past two decades, have generated much evidence that a relatively high intake of added sugar, especially SSBs, plays a significant role in several chronic conditions. We now have overwhelming evidence of a close association between consumption of SSBs and obesity, the metabolic syndrome, T2D, CHD, and dental caries. One important mechanism by which SSBs harm health is by displacing nutritious foods from the diet and thereby lowering the intake of various nutrients. Both adults and children should limit consumption of SSBs to one can per day or the equivalent amount of added sugar from other foods.

References

1. Yudkin J. Pure, white and deadly. London: Davis-Poynter; 1972.
2. Yudkin J. Sugar and disease. Nature. 1972;239:197–9.
3. Yudkin J. Sucrose and cardiovascular disease. Proc Nutr Soc. 1972;31:331–7.

4. Marriott BP, Olsho L, Hadden L, Connor P. Intake of added sugars and selected nutrients in the United States, National Health and Nutrition Examination Survey (NHANES) 2003–2006. Crit Rev Food Sci Nutr. 2010;50:228–58.
5. Duffey KJ, Popkin BM. Shifts in patterns and consumption of beverages between 1965 and 2002. Obesity. 2007;15:2739–47.
6. Kit BK, Fakhouri TH, Park S, Nielsen SJ, Ogden CL. Trends in sugar-sweetened beverage consumption among youth and adults in the United States: 1999–2010. Am J Clin Nutr. 2013;98:180–8.
7. Hu FB, Malik VS. Sugar-sweetened beverages and risk of obesity and type 2 diabetes: epidemiologic evidence. Physiol Behav. 2010;100:47–54.
8. Malik VS, Pan A, Willett WC, Hu FB. Sugar-sweetened beverages and weight gain in children and adults: a systematic review and meta-analysis. Am J Clin Nutr. 2013;98:1084–102.
9. Malik VS, Popkin BM, Bray GA, Després JP, Willett WC, Hu FB. Sugar-sweetened beverages and risk of metabolic syndrome and type 2 diabetes. Diabetes Care. 2010;33:2477–83.
10. de Koning L, Malik VS, Rim EB, Willet WC, Hu FB. Sugar-sweetened beverages and artificially sweetened beverage consumption and risk of type 2 diabetes in men. Am J Clin Nutr. 2011;93:1321–7.
11. Schulze MB, Hoffmann K, Manson JE, et al. Dietary pattern, inflammation, and incidence of type 2 diabetes in women. Am J Clin Nutr. 2005;82:675–84.
12. Chen L, Caballero B, Mitchell DC, et al. Reducing consumption of sugar-sweetened beverages is associated with reduced blood pressure: a prospective study among United States adults. Circulation. 2010;121:2398–406.
13. Dhringa R, Sullivan L, Jacques PF, et al. Soft drink consumption and risk factors of developing cardiometabolic risk factors and metabolic syndrome in middle-aged adults in the community. Circulation. 2007;116:480–8.
14. Huang C, Huang J, Tian Y, Yang X, Gu D. Sugar sweetened beverages consumption and risk of coronary heart disease: a meta-analysis of prospective studies. Atherosclerosis. 2014;234:11–6.
15. Office of Disease Prevention and Health Promotion. Healthy People 2020. Oral Health. 2010. http://www.healthypeople.gov/2020/topicsobjectives2020/overview.aspx?topicid=32. Accessed 30 Aug 2014.
16. Touger-Decker R, van Loveren C. Sugars and dental caries. Am J Clin Nutr. 2003;78:881S–92.
17. Sohn W, Burt BA, Sowers MR. Carbonated soft drinks and dental caries in the primary dentition. J Dent Res. 2006;85:262–6.
18. Bernabé E, Vehkalahti MM, Sheiham A, Aromaa A, Souminen AL. Sugar-sweetened beverages and dental caries in adults: a four-year prospective study. J Dent. 2014;42:952–8.
19. Rennie KL, Livingstone MB. Associations between dietary added sugar intake and micronutrient intake: a systematic review. Br J Nutr. 2007;97:832–41.
20. Joyce T, Gibney MJ. The impact of sugar consumption on overall dietary quality in Irish children and teenagers. J Hum Nutr Diet. 2008;21:438–50.
21. Gibson S, Boyd A. Associations between added sugars and micronutrient intakes and status: further analysis of data from the national diet and nutrition survey of young people aged 4 to 18 years. Br J Nutr. 2009;101:100–7.
22. Vartanian LR, Schwartz MB, Brownell KD. Effects of soft drink consumption on nutrition and health: a systematic review and meta-analysis. Am J Pub Health. 2007;97:667–75.
23. Johnson RK, Appel LJ, Brands M, et al. Dietary sugars intake and cardiovascular health: a scientific statement from the American Heart Association. Circulation. 2009;120:1011–20.
24. World Health Organization. WHO opens public consultation on draft sugars guideline. 2014. http://www.who.int/mediacentre/news/notes/2014/consultation-sugar-guideline/en/. Accessed 5 Sept 2014.
25. Foster-Powell K, Holt SH, Brand-Miller JC. International table of glycemic index and glycemic load values: 2002. Am J Clin Nutr. 2002;76:5–56.
26. Andreyeva T, Chaloupka FJ, Brownell KD. Estimating the potential of taxes on sugar-sweetened beverages to reduce consumption and generate revenue. Prev Med. 2011;52:413–6.

Chapter 20
High-Fructose Corn Syrup Use in Beverages: Composition, Manufacturing, Properties, Consumption, and Health Effects

John S. White and Theresa A. Nicklas

Keywords Nutritive sweeteners • High-fructose corn syrup, HFCS • Soft drinks • Flavored milk • Energy drinks

Key Points

1. High-fructose corn syrup (HFCS) replaced most of the sucrose (table sugar) in US beverages 30 years ago. Today, about 70 % of HFCS production is used in beverages.
2. HFCS and sucrose are similar in composition, manufacturing, beverage functionality, nutritional value, metabolism, and health effects.
3. HFCS is often confused with pure fructose (100 % fructose) and regular corn syrup (100 % glucose and glucose polymers); it is neither. It is comprised of near-equivalent amounts of glucose and fructose, much like sucrose, honey, and fruit juice concentrates.
4. HFCS is primarily a US sweetener. Sucrose accounts for more than 90 % of global caloric sweetener use.
5. The FDA GRAS (generally recognized as safe) process affirmed the safety of HFCS on two occasions.
6. There is scant scientific evidence to support unique health effects of HFCS in humans. Reports of untoward effects are largely based on low-evidentiary value epidemiologic and animal experiments or exaggerated human studies comparing pure fructose with pure glucose at doses above normal human consumption.

J.S. White, Ph.D. (✉)
White Technical Research, 8895 Hickory Hills Drive, Argenta, IL 62501, USA
e-mail: white.tech.res@gmail.com

T.A. Nicklas, Dr.P.H.
Department of Pediatrics, Children's Nutrition Research Center, Baylor College of Medicine, 1100 Bates Street, Houston, TX 77030, USA
e-mail: tnicklas@bcm.edu

© Springer International Publishing Switzerland 2016
T. Wilson, N.J. Temple (eds.), *Beverage Impacts on Health and Nutrition*, Nutrition and Health, DOI 10.1007/978-3-319-23672-8_20

7. Reformulating a beverage sweetener from HFCS to sucrose does not improve its nutritional value. Expert scientific panels have repeatedly acknowledged the metabolic and nutritional equivalence of HFCS and sucrose.

Introduction

High-fructose corn syrup (HFCS) has been used in beverages for more than 30 years. Technology to produce it was developed in the 1960s, it was introduced to the food and beverage industry as a liquid sweetener alternative to sucrose (sugar) in the 1970s, and it fully replaced sucrose in the USA in most beverages by the mid-1980s. Made from abundant and relatively price-stable domestic corn, HFCS has been a safe and reliable sweetener for the beverage industry. All of that changed in 2004, with the publication of a commentary promoting the hypothesis that HFCS-sweetened beverages held significant and unique responsibility for the current obesity epidemic [1]. While the ecological data suggested a possible relationship between HFCS and obesity, the population-based association utilized crude estimates of sugar consumption and did not control for confounding effects of other relevant variables.

Consumption of HFCS has been in decline since the turn of the century, whereas obesity rates continued to increase and in some cases may show signs of leveling off [2]. Despite this trend, much attention has continued to focus on sugars, or more specifically, the fructose moiety in HFCS, as the agent in food that somehow alters the body's ability to maintain energy balance and may also affect aspects of cell metabolism that may promote an increase in additional disease states. This hysteria in the scientific community has promoted some beverage manufacturers to reformulate products away from HFCS and back to sucrose.

This chapter will compare vis-à-vis sucrose the composition, manufacturing, beverage properties, consumption, and the purported health effects of HFCS. This chapter will also discuss whether reformulation from HFCS to sucrose is defensible from a health or marketing perspective.

Composition

Composition: HFCS vs. Sucrose

HFCS and sucrose are biochemically classified as carbohydrate sugars (saccharides). HFCS consists primarily of the monosaccharide sugars glucose and fructose in the free or unbonded state, while sucrose is a disaccharide sugar in which glucose and fructose are covalently linked through a glycosidic bond. Two of several structural forms (anomers) of monosaccharide glucose and fructose are shown in Fig. 20.1, along with their bonded counterpart, disaccharide sucrose. Although the

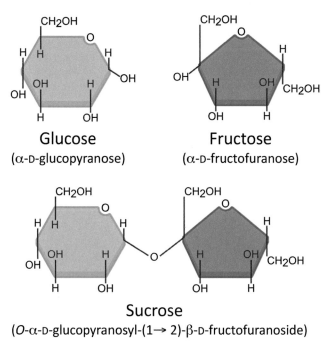

Fig. 20.1 Chemical structures of glucose, fructose, and sucrose

Table 20.1 Comparison of HFCS and sucrose composition (pre- and post-digestion)

Component (% total sugars)	HFCS-42	Sucrose	Total invert sugar	HFCS-55
Predigestion				
Sucrose		100	6	
Fructose	42	<0.01	47	55
Glucose	52	<0.01	47	41
Oligosaccharides	6			4
Physical form	Syrup	Crystalline	Syrup	Syrup
Post-digestion				
Sucrose		0	0	
Fructose	42	50	50	55
Glucose	58	50	50	45
Oligosaccharides	0			0

glycosidic bond of sucrose locks glucose and fructose in a fixed 1:1 ratio, HFCS manufacturers can vary this ratio since the monosaccharides are unbonded. Accordingly, HFCS is commonly made in two forms: HFCS-55 (containing 55 % fructose) and HFCS-42 (42 % fructose). As detailed in Table 20.1 (*predigestion*), the remaining carbohydrate in HFCS (45 % or 58 %, respectively) contains glucose and minor amounts of oligosaccharides (principally maltose, maltotriose, and maltotetraose), short-chain glucose polymeric remnants of the cornstarch from which HFCS is made. Both forms of HFCS thus contain appreciable amounts of glucose.

Enzymes in the mouth and small intestine (amylases) break oligosaccharide bonds during digestion, liberating free glucose; intestinal sucrase splits the glycosidic bond in sucrose, releasing free fructose and free glucose. Sucrase is a plentiful and fast-acting enzyme, so sucrose hydrolysis is rarely an issue. Invert sugar is a syrup sweetener similar in composition to HFCS, made by hydrolyzing sucrose with acid or enzymes. While there are certainly differences in the chemical compositions of HFCS and sucrose prior to digestion—monosaccharides in HFCS vs. the disaccharide sucrose—these initial differences disappear once digestion is completed (Table 20.1, *post-digestion*). Thus, digestion of both HFCS and sucrose delivers the same sugars in roughly the same ratios to the same tissues within the same time frame to the same metabolic pathways [3].

It should be noted that the name *high-fructose* corn syrup, coined by the corn wet milling industry to differentiate the fructose-containing sweetener from *regular* all-glucose corn syrup, is really an unfortunate and misleading description of the product. The name implies a sweetener with high amounts of fructose in comparison with other sweeteners, when, in reality, it contains a little more (HFCS-55) or a little less (HFCS-42) fructose than sucrose. An FDA petition from the Corn Refiners Association to allow manufacturers the option of using *corn sugar* on package labels in lieu of high-fructose corn syrup was denied in 2012 [4], so the name will likely continue as a source of confusion despite the close similarity in composition between HFCS and sucrose.

Is the Level of Fructose in HFCS-Sweetened Carbonated Beverages Higher than That Claimed by Manufacturers and Required by Regulation?

The fructose level in HFCS is widely advertised as 42 % or 55 % for HFCS-42 and HFCS-55, respectively, in manufacturer technical specification brochures [5, 6] and numerous descriptions in the scientific literature [3, 7–10]. However, US Federal standards in the *Food Chemicals Codex* [11] and incorporated into the *Code of Federal Regulations* [12] stipulate that 42 % and 55 % are the *minimum* permissible fructose percentages for these sweeteners. To ensure the government requirement is met and customers do not reject product formulations, manufacturers routinely target fructose levels slightly above these minima.

Manufacturers of HFCS and bottlers of carbonated soft drinks were surprised when concern was raised that the level of fructose in beverages was higher than that claimed by manufacturers and required by regulation. Ventura et al. [13] analyzed the fructose content in 23 HFCS-sweetened beverages by high-pressure liquid chromatography. The mean fructose content reported was 59 % (range 47–65 %), a significant variance from that claimed by manufacturers of HFCS-55. The authors proposed that the unexpected fructose differential vis-à-vis sucrose could be uniquely contributing to higher consumption than generally believed and subsequently implicated HFCS in the increased incidence of obesity during early development, fatty liver disease among US Hispanics, and global diabetes [14–16]. In reviewing the paper, Hobbs and Krueger [17, 18] determined that the elevated fructose levels in HFCS-sweetened beverages reported by Ventura et al. were due to the use of a method that was not intended to be used for HFCS or carbonated beverages. A subsequent study, funded by the International Society of Beverage Technologists (ISBT) and using analytical methodology verified for HFCS in carbonated beverages, found the fructose percentage in pooled data (160 total measurements by two independent laboratories of 80 randomly selected carbonated beverages sweetened with HFCS-55) to be 55.58 % of total sugars (SD 0.47 %, 95 % confidence interval 55.51–55.65 %) [19]. This value is in close agreement with industry-published values and satisfies government regulatory and labeling requirements. The concern raised and implications made by Ventura et al. were therefore unfounded, leading to continued misperceptions about HFCS suitability in beverages.

Manufacturing of HFCS and Sucrose

The sweetener made in the USA from corn is called high-fructose *corn* syrup. Outside the USA, it is called by other names (high-fructose syrup, isoglucose, glucose-fructose syrup, and fructose-glucose syrup) since it can be made from whatever abundant starch crop is available, including wheat, potato, rice, and tapioca. For comparison, sugarcane and sugar beets are the common botanical sources for sucrose in the USA.

The processes used in manufacturing HFCS and sucrose are compared in Table 20.2. The processing of the two sweeteners overlaps in many ways because both are derived from botanical sources. The desirable carbohydrate fractions must be extracted and purified away from the complex biochemical background of protein/fat/nucleic acid/fiber/minerals and competing flavored/colored/aromatic organic compounds. Both processes take advantage of the limited number of available refining techniques for carbohydrate extraction, purification, and carbohydrate enrichment.

Critics of HFCS have discussed the use of enzymes to carry out "molecular transformations" as a processing feature distinguishable from sucrose processing. This ignores the realities of modern, real-world food and beverage production. Enzymes are used for a variety of purposes in many of the foods and beverages we consume on a daily basis: cheese and yogurt; baked goods; beer, wine, and spirits; meat preparations; fruit juices; and fermented sauces, to name just a few [20]. It is true that amylases are used to hydrolyze starch to glucose and that isomerase then converts about half of the glucose to fructose. But it is equally true that enzymes

Table 20.2 Comparison of HFCS and sucrose processing

Processing step	HFCS	Sucrose
Source	Botanical: corn	Botanical: cane or beet
Preprocessing	Harvest-ship-clean	Harvest-ship-clean
Preparation	Steeping (*water, SO2*)	Chipping/milling/pulping soaking (*water*)
Carbohydrate extraction	Wet milling (*grind/mill/centrifuge/wash*)	Sulfitation (*SO2, lime*) (*clarify, evaporate, crystallize, centrifuge*)
Purification	Filtration	Affination (*crystallize, melt*)
	Carbon	Carbonatation (*CO2, lime*) or phosphatation (*H3PO4, lime*)
	Ion exchange	Bone char (*carbon*)
		Ion exchange
Carbohydrate enrichment	Fractionation	Evaporation
	Evaporation	Crystallization
Enzyme conversions	Carbohydrate polymer hydrolysis (*α-amylase, glucoamylase*)	Carbohydrate polymer hydrolysis (*dextranase, α-amylase*)
	Glucose-to-fructose isomerization (*glucose isomerase*)	Sucrose-to-invert sugar inversion (*invertase*)

are frequently employed in sucrose production to carry out molecular transformations, like depolymerization of high molecular weight carbohydrates via carbohydrases to facilitate sugars extraction and hydrolysis of sucrose via yeast invertase to free glucose and fructose in the production of medium and total invert sugar. Viewed side-by-side in Table 20.2, it becomes apparent that HFCS and sucrose manufacturers both use sophisticated separations and refining technology to produce the highly purified sweeteners required for use by the food and beverage industry.

Properties of HFCS and Sucrose

Prior to the introduction of HFCS, sucrose was the only viable choice in nutritive (caloric) sweeteners for high-volume use in foods and beverages. Manufacturers were satisfied with sucrose—other than periodic spikes in price and availability—as it was a versatile sweetener with physical and functional properties well suited for use in a wide variety of products. But it is certainly fair to say that the beverage industry was on the lookout for a new sweetener with properties similar to sucrose but without the problems of supply and price fluctuations.

More than 70 % of HFCS annual production is used in beverages [21, 22] for two primary reasons. First, its production is based not on offshore sugarcane subject to political and weather upsets, but on stable and abundant homegrown corn. And second, it has a unique set of properties due to its composition that are especially well suited to beverage applications.

Table 20.3 Sweetness comparison of HFCS, sucrose, and component sugars

Sugar	Relative sweetness (10 % solution)
Fructose	117
Sucrose	100 (standard)
HFCS-55	99
HFCS-42	90
Glucose	65

Sweetness

The sweetness of HFCS, sucrose, and their component sugars is compared in Table 20.3 [3]. Sweetness intensity is commonly measured in a solution (10 % dry solids basis) at room temperature relative to sucrose (the standard). Fructose is the sweetest nutritive sugar with a relative sweetness in a 10 % solution of 117 compared with sucrose. Glucose is the least sweet of the sugars listed with a relative sweetness of 65. HFCS-55 was designed to have the same relative sweetness as sucrose so it could simply replace sucrose in beverages on a one-to-one (dry) basis. Because of its proportionately lower fructose and greater glucose composition, HFCS-42 is less sweet than HFCS-55, sucrose, and honey.

Flavor Enhancement

Every sugar has a unique sweetness perception profile. The profile for sucrose is broad and bell shaped, slow to develop and slow to decay. Although this profile is compatible with use in many foods and beverages, sucrose does have a tendency to mask sensitive and delicate flavors such as the fruit and spice found in beverages. The profile for HFCS is actually the sum of the two overlapping profiles of fructose and glucose. The fructose profile is quick to develop and quick to decay, with an intensity peak greater than sucrose. The peak for glucose is of lower intensity and develops after fructose but before sucrose. The sum of these two peaks gives an earlier sweetness perception that is shorter in duration than sucrose. For this reason, HFCS is said to enhance flavors more—or mask them less—than sucrose [23].

Stability in Acid

Many sweetened beverages are fairly acidic; carbonated cola beverages, for example, are commonly around pH 3.5. Under acidic conditions, the glycosidic bond in sucrose is readily hydrolyzed (inverted) in a reaction that is accelerated with increasing ambient storage temperature [24]. For example, it takes about 200 days at 68°F for half the original sucrose in a carbonated beverage to invert to free glucose and fructose, but just 10 days at 104°F. Because of inversion, the composition of sugars in sucrose-sweetened beverages is always in flux, with ever-shifting ratios of diminishing sucrose and increasing free glucose and fructose between bottling and consumption. One reason bottlers turned to HFCS was because its composition is unaffected by beverage pH, resulting in a more consistent product quality and taste.

Physical Form

As the name indicates, HFCS is a syrup product in which the sugars are essentially pre-dissolved in water. This is a big advantage to manufacturers who can unload HFCS from a delivery truck or railcar and convey it around the plant to holding and makeup tanks, all with the use of pumps and at minimal labor and energy cost [3]. In contrast to sucrose, there is no bagged sugar to manually dump, heat, and dissolve; no waste bags to dispose of; and fewer pest, vermin, and microbial contamination issues. Reductions in the risk of contamination by using HFCS in a closed storage system benefit both the consumer and manufacturer.

Consumption of HFCS and Sucrose

HFCS and Sucrose Are the Dominant Caloric Sweeteners in the USA; HFCS Has Been in Decline since 1999

US per capita availability of caloric sweeteners (adjusted for loss) is shown in Fig. 20.2 for the years 1970–2011 [25]. These data are collected annually from sweetener producers by the USDA-ERS. Availability provides a good estimate of actual consumption if production figures are adjusted downward to account for losses during ingredient shipment, food manufacture, food shipment and warehousing, in-home preparation, and table waste. Several conclusions may be drawn from Fig. 20.2:

- Following a short lag time after the introduction of HFCS in the late 1960s, its use rapidly increased from 1970 to 1985, when total substitution of HFCS for sucrose in much of the beverage industry was complete. Growth continued thereafter at a slower rate until 1999, the peak year for HFCS use.
- HFCS use has been in significant decline for 15 years. The reasons for this are many, including declining sugar-sweetened soft drink sales, a shift in preference to unsweetened beverages such as bottled water, increasing health consciousness among Americans, and the negative publicity HFCS has received.

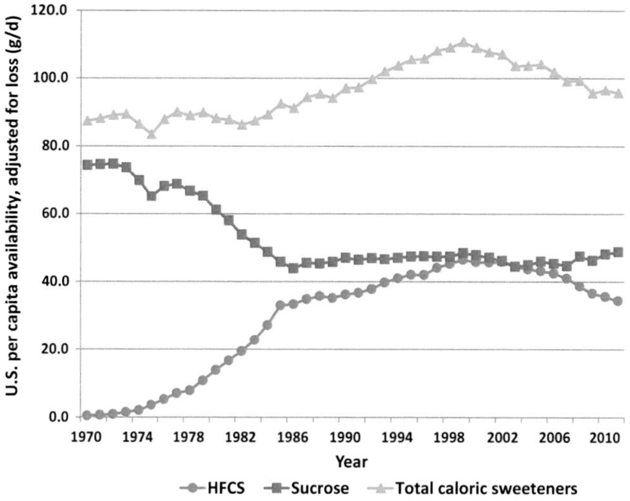

Fig. 20.2 US per capita availability of HFCS, sucrose, and total caloric sweeteners, 1970–2011 (USDA-ERS, adjusted for loss)

- HFCS and sucrose consumption were mirror images between 1970 and 1998: sucrose consumption declined at about the same rate HFCS increased. This was a direct result of the many functional similarities between the two sweeteners, allowing a roughly one-for-one (dry basis) substitution of HFCS for sucrose.
- Sucrose has benefitted from the recent decline in HFCS use: HFCS consumption levels are now back where they were about 30 years ago, while sucrose consumption has trended upward the past few years.
- Related to the HFCS trend, total caloric sweeteners consumption peaked in 1999 and has been in decline ever since. This has occurred in part due to increased consumption of diet beverages and bottled water and increased health consciousness among consumers.

HFCS Is Primarily a US Sweetener: We Live in a Sucrose-Sweetened World

Although HFCS is a prominent sweetener in the USA, it is not widely used elsewhere in the world. As shown in Fig. 20.3, sucrose use dominated HFCS on a global scale by >9:1 from 1980 to 2012, a ratio that shows no sign of changing [26]. The reasons are straightforward: HFCS manufacturing requires dedicated and abundant starch and water, refining knowledge and equipment, and a non-sucrose centric economy. There are not many locations in the world where these conditions are met. In Brazil, for example, corn is simply not as cost-effective for sweetener production. Consequently, most sugar-sweetened beverages outside the USA are sweetened with sucrose, whereas HFCS predominates in the USA.

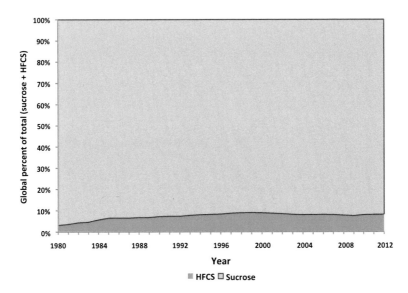

Fig. 20.3 Worldwide comparison of HFCS and sucrose use, 1980–2012 (LMC Sweetener Analysis)

Health Effects

There has been much conjecture over the past decade about purported health effects of HFCS. But does HFCS really constitute a unique health risk versus other sugars?

How HFCS Became the Focus of Attention

In the absence of evidence to the contrary, HFCS was understood by the food and beverage industry to be a safe ingredient based on similarities in composition to sucrose (as discussed above), authoritative reviews [27, 28], and FDA GRAS (generally recognized as safe) status [29]. All of that changed in 2004 with publication of a commentary in the *American Journal of Clinical Nutrition* that hypothesized, "the overconsumption of HFCS in calorically sweetened beverages may play a role in the epidemic of obesity" [1]. This hypothesis was formulated on the basis of ecological data, whereby observed trends were translated into an association between increased use of HFCS from 1970 to 2000 (see Fig. 20.2) and concurrent rising rates of obesity. However, ecological data or time trend data cannot be relied upon to prove or disprove a hypothesis.

Since overconsumption of any caloric compound in any food or beverage will likely lead to overweight and obesity, it is hard to accept the HFCS hypothesis for the following reasons:

- Correlation is not causation, a basic tenet in science.

- Sucrose was excluded from the hypothesis despite its striking similarities to HFCS in caloric value, consumption level, food uses, post-digestion composition, and delivery of sugars to the bloodstream. Why wasn't it included? Because the 1970–2000 association between sucrose and obesity showed a *negative* trend (Fig. 20.2).
- Association between HFCS and obesity was lost after 1999: HFCS availability declined, while obesity rates continued to increase. There is no association today between HFCS and obesity [2].
- Obesity is also a serious public health problem in countries outside the USA, but HFCS simply cannot be a unique or significant contributor. Sucrose is the dominant global sweetener outside of the USA, and obesity rates have increased as well in many of these sucrose-dominant countries.

Despite these obvious inconsistencies, the HFCS hypothesis drew the attention of scientists and the public alike, ignorance about sweeteners and the social media explosion blurred the line between fact and fiction, sucrose was informally accorded "healthy sweetener" status, and HFCS achieved a level of notoriety seldom seen among food ingredients.

HFCS Does Not Uniquely Contribute to Human Disease Differently from Sucrose

It has been suggested that the 5 % additional fructose in HFCS-55 relative to sucrose may be metabolically relevant and carry added health risks in comparison to sucrose [15, 30]. This argument ignores the substantial HFCS-42 (8 % *less* fructose than sucrose) used annually in foods and beverages. Nevertheless, a number of randomized controlled studies (RCTs) have compared HFCS-55 with sucrose in human subjects [31–34]. While the studies were all of short duration (10 weeks or less), they provide the highest quality data available comparing HFCS with sucrose. To date, the majority of comparisons conducted at typical consumption levels observed no significant differences between HFCS and sucrose on the following metabolic or endocrine responses and health-related effects in human subjects [35]:

Glucose	Uric acid	Ectopic fat (muscle)
Insulin	Weight loss	Postprandial triglycerides
Leptin	Body mass	
Ghrelin	Fat mass	Waist circumference
Energy intake	BMI	Blood pressure
Appetite	% Body fat	Hypothalamic blood flow
Satiety	Liver fat	

Based on this body of evidence, numerous expert panels convened in the past 10 years—including those by the American Medical Association and the Academy of Nutrition and Dietetics—concluded HFCS and sucrose are processed similarly by the human body [36–43], given their compositional similarity.

Why the Controversy Persists

With the realization that HFCS and sucrose do not affect the body differently and do not cause unwanted metabolic effects over the range of usual human consumption, attention turned to the fructose component that is common to both. It has been known for more than a century that fructose and glucose, component sugars of both HFCS and sucrose, are absorbed and metabolized using distinct but overlapping mechanisms. The chief differences are threefold [44]:

1. Sugars absorption

    a. Sucrose requires hydrolysis at the lumen of the small intestine before absorption, while the free fructose and glucose in HFCS are available for immediate absorption—in practice, sucrose hydrolysis is rapid and quantitative and has never been demonstrated to be rate limiting.
    b. Three transport mechanisms (SGLT-1, GLUT5, and GLUT2) are available to move the free sugars into enterocytes, the cells comprising the intestinal wall.
    c. Fructose and glucose both pass from the enterocyte into the portal bloodstream via the GLUT2 transporter.

2. Site of metabolism—fructose is largely removed from the blood and metabolized by the liver, while glucose is utilized not only in the liver but also throughout the body.
3. Regulatory control—fructose metabolism lacks the regulatory controls of glucose and is therefore rapidly processed in the liver.

It is to be expected, then, that experimental studies comparing the metabolism of pure glucose and fructose will nearly always show a difference.

A popular contemporary experimental model compares fructose vs. glucose effects at high intake levels on metabolic endpoints. It is argued that this model effectively isolates specific fructose effects from those of other dietary sugars. Accordingly, fructose and glucose are tested independently at levels most often exceeding 20 % and 50 % of total energy in human and animal subjects, respectively. Based on results from similar experimental designs, fructose has been labeled a risk factor for cardiovascular disease, hypertension, obesity, diabetes, kidney disease, the metabolic syndrome [45], cancer [46, 47], and nonalcoholic fatty liver disease [48]. But is this correct?

Fructose vs. glucose research must be carefully evaluated for relevance to the human diet. Humans nearly always consume fructose concurrently with equivalent amounts of glucose, whether from natural (fruits, vegetables, and nuts) or added (sweeteners—sucrose, HFCS, honey, and fruit juice concentrate) sources. It is not widely recognized that fructose consumed from these sources is dwarfed by the large background surplus of starch-derived glucose in the typical diet, which surpasses fructose by a ratio exceeding 3:1 [2, 49]. Furthermore, the best reported estimate of whole-diet fructose exposure in humans was 9.1 % and 14.6 % of energy, respectively, for the 50th and 95th population percentiles [50]. Thus, popular fructose models exaggerate not only the consumption pattern (single vs. mixed sugars) but also the fructose exposure, exceeding the typical human intake range

(<17.9 % of energy for the highest consumers, males and females aged 19–22) and shifting the normal glucose/fructose ratio in the diet.

A recent series of meta-analyses by Sievenpiper et al. [51–56] of RCTs provides further evidence that exaggerated experimental designs are not reliable predictors of human outcomes. They determined that only when fructose was provided as excess energy (hypercaloric) were undesirable effects observed for metabolic markers of body weight, diabetes, cardiometabolic risk, blood pressure, blood lipids, and uric acid. Isocaloric exchange of fructose for other carbohydrates was actually observed to improve glycemic control without affecting insulin in diabetics [57, 58].

Finally, it must be recognized that per capita fructose consumption (availability) from added sugars has remained relatively constant for nearly a century at 39 ± 4 g/day/person [2, 59]. Although fructose intake increased between 1983 and 1998, there has been a decline since 1999; current intake levels are comparable to those from the early 1920s. Thus, fructose cannot rationally be held responsible for escalating rates of contemporary disease if (1) intake levels have been in decline for more than a decade and (2) historical intake has shown little variation over the past century.

Added Sugars Have Not Increased Disproportionately in the Diet over the Past 40 Years

The premature attention given to added sugars as the *cause du jour* of obesity and attendant diseases has carried with it the tacit belief that added sugars have increased disproportionately in the diet with the advent of HFCS. They have not. While true that the introduction of HFCS around 1970 in the USA heralded a 40-year period in which per capita energy intake increased by 450 kcal/day, added sugars actually played a minor role, accounting for <8 % of the daily energy increase, and added fats and flour/cereal products accounted for >90 % of the increase [2, 60]. Thus, added fats and flour/cereal products may reasonably be said to have accounted for a disproportionately large portion of the energy increase; the same cannot be said for added sugars.

Conclusion

To reformulate or not to reformulate: that is the question

This chapter has compared HFCS and sucrose composition, manufacturing, beverage properties, consumption, and health effects. These two principal sweeteners are very similar and broadly interchangeable in many beverage applications—after all, it was only in the 1980s that HFCS successfully supplanted sucrose as the principal sweetener in carbonated and other beverages in the USA.

Although there is no scientific rationale to support the belief that HFCS poses a unique health threat, that HFCS is processed any differently by the body than sucrose, or that added sugars are primarily responsible for increased risk of chronic diseases, some food and beverage manufacturers have reformulated products to remove HFCS. In nearly all cases, it was replaced with…no surprise…sucrose, essentially reversing the sweetener reformulation process of the 1980s. As documented above, replacing HFCS with sucrose is a metabolic wash—there are no metabolic or nutritional advantages to be gained.

If there is no scientific rationale for reformulation, why else might food and beverage companies switch sweeteners? Some manufacturers seek market share by appealing to consumers who are confused, uncertain, and concerned about HFCS, believing there is a significant customer base demanding HFCS-free products. Consumer and market data do not support this strategy. Recent research from Mintel reveals that on an unaided basis, far more consumers express concern about the level of added sugar in carbonated beverages (60 %) than whether the sweetener used is HFCS (2.2 %) [61]. Nielsen retail scan data show little change in sales trend lines when sucrose replaces HFCS in a variety of foods and beverages: products with declining sales continue to falter, while those with flat sales do not gain market share after reformulation [62]. Beverage manufacturers are thus better off focusing on reducing calories of existing product lines—which can be accomplished with either HFCS or sucrose—than by swapping sweeteners. Although consumer and marketing data are not science based, they do inform decisions being made about sweetener reformulation.

HFCS has been a safe, dependable, functional, and valued ingredient to the beverage industry for more than 40 years. When the furor surrounding it subsides and proper scientific and public perspective is restored, HFCS will once again be recognized for what it is: a functional, dependable, and valued beverage sweetener.

References

1. Bray GA, Nielsen SJ, Popkin BM. Consumption of high-fructose corn syrup in beverages may play a role in the epidemic of obesity. Am J Clin Nutr. 2004;79:537–43.
2. White JS. Challenging the fructose hypothesis: new perspectives on fructose consumption and metabolism. Adv Nutr. 2013;4:246–56.
3. White JS. Straight talk about high-fructose corn syrup: what it is and what it ain't. Am J Clin Nutr. 2008;88:1716S–21.
4. Food and Drug Administration, Department of Health & Human Services. Response to petition from corn refiners association to authorize "Corn Sugar" as an alternative common or usual name for high fructose corn syrup (HFCS). Docket No FDA-2010-P-0491. College Park. 2012. http://www.fda.gov/AboutFDA/CentersOffices/OfficeofFoods/CFSAN/CFSANFOIA ElectronicReadingRoom/ucm305226.htm. Accessed 15 Jan 2014.
5. ADM Corn Processing. Technical Data Sheet: Typical data information for CornSweet 42, Product code 010042. Decatur: Archer Daniels Midland Company. http://www.adm.com/_layouts/ProductDetails.aspx?productId=8. Accessed 30 Oct 2013.
6. ADM Corn Processing. Technical Data Sheet: Typical data information for CornSweet 55, Product code 010055. Decatur: Archer Daniels Midland Company. http://www.adm.com/_layouts/ProductDetails.aspx?productId=10. Accessed 30 Oct 2013.
7. White JS. Fructose syrup: production, properties, and applications. In: Schenck FW, Hebeda RE, editors. Starch hydrolysis products: worldwide technology, production, and application. New York: VCH; 1992. p. 177–99.

8. Hanover LM, White JS. Manufacturing, composition, and applications of fructose. Am J Clin Nutr. 1993;58(5 Suppl):724S–32.

9. White JS. Misconceptions about high-fructose corn syrup: is it uniquely responsible for obesity, reactive dicarbonyl compounds, and advanced glycation endproducts? J Nutr. 2009;139:1219S–27.

10. Buck AW. High fructose corn syrup. In: O'Brien-Nabors L, editor. Alternative sweeteners. 4th ed. Boca Raton: CRC; 2011.

11. Institute of Medicine of the National Academies. Food Chemicals Codex. 5th ed. Washington: The National Academies Press; 2003.

12. U.S. Food and Drug Administration. Code of Federal Regulations: high fructose corn syrup. Federal Register 2009;21 CFR 184.1866:574.

13. Ventura EE, Davis JN, Goran MI. Sugar content of popular sweetened beverages based on objective laboratory analysis: focus on fructose content. Obesity (Silver Spring). 2011;19:868–74.

14. Goran MI, Dumke K, Bouret SG, Kayser B, Walker RW, Blumberg B. The obesogenic effect of high fructose exposure during early development. Nat Rev Endocrinol. 2013;9:494–500.

15. Goran MI, Ulijaszek SJ, Ventura EE. High fructose corn syrup and diabetes prevalence: A global perspective. Glob Public Health. 2013;8:55–64.

16. Goran MI, Ventura EE. Genetic predisposition and increasing dietary fructose exposure: the perfect storm for fatty liver disease in Hispanics in the U.S. Dig Liver Dis. 2012;44:711–3.

17. Hobbs LJ, Krueger D. Response to "Sugar content of popular sweetened beverages based on objective laboratory analysis: focus on fructose content". Obesity (Silver Spring) 2011;19:687; author Goran reply -8; Hobbs & Krueger reply to Goran 8.

18. Hobbs LJ, Krueger D. Response to "Response to the letter regarding 'Sugar content of popular sweetened beverages'". Obesity (Silver Spring) 2011;19:688.

19. White JS, Hobbs LJ, Fernandez S. Fructose content and composition of commercial HFCS-sweetened carbonated beverages. Int J Obes (Lond). 2015;39:176–82.

20. Wong DWS. Food enzymes: structure and mechanism. New York: Chapman & Hall; 1995.

21. USDA-ERS. Sugar & sweeteners: background. USDA-ERS; 2012. http://www.ers.usda.gov/topics/crops/sugar-sweeteners/data.aspx.

22. USDA-ERS. Table 30 – U.S. high fructose corn syrup (HFCS) supply and use. USDA-ERS; 2013. http://www.ers.usda.gov/datafiles/Sugar_and_Sweeteners_Yearbook_Tables/Corn_Sweetener_Supply_Use_and_Trade/TABLE30.XLS.

23. White JS, Parke DW. Fructose adds variety to breakfast. Cereal Foods World. 1989;34:392–8.

24. Wienen W, Shallenberger R. Influence of acid and temperature on the rate of inversion of sucrose. Food Chem. 1988;29:51–5.

25. USDA/Economic Research Service. USDA-ERS. Food availability (per capita) data system: loss-adjusted food availability. Sugar and Sweeteners (added), 2013.

26. LMC Sweetener Analysis. World sugar and HFCS consumption. New York: LMC International, p. 1989–2013.

27. Glinsmann WH, Bowman BA. The public health significance of dietary fructose. Am J Clin Nutr. 1993;58(5 Suppl):820S–3.

28. Glinsmann WH, Irausquin H, Park YK. Evaluation of health aspects of sugars contained in carbohydrate sweeteners. Report of Sugars Task Force, 1986. J Nutr. 1986;116(11 Suppl):S1–216.

29. Food and Drug Administration, Department of Health and Human Services. Direct food substances affirmed as generally recognized as safe: high fructose corn syrup. Code of Federal Regulations. 2013. (Revised);21CFR184.1866.

30. Bray GA, Popkin BM. Calorie-sweetened beverages and fructose: what have we learned 10 years later? Pediatr Obes. 2013;8:242–8.

31. Melanson KJ, Zukley L, Lowndes J, Nguyen V, Angelopoulos TJ, Rippe JM. Effects of high-fructose corn syrup and sucrose consumption on circulating glucose, insulin, leptin, and ghrelin and on appetite in normal-weight women. Nutrition. 2007;23:103–12.

32. Zukely L, Lowndes J, Nguyen V, et al. Consumption of beverages sweetened with high fructose corn syrup and sucrose produce similar levels of glucose, leptin, insulin and ghrelin in obese females. FASEB J. 2007;21:538.
33. Stanhope KL, Griffen SC, Bair BR, Swarbrick MM, Keim NL, Havel PJ. Twenty-four-hour endocrine and metabolic profiles following consumption of high-fructose corn syrup-, sucrose-, fructose-, and glucose-sweetened beverages with meals. Am J Clin Nutr. 2008;87:1194–203.
34. Soenen S, Westerterp-Plantenga MS. No differences in satiety or energy intake after high-fructose corn syrup, sucrose, or milk preloads. Am J Clin Nutr. 2007;86:1586–94.
35. Rippe JM, Angelopoulos TJ. Sucrose, high-fructose corn syrup, and fructose, their metabolism and potential health effects: what do we really know? Adv Nutr. 2013;4:236–45.
36. Rippe JM, Kris Etherton PM. Fructose, sucrose, and high fructose corn syrup: modern scientific findings and health implications. Adv Nutr. 2012;3:739–40.
37. Forshee RA, Storey ML, Allison DB, et al. A critical examination of the evidence relating high fructose corn syrup and weight gain. Crit Rev Food Sci Nutr. 2007;47:561–82.
38. Fulgoni 3rd V. High-fructose corn syrup: everything you wanted to know, but were afraid to ask. Am J Clin Nutr. 2008;88:1715S.
39. Murphy SP. The state of the science on dietary sweeteners containing fructose: summary and issues to be resolved. J Nutr. 2009;139:1269S–70.
40. Jones JM. Dietary sweeteners containing fructose: overview of a workshop on the state of the science. J Nutr. 2009;139:1210S–3.
41. Rippe JM, Saltzman E. Sweetened beverages and health: current state of scientific understandings. Adv Nutr. 2013;4:527–9.
42. American Medical Association. Report 3 of the Council on Science and Public Health (A-08): the health effects of high fructose syrup. Chicago: American Medical Association; 2008.
43. Fitch C, Keim KS, Academy of N, Dietetics. Position of the Academy of Nutrition and Dietetics: use of nutritive and nonnutritive sweeteners. J Acad Nutr Diet. 2012;112:739–58
44. Tappy L, Le KA. Metabolic effects of fructose and the worldwide increase in obesity. Physiol Rev. 2010;90:23–46.
45. Johnson RJ, Segal MS, Sautin Y, et al. Potential role of sugar (fructose) in the epidemic of hypertension, obesity and the metabolic syndrome, diabetes, kidney disease, and cardiovascular disease. Am J Clin Nutr. 2007;86:899–906.
46. Annema N, Heyworth JS, McNaughton SA, Iacopetta B, Fritschi L. Fruit and vegetable consumption and the risk of proximal colon, distal colon, and rectal cancers in a case-control study in Western Australia. J Am Diet Assoc. 2011;111:1479–90.
47. Aune D, Chan DS, Vieira AR, et al. Dietary fructose, carbohydrates, glycemic indices and pancreatic cancer risk: a systematic review and meta-analysis of cohort studies. Ann Oncol. 2012;23:2536–46.
48. Lim JS, Mietus-Snyder M, Valente A, Schwarz JM, Lustig RH. The role of fructose in the pathogenesis of NAFLD and the metabolic syndrome. Nat Rev Gastroenterol Hepatol. 2010;7:251–64.
49. Carden TJ, Carr TP. Food availability of glucose and fat, but not fructose, increased in the US between 1970 and 2009: analysis of the USDA food availability data system. Nutr J. 2013;12:130.
50. Marriott BP, Cole N, Lee E. National estimates of dietary fructose intake increased from 1977 to 2004 in the United States. J Nutr. 2009;139:1228S–35.
51. Ha V, Sievenpiper JL, de Souza RJ, et al. Effect of fructose on blood pressure: a systematic review and meta-analysis of controlled feeding trials. Hypertension. 2012;59:787–95.
52. Sievenpiper JL, Carleton AJ, Chatha S, et al. Heterogeneous effects of fructose on blood lipids in individuals with type 2 diabetes: systematic review and meta-analysis of experimental trials in humans. Diabetes Care. 2009;32:1930–7.
53. Sievenpiper JL, de Souza RJ, Mirrahimi A, et al. Effect of fructose on body weight in controlled feeding trials: a systematic review and meta-analysis. Ann Intern Med. 2012;156:291–304.

54. Sievenpiper JL, Wang DD, De Souza RJ, et al. Effect of fructose on postprandial triglycerides: a systematic review and meta-analysis of controlled feeding trials. Can J Diabetes. 2012;36:S19.
55. Wang D, Sievenpiper JL, de Souza RJ, et al. Effect of fructose on postprandial triglycerides: a systematic review and meta-analysis of controlled feeding trials. Atherosclerosis. 2014;232:125–33.
56. Wang DD, Sievenpiper JL, de Souza RJ, et al. The effects of fructose intake on serum uric acid vary among controlled dietary trials. J Nutr. 2012;142:916–23.
57. Cozma AI, Sievenpiper JL, de Souza RJ, et al. Effect of fructose on glycemic control in diabetes: a systematic review and meta-analysis of controlled feeding trials. Diabetes Care. 2012;35:1611–20.
58. Sievenpiper JL, Chiavaroli L, de Souza RJ, et al. 'Catalytic' doses of fructose may benefit glycaemic control without harming cardiometabolic risk factors: a small meta-analysis of randomised controlled feeding trials. Br J Nutr. 2012;108:418–23.
59. USDA/Economic Research Service. USDA-ERS. Food availability (per capita) data system: food availability. Sugar and sweeteners (added). 2012.
60. USDA/Economic Research Service. Food availability (per capita) data system: loss-adjusted food availability. http://www.ers.usda.gov/data-products/food-availability-%28per-capita%29-data-system.aspx,Calories.xls. Accessed 13 July 2011.
61. Mintel Research Consultancy. http://www.cornnaturally.com/Consumer-Research/mintel-research-on-hfcs. Accessed 10 Feb 2014.
62. Nielsen Company. http://www.cornnaturally.com/Consumer-Research/Nielsen-Shopper-Data. Accessed 10 Feb 2014.

Part VII
Beverage Mechanics: Color, Taste, Labeling, and Ingredient Function

Chapter 21
The Crucial Role of Color in the Perception of Beverages

Charles Spence

Keywords Color • Taste • Flavor • Visual dominance • Disconfirmed expectation • Multisensory integration

Key Points

1. Color is not included in most definitions of flavor.
2. That said, there can be no doubt but that what we see exerts a profound influence on our perception of, and responses toward, beverages.
3. Color is used in beverages by marketers to capture the attention of the shopper on the supermarket shelf (just think of those transparent blue raspberry-flavored drinks).
4. Color cues also provide an indication as to the likely identity and intensity of the flavor of a beverage.
5. Get the color right, and the consumers' expectations will be met, normally a good thing.
6. Get the color wrong, and consumers may experience a negatively valenced disconfirmation of expectation—rarely a good idea.
7. Beverage color is a crucial aspect of the consumer's overall multisensory product experience. In fact, it can be all that stands between long-term success and failure in the highly competitive marketplace for beverages.

C. Spence (✉)
Crossmodal Research Laboratory, Department of Experimental Psychology, Oxford University, South Parks Road, Oxford OX1 3UD, UK
e-mail: charles.spence@psy.ox.ac.uk

© Springer International Publishing Switzerland 2016 305
T. Wilson, N.J. Temple (eds.), *Beverage Impacts on Health and Nutrition*,
Nutrition and Health, DOI 10.1007/978-3-319-23672-8_21

Introduction

It has been known for many years that visual cues play an important role in multi-sensory flavor perception and this can be critical in the beverage choices made by the consumer. What we see also profoundly influences our food choices and consumption behaviors [2]. Something like 200 studies have been published on this topic since the original report appeared back in 1936 (see [33], for a review of this extensive literature). By and large, the research that has been published to date shows that people's judgment of the identity of a beverage's taste, aroma (or bouquet), and flavor can all be influenced by changing the color (either appropriate, inappropriate, or absent) of the drink that they happen to be evaluating. Additionally, many (but by no means all) of the studies that have investigated the effect of varying the intensity of the color added to a beverage have shown an effect on the intensity of taste and/or flavor perception (see [33], for a review). Color also influences appetitive behaviors [35].

Color and Flavor Perception

One of the classic studies demonstrating the influence of color on *taste* sensitivity in humans was conducted by Maga [17]. He investigated the consequences on perceptual thresholds of coloring aqueous solutions of the four basic tastes (e.g., sweet, sour, bitter, and salty) red, yellow, or green using tasteless and odorless food dyes (hence avoiding any chemical "masking" by colorant molecules). Maga found that the concentration of the tastant often had to be increased in order for participants to correctly detect its presence in a colored, as compared to an uncolored, solution. So, for example, adding yellow coloring to a sweet solution significantly decreased taste sensitivity, whereas the addition of green color increased it. Meanwhile, coloring a solution red was found to result in a significant lowering of participants' sensitivity to bitterness. Finally, coloring a solution yellow or green significantly decreased participants' sensitivity to sourness (see also [43]).

Elsewhere, Morrot et al. [18] investigated the effects of color on people's perception of the aroma (or bouquet) of wine. These researchers fooled the students enrolled on a university wine degree course in Bordeaux, France, into believing that they were holding a glass of red wine, simply by coloring a white Bordeaux wine red with an odorless food dye! The participants in this now classic study were initially instructed to evaluate the aroma of a glass of white wine while sniffing it. Next, they did the same with a glass of red. As one might have expected, completely different odor descriptors were used when describing the aromas of the two wines: e.g., notes such as citrus, lychee, straw, and lemon when describing the white wine and notes like chocolate, berry, tobacco, etc., when describing the red.

Finally, the students were given a third glass of wine and were asked to decide whether the bouquet displayed aroma notes that were typical of red or white wine.

(The third glass looked like a glass of red wine but was, in fact, the same white wine that they had been given originally, but now colored so as to be indistinguishable in color from a red.) Surprisingly, when forced to choose, the students went for the red (rather than white) wine odor descriptors. That is, they were unable to pick out the aromas in the miscolored wine that they had previously reported when sniffing the original white wine. Results such as these therefore demonstrate just how powerful visual cues can dominate over people's orthonasal olfactory experience of a drink (see also [21], for early research on coloring wine, and [30], for a review). Subsequently, Parr et al. [22] reported similar results with New Zealand wine experts who, in this case, were allowed to taste (and not just sniff) the wine.

Outside of the world of wine, many researchers have demonstrated similar effects of beverage color on people's ability to identify the flavor of various drinks (e.g., [1, 26, 28, 47, 49]), as well as on their ratings of odor intensity [50, 51].

The story regarding vision's influence over odor perception is complicated somewhat by the results of a study by Koza et al. [15]. These researchers demonstrated that color has a qualitatively different effect on the perception of the orthonasally versus retronasally presented odors associated with a commercial tangerine-pineapple-guava-flavored water drink. *Orthonasal* olfaction refers to the inhalation of external odors when sniffing. *Retronasal* olfaction involving the posterior nares is associated with the detection of those olfactory stimuli that are periodically forced out of the nasal cavity whenever we swallow. Koza et al. [15] found that adding the red food coloring led to the intensity of the drink's aroma being rated as higher in those participants who sniffed the drink orthonasally. By contrast, it was rated as less intense in the presence (vs. absence) of color when the same drinks were experienced retronasally by another group of participants.

Koza et al. [15] accounted for this surprising pattern of results by highlighting the fact that it may be more important for us to correctly evaluate a drink once it has entered our mouth, since that is the time when it will pose a much greater risk of potentially poisoning us. Should Koza et al.'s intriguing results be replicated in future research (preferably using a within-participants experimental design), it would certainly add weight to the suggestion that qualitatively different patterns of multisensory integration/perception can be observed following the presentation of odors orthonasally as compared to retronasally. It would also draw attention to the need to pay careful attention to the methodological details of stimulus presentation in those studies of colored beverages that have been published to date.

Given the significant effect that color exerts both on taste sensitivity [17] and on various aspects of odor perception (e.g., [1, 15, 18, 28]), it should come as little surprise that color cues have also been shown to exert a robust effect on people's flavor identification responses. The participants in a classic study by DuBose et al. [4] had to try and identify the flavors of various differently colored fruit-flavored drinks. Certain of the color-flavor pairings were "appropriate" (such as a cherry-flavored drink colored red), while others were "inappropriate" (such as a lime-flavored drink that had been colored red). The participants had to try to identify 16 different beverages resulting from the crossing of four flavors (cherry-, orange-, or lime-flavored, or flavorless) and four colors (red, orange, green, or colorless). The

Reported	Color of cherry-flavoured drink			
Flavour	Red	Orange	Green	Colourless
Cherry	70%	41%	33%	37%
Orange	0%	19%	0%	0%
Lime	0%	0%	26%	7%

Table 21.1 Partial summary of the results of a classic study by DuBose et al. [4], highlighting the effect of food coloring on the perception of the identity of a beverage's flavor. The table highlights the distribution of the three most common flavor responses when tasting the cherry-flavored drink. The numerical values indicate the percentages of each flavor response for each color

participants were given a list of 14 possible flavors (strawberry, raspberry, lemon, lime, grape, apple, cherry, orange, blueberry, lemon-lime, grapefruit, apricot, other, or no flavor) to choose from. They misidentified the flavors of a number of the drinks when colored inappropriately. Often, incorrect responses appeared to have been driven by the colors of the drinks themselves. So, for example, 26 % of the participants reported that a cherry-flavored drink tasted of lemon/lime when colored green, as compared to no lime-flavor responses when the drink was colored red (see Table 21.1 for a selective summary of the results).

Similar results have been reported in many other studies over the years (see [33], for a review). An interesting, *though* as yet unanswered, question here is why only a proportion of participants' responses were influenced by the color of the drinks in the study carried out by DuBose et al. [4]. One suggestion is that people may simply differ in the degree to which particular colors induce specific flavor expectations [28, 29, 40, 41, 45]. The existence of such individual differences (often culturally determined) in color-based flavor expectations helps to explain why it is that there is such significant interindividual variation in the extent to which particular colors affect flavor identification responses.

One particularly interesting finding to have emerged in this area comes from research demonstrating that the taster status of the participants modulates the extent to which visual cues influence flavor perception [46]. Supertasters generally have more taste buds on their tongue than nontasters. In fact, it has been suggested that some supertasters may have as many as 16 times more taste buds than certain other nontasters. An individual's taster status has been shown to affect their perception of all the basic tastes (e.g., sweet, sour, bitter, salty). The participants in Zampini et al.'s [46] study had to try to identify the flavor of fruit-flavored drinks presented among flavorless drinks. The drinks were colored red, orange, yellow, and gray or else presented as colorless solutions. Overall, the *nontasters* among the participants correctly identified 19 % of the solutions, the *medium tasters* 31 %, and the *supertasters* 67 %. Coloring the orange-flavored solutions orange led to a significant increase in the accuracy of participants' flavor identification responses (see Fig. 21.1). Similarly, coloring the blackcurrant-flavored solutions grayish purple also led to a significant facilitation of performance. Note here that many blackcurrant-flavored beverages, including drinkable yogurts, are typically colored grayish purple.

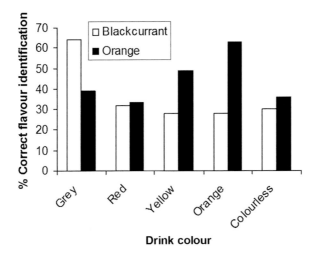

Fig. 21.1 Results of a study by Zampini et al. [46] highlighting the influence of color on people's ability to correctly identify orange- and blackcurrant-flavored solutions. Note that the participants tasted the drinks but did not swallow (cf. [15])

What is more, the participants in Zampini et al.'s [46] study rated the congruently colored drinks as having a more intense flavor than when presented either with no color or with an incongruent color. By contrast, no such effect of congruent coloring was reported on participants' judgments of sourness or sweetness. Interestingly, Zampini et al. found that the addition of color to a beverage had the largest effect on the flavor identification responses of the nontasters, less of an effect on the medium tasters, and very little effect on the color identification responses of the supertasters.

In summary, the addition of color (be it appropriate, inappropriate, or absent) can exert a significant effect on people's flavor identification responses. By contrast, the manipulation of the *intensity* of the color added to a foodstuff does not, however, appear to have such a clear-cut effect on people's judgments of flavor (or, for that matter, taste) intensity (see [33], for a review).

Sensory Incongruency in the Beverage Sector

The disconfirmation of expectation that often results when the expected and actual flavor of a commercial beverage differs too much is normally an undesirable quality for consumers. Here one need only think of the clear cola drinks—Tab Clear and Crystal Pepsi—that failed miserably when they were launched some years ago (e.g., [39, 42]). That said, there are a few situations in which the consumer may be happy to be surprised. Think here only of a dinner served at a modernist restaurant or having a drink in a cocktail bar (see [35]). In terms of incongruously colored cocktail drinks, one need only mention the orange-flavored blue Curaçao. Incongruently colored products also seem to be appreciated by children, just think of the green tomato ketchup or Confused Skittles (see [31], for a review).

Off Colors in Beverages

One aspect of beverage color that can have a particularly detrimental impact on consumer perception is when a drink takes on the visual appearance that makes the consumer think that it may have gone off or be in some other way of poor quality (e.g., [38]). Crumpacker [3] has provided an informative anecdote that is relevant to this theme: She describes the case of a batch of 26,000 quarts of Tropicana grapefruit juice that had been donated to a food bank back in 1981. People apparently refused to drink the juice because of its abnormal brown color (even though those who tried it reported that it tasted just fine). Given the importance of the visual appearance of a beverage to its acceptance by consumers, it should come as little surprise that many researchers/companies spend a lot of time trying to make sure that the colors of their beverages have been optimized. This is especially true for those drinks, such as orange juice, that are subject to natural variation, e.g., in the raw materials from one season to the next, and from one fruit-growing region to another (see [5, 43]).

Cross-Cultural Differences in the Meaning of Beverage Color

Oftentimes, there simply isn't a one-to-one mapping between beverage color (hue) and flavor. For instance, the same red drink might signify (and hence set up an expectation of) strawberry flavor in one individual while being associated with the flavor of watermelon in another. In our own cross-cultural research (e.g., [27, 40]), we often find that people from different parts of the world sometimes associate very different flavors with one and the same color in a beverage. So, for example, in one study, we found that the red drink shown in Fig. 21.2a was associated with the flavor of raspberry by young British consumers, but with a cherry flavor by young Taiwanese participants. In this case, both flavors are naturally associated with the same red color. By contrast, when we showed the blue drink displayed in Fig. 21.2b to participants, the Brits thought that it would taste of raspberry, while the Taiwanese participants thought of a mint-flavored product. In this case, the British participants have presumably internalized the arbitrary crossmodal link that certain drink brands have managed to establish between blue coloring and raspberry-flavored soft drinks such as Gatorade and Slush Puppie.

While such individual differences in the meaning of beverage color are frequently observed in cross-cultural research, it is important to note that similar differences have also been demonstrated within apparently homogenous groups of participants (i.e., who all come from the same cultural background; see [27–29, 45]). Thus, ultimately, it may be more important to establish the flavor expectations

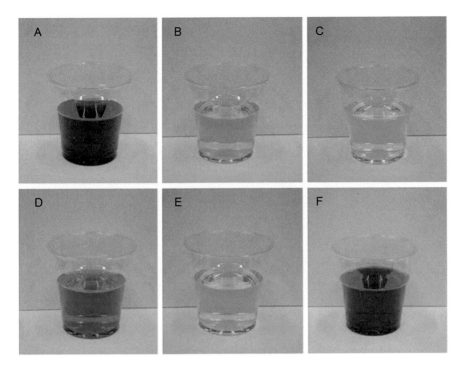

Fig. 21.2 For many years, researchers have known that changing the color of a beverage can change its perceived taste and flavor. In much of our current research here at the Crossmodal Research Laboratory at Oxford University, we try to establish the specific taste/flavor expectations that are elicited by particular food colors. Oftentimes, this is done by presenting pictures of a series of beverages to participants from different parts of the world and assessing their flavor expectations. For example, the six beverage colors shown here were presented to young participants in Taiwan and the UK [28]. Several of these beverages (e.g., those shown in panels *B* and *F*) were associated with different flavors by the participants in the two countries (see the text for details)

that are held by a given group of consumers on seeing a particular beverage color than many researchers previously gave credit for [14]. It is often these automatically generated flavor expectations (or predictions) that determine what flavor an individual identifies on tasting a drink. Such visually determined flavor expectations can also play a major role in determining whether a consumer experiences a disconfirmation of expectation. As mentioned already, this is normally a negatively valenced experience for consumers (see [35, 44]).

Product-Extrinsic Color

Beyond the color of the drink itself, it is important to note that the color of the packaging, not to mention the color of the cup in which a consumer drinks the product, can also impact on people's flavor experiences ([24]; see [34], for a review; see also [9]). And beyond that, Oberfeld et al. [19] have reported that ambient color can

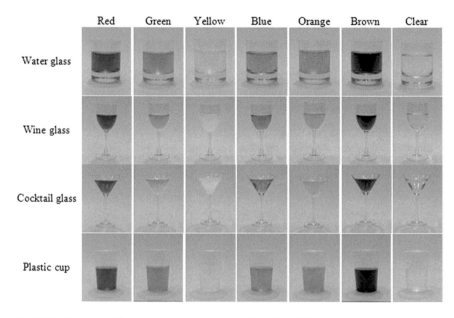

Fig. 21.3 The seven different beverage colors shown in the four different receptacles (water glass, wine glass, cocktail glass, and plastic cup) used in a recent study by Wan et al. [40]

affect people's taste and flavor ratings. In an intriguing series of experiments conducted in a winery on the Rhine and in the psychology laboratory, these German researchers were able to demonstrate that changing the color of the ambient lighting in which people tasted a white wine (specifically changing it from white to red, blue, or green) exerted a significant effect on the its perceived taste and flavor (specifically its sweetness and spiciness; a Reisling wine was used in this study).[1] The ambient lighting even affected how much people were willing to pay for the wine (being 50 % higher under one lighting condition than another). Elsewhere, researchers have shown that people who like strong coffee tend to drink more of it under brighter ambient lighting conditions, whereas those who like their coffee weaker consume more under dimmer lighting [7].

The taste and flavor expectations that a consumer generates on seeing a particular beverage color can also be modulated by the type of receptacle in which that drink happens to be presented (see [40]). So, for example, in our latest research, we have demonstrated that the flavor associations that are generated for a given beverage color sometimes change as function of the shape of the glass in which that drink is presented (see Fig. 21.3).

[1] Note that the wine was tasted from black tasting glasses so that any change in the ambient lighting didn't influence the visual appearance properties of the wine itself.

On the Ecological Validity of Laboratory-Based Research on Colored Beverages

Over the years, some researchers have questioned the ecological validity of much of the laboratory-based research on beverage color (e.g., [8]). One pertinent criticism is that the within-participants experimental design (which represents a particularly popular approach to testing beverage color among academic researchers) likely draws the attention of the participants involved to the salient color changes that they are testing, more than might otherwise (i.e., normally) be the case. What is more, in the majority of our real-world interactions with beverage products, there is normally a variety of additional information (e.g., packaging or written/verbal descriptions) available to the consumer to help them predict what a given beverage color means in a specific context. It is important to bear in mind that such cues are normally denied to the participants in the majority of laboratory studies.

Nevertheless, despite these caveats, it should be noted that beverage color influences people's flavor perception automatically, even when they know that the coloring of the beverages that they are tasting has been designed to trick them [45]. One likely explanation for the existence of such crossmodal effects of sight on taste and flavor perception is that our brains automatically makes predictions about the likely taste, flavor, and potential nutritional qualities of food and beverage products as soon as we set eyes on them (see [32]).

Conclusion

The evidence published to date clearly demonstrates that beverage color exerts a powerful influence over people's flavor *identification* responses (e.g., [4, 36, 42, 45, 46]). This visual dominance over (or modification of) flavor perception has been demonstrated across the age spectrum, from childhood to old age (e.g., [16, 20, 23]; see [31], for a review). Changing the intensity of a beverage's coloring can also influence people's ratings of taste/flavor intensity as well [10–13, 25, 37]. However, it should be remembered here that such color intensity effects are not always observed (e.g., [6]); in fact, much may depend on people's sensory expectations (based on their prior experience) regarding the taste/flavor intensity of a beverage given a certain level of color intensity.

Many consumers appear to associate very bright food coloring with artificial-tasting products. At the other extreme, a number of companies have failed when they have launched clear, flavored beverages into the marketplace—just think of Tab Clear and Crystal Pepsi [39, 42]. Although beyond the scope of the present review, it is worth mentioning that food coloring can also influence the perceived refreshment value of beverage products [48, 49]; color can even affect people's consumption behaviors, not to mention playing a role in modulating their acceptance of a beverage product [2, 35]. Ultimately, then, both the hue and intensity of a beverage's color has a profound effect on the consumer's perception and behavior. Color, therefore, is crucial to the perception of beverages.

References

1. Blackwell L. Visual clues and their effects on odour assessment. Nutr Food Sci. 1995;5:24–8.
2. Clydesdale FM. Color as a factor in food choice. Crit Rev Food Sci Nutr. 1993;33:83–101.
3. Crumpacker B. The sex life of food: when body and soul meet to eat. New York: Thomas Dunne Books; 2006.
4. DuBose CN, Cardello AV, Maller O. Effects of colorants and flavorants on identification, perceived flavor intensity, and hedonic quality of fruit-flavored beverages and cake. J Food Sci. 1980;45:1393–9, 1415.
5. Fernández-Vázquez R, Hewson L, Fisk I, Vila D, Mira F, Vicario IM, Hort, J. Colour influences sensory perception and liking of orange juice. Flavour. 2014:3:1.
6. Frank R, Ducheny K, Mize S. Strawberry odor, but not red color, enhances the sweetness of sucrose solutions. Chem Senses. 1989;14:371–7.
7. Gal D, Wheeler SC, Shiv B. Cross-modal influences on gustatory perception. 2007. http://ssrn.com/abstract=1030197 unpublished manuscript.
8. Garber Jr LL, Hyatt EM, Starr Jr RG. Placing food color experimentation into a valid consumer context. J Food Prod Market. 2001;7(3):3–24.
9. Guéguen N, Jacob C. Coffee cup color and evaluation of a beverage's "warmth quality". Color Res Appl. 2012. doi:10.1002/col.21757.
10. Hyman A. The influence of color on the taste perception of carbonated water preparations. Bull Psychon Soc. 1983;21:145–8.
11. Johnson J, Clydesdale FM. Perceived sweetness and redness in colored sucrose solutions. J Food Sci. 1982;47:747–52.
12. Johnson JL, Dzendolet E, Clydesdale FM. Psychophysical relationships between perceived sweetness and redness in strawberry-flavored beverages. J Food Prot. 1983;46:21–5. 28.
13. Johnson JL, Dzendolet E, Damon R, Sawyer M, Clydesdale FM. Psychophysical relationships between perceived sweetness and color in cherry-flavored beverages. J Food Prot. 1982;45:601–6.
14. Koch C, Koch EC. Preconceptions of taste based on color. J Psychol Interdisc Appl. 2003;137:233–42.
15. Koza BJ, Cilmi A, Dolese M, Zellner DA. Color enhances orthonasal olfactory intensity and reduces retronasal olfactory intensity. Chem Senses. 2005;30:643–9.
16. Lavin J, Lawless H. Effects of color and odor on judgments of sweetness among children and adults. Food Qual Pref. 1998;9:283–9.
17. Maga JA. Influence of color on taste thresholds. Chem Senses Flav. 1974;1:115–9.
18. Morrot G, Brochet F, Dubourdieu D. The color of odors. Brain Lang. 2001;79:309–20.
19. Oberfeld D, Hecht H, Allendorf U, Wickelmaier F. Ambient lighting modifies the flavor of wine. J Sens Stud. 2009;24:797–832.
20. Oram N, Laing DG, Hutchinson I, et al. The influence of flavor and color on drink identification by children and adults. Dev Psychobiol. 1995;28:239–46.
21. Pangborn RM, Berg HW, Hansen B. The influence of color on discrimination of sweetness in dry table-wine. Am J Psychol. 1963;76:492–5.
22. Parr WV, White KG, Heatherbell D. The nose knows: influence of colour on perception of wine aroma. J Wine Res. 2003;14:79–101.
23. Philipsen DH, Clydesdale FM, Griffin RW, Stern P. Consumer age affects response to sensory characteristics of a cherry flavoured beverage. J Food Sci. 1995;60:364–8.

24. Piqueras-Fiszman B, Spence C. Does the color of the cup influence the consumer's perception of a hot beverage? J Sens Stud. 2012;27:324–31.
25. Roth HA, Radle LJ, Gifford SR, Clydesdale FM. Psychophysical relationships between perceived sweetness and color in lemon- and lime-flavored drinks. J Food Sci. 1988;53:1116–9, 1162.
26. Schutz HG. Color in relation to food preference. In: Farrell KT, Wagner JR, Peterson MS, MacKinney G, editors. Color in foods: a symposium sponsored by the quartermaster food and container institute for the armed forces quartermaster research and development command. Washington: U.S. Army Quartermaster Corps. National Academy of Sciences – National Research Council; 1954, p. 16–23.
27. Shankar MU, Levitan C, Spence C. Grape expectations: the role of cognitive influences in color-flavor interactions. Consc Cogn. 2010;19:380–90.
28. Shankar M, Simons C, Levitan C, Shiv B, McClure S, Spence C. An expectations-based approach to explaining the crossmodal influence of color on odor identification: the influence of temporal and spatial factors. J Sens Stud. 2010;25:791–803.
29. Shankar M, Simons C, Shiv B, Levitan C, McClure S, Spence C. An expectations-based approach to explaining the influence of color on odor identification: the influence of degree of discrepancy. Att Perc Psychophys. 2010;72:1981–93.
30. Spence C. The color of wine – Part 1. World Fine Wine. 2010;28:122–9.
31. Spence C. The development and decline of multisensory flavour perception. In: Bremner AJ, Lewkowicz D, Spence C, editors. Multisensory development. Oxford: Oxford University Press; 2012. p. 63–87.
32. Spence C. Eating with our eyes: on the colour of flavour. In: Elliott A, Fairchild M, editors. The handbook of color psychology. Cambridge: Cambridge University Press; 2015. p. 603–618.
33. Spence C, Levitan C, Shankar MU, Zampini M. Does food color influence taste and flavor perception in humans? Chemosens Percept. 2010;3:68–84.
34. Spence C, Piqueras-Fiszman B. The multisensory packaging of beverages. In: Kontominas MG, editor. Food packaging: procedures, management and trends. Hauppauge: Nova Publishers; 2012. p. 187–233.
35. Spence C, Piqueras-Fiszman B. The perfect meal: the multisensory science of food and dining. Oxford: Wiley-Blackwell; 2014.
36. Stillman J. Color influences flavor identification in fruit-flavored beverages. J Food Sci. 1993;58:810–2.
37. Strugnell C. Colour and its role in sweetness perception. Appetite. 1997;28:85.
38. Tepper BJ. Effects of a slight color variation on consumer acceptance of orange juice. J Sens Stud. 1993;8:145–54.
39. Triplett T. Consumers show little taste for clear beverages. Market News. 1994;28(11):2. 11.
40. Wan X, Velasco C, Michel C, Mu B, Woods AT, Spence C. Does the shape of the glass influence the crossmodal association between colour and flavour? A cross-cultural comparison. Flavour. 2014;3:3.
41. Wan X, Zhou X, Mu B, Du D, Velasco C, Michel C, Spence C. Crossmodal expectations of tea colour based on its flavour. J Sens Stud. 2014;29:285–293.
42. Watson E. We eat with our eyes: Flavor perception strongly influenced by food color, says DDW.2013.http://www.foodnavigator-usa.com/Science/We-eat-with-our-eyes-Flavor-perception-strongly-influenced-by-food-color-says-DDW.
43. Wei S-T, Ou L-C, Luo MR, Hutchings JB. Optimization of food expectations using product colour and appearance. Food Qual Pref. 2012;23:49–62.
44. Yeomans M, Chambers L, Blumenthal H, Blake A. The role of expectancy in sensory and hedonic evaluation: the case of smoked salmon ice-cream. Food Qual Pref. 2008;19:565–73.
45. Zampini M, Sanabria D, Phillips N, Spence C. The multisensory perception of flavor: assessing the influence of color cues on flavor discrimination responses. Food Qual Pref. 2007;18:975–84.

46. Zampini M, Wantling E, Phillips N, Spence C. Multisensory flavor perception: assessing the influence of fruit acids and color cues on the perception of fruit-flavored beverages. Food Qual Pref. 2008;19:335–43.
47. Zellner DA, Bartoli AM, Eckard R. Influence of color on odor identification and liking ratings. Am J Psychol. 1991;104:547–61.
48. Zellner DA, Durlach P. What is refreshing? An investigation of the color and other sensory attributes of refreshing foods and beverages. Appetite. 2002;39:185–6.
49. Zellner DA, Durlach P. Effect of color on expected and experienced refreshment, intensity, and liking of beverages. Am J Psychol. 2003;116:633–47.
50. Zellner DA, Kautz MA. Color affects perceived odor intensity. J Exp Psychol Hum Perc Perf. 1990;16:391–7.
51. Zellner DA, Whitten LA. The effect of color intensity and appropriateness on color-induced odor enhancement. American J Psychol. 1999;112:585–604.

Chapter 22
Functions of Common Beverage Ingredients

Heather N. Nelson, Kelli L. Rush, and Ted Wilson

Keywords Additive • Food processing • Acidity regulator • Antioxidant • Synergist • Preservative • Sequestrant • Emulsifier • Stabilizer • Thickener

Key Points

1. Beverages contain added ingredients that work to enhance flavor, color, nutritional value, texture, and/or shelf stability.
2. Beverages commercially sold must comply with FDA guidelines that require food safety barriers such as thermal processing.
3. Beverage requirements may be met by techniques such as thermal processing or by use of preservative systems such as added ingredients to prevent microbial growth or to prevent quality loss from heating or time prior to sale.
4. Organic acids impart tart taste and have antioxidant and preservative qualities.
5. Fatty acids serve as emulsifiers and hydrocolloids provide thickness.
6. Salts provide electrolytes, fluid stability, and/or microbiological control (preservative).
7. Sweeteners affect taste characteristics and caloric content.

Introduction

The numerous beverage brands, flavors, and products that include regular and diet carbonated soft drinks, juices, sports drinks, energy drinks, teas, coffees, beers, wines, and other alcoholic beverages represent a vast industry in the USA. Each beverage represents a unique profile of ingredients (chemicals) that are critical to

H.N. Nelson • K.L. Rush • T. Wilson, Ph.D. (✉)
Department of Biology, Winona State University, 232 Pasteur Hall, Winona, MN 55987, USA
e-mail: ewilson@winona.edu

© Springer International Publishing Switzerland 2016
T. Wilson, N.J. Temple (eds.), *Beverage Impacts on Health and Nutrition*,
Nutrition and Health, DOI 10.1007/978-3-319-23672-8_22

defining the taste, function, and shelf-life of these products. By itself, the nonalcoholic beverage industry commands an impressive $141 billion direct economic impact and provides 233,000 jobs [1].

In order for these products to resist spoilage and maintain their original flavor and consistency during transportation and shelf-life prior to sale, a wide range of ingredients with a numerous functions are used to formulate nonalcoholic beverages. All of the ingredients used by US manufacturers are deemed safe for use in foods by the FDA. Ingredients have to be deemed GRAS (generally recognized as safe) in order to be legally used in foods. Flavors have either been assessed by FDA as GRAS or are deemed GRAS by FEMA (The Flavor and Extract Manufacturers Association of the United States (https://www.femaflavor.org/gras). However, while the safety of ingredients has been well characterized, other ingredient characteristics are not well determined. For example, FDA has no specific guidance to define the term "natural" for most ingredients. They do, however, have definitions for natural flavors and natural colors.

Some of the functions of ingredients found in nonalcoholic beverages are to impart taste characteristics, reduce caloric intake, add color, add flavor, act as a preservative, and regulate the appearance and consistency of the beverage. Manufacturers may choose to add fortificants, or other functional ingredients including vitamins, minerals, botanicals, and electrolytes. Ingredients that are often added to nonalcoholic beverages include organic acids, fatty acids, starches, gums, salts, sweeteners, flavors, and colors. This chapter identifies some of the more common additives used in nonalcoholic beverages and provides an explanation of their functions.

Organic Acids

Organic acids, including citric, fumaric, and malic acids, are naturally found in fruits and vegetables, such as grapes, peaches, lemons, tomatoes, and red peppers [2]. In nonalcoholic beverages, organic acids are added to impart sour or tart taste, provide or stabilize pH dependent colors, and provide antioxidant properties that also stabilize colors and flavor systems and for preservative or antimicrobial qualities. While organic acids can be directly added to beverages, some are produced as by-products of fermentation, although this is mostly true for alcoholic drinks and some nonalcoholic beverages such as kombucha tea, and probiotic-cultured beverages are also fermented. While some suggest that organic acids can harm tooth enamel, this effect requires prolonged contact of the acid with the tooth. Thus, bathing teeth over a long period of time with soda and certain juices, including lime, lemon, and orange, can theoretically lead to this effect, but when normally consumed the saliva neutralizes this acidity rapidly [3].

Organic acids are often termed *acidity regulators* or *buffers* in industry because they allow manufacturers to control the pH of their products. This is an important consideration with thermal processing, where pH will change with temperature and severe changes in pH can deteriorate the beverage quality or taste. For example, the stabilization of pH can be critical in protein-containing beverages. Many organic acids can function as *antioxidants*, prolonging shelf-life by preventing the oxidation of lipids, including some pigments and natural flavor oils. In addition, certain organic acids function as *synergists*, enhancing the ability of antioxidants to control free radicals. When consumed by humans, drinks containing these antioxidants and synergists may also aid in the control of free radicals in the human system. As a result, the marketability of some beverages can be improved by including the word "antioxidant" on the product label to attract consumer interest for perceived health benefits. However, most organic acids are in beverages for their function properties and not to confer any specific health benefit.

Because organic acids create an acidic environment, they have antibiological qualities that are bacteriostatic to many microorganisms and thereby function as *preservatives*. Additionally, organic acids also function as *sequestrants*, or *chelating agents*, due to their ability to form several bonds to a single metal ion. Free metal ions are undesirable as they have the ability to react with other compounds, producing insoluble and/or colored compounds. Organic acids form water-soluble chelates with these metal ions, preventing them from negatively affecting the quality and aftertaste of the product in which they are contained [4].

Citric Acid, Fumaric Acid, and Malic Acid

Citric acid contributes to the sour taste of some fruits, including lemons. Citric acid is a chelating agent and a synergist to antioxidants. At an alkaline pH, the citrate ion increases the solubility of calcium by forming a soluble, negatively charged calcium-citrate complex [5]. Fumaric acid and malic acid are derivatives of citric acid with a similar function, although the degree to which each contributes to the sourness of a product is different (Fig. 22.1).

Ascorbic Acid and Erythorbic Acid

Ascorbic acid (vitamin C) is a water-soluble vitamin that aids in the repair and growth of tissues; repair and maintenance of bones, teeth, and cartilage; facilitates collagen creation; and acts as an antioxidant [4, 6]. The nutritional importance of

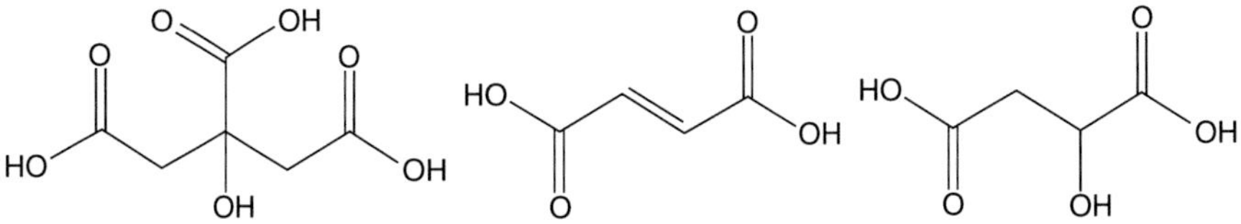

Fig. 22.1 Chemical structures of common organic acids

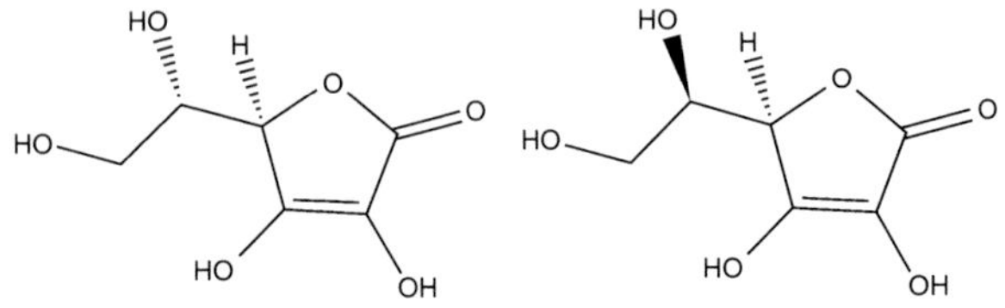

Fig. 22.2 Organic acid stereoisomers

this vitamin prompts beverage manufacturers to add it to their products. Additionally, most beverage processing may lead to the degradation of the ascorbate content of the original fresh fruit. As a result, ascorbate is commonly added back to make up for degradation of the original ascorbate. Erythorbic acid is a stereoisomer of ascorbic acid and also functions as an antioxidant. It is used in beverages due to its comparatively low price (Fig. 22.2).

Calcium Disodium EDTA and Tartaric Acid

Calcium disodium EDTA (the salt complex formed from ethylenediaminetetraacetic acid/edetic acid) is a good chelating agent that is used to sequester metal ions in aqueous solutions [4] and consequently has the ability to preserve color and retain flavor. Beverages that contain both benzoate salts and ascorbic (or erythorbic) acids can potentially form carcinogenic benzene; however, EDTA salts can prevent benzene formation [7]. Tartaric acid acts as an antioxidant and metal chelating agent [4].

Carbonated Water

Carbon dioxide gas dissolved in water creates carbonic acid (see equation). The carbonated water that is present in beverages can be found naturally in spring water or artificially created by the addition of carbon dioxide gas. The process of fermentation that is so critical to kombucha tea, kefir, and champagne is another way that a beverage can become carbonated.

$$H_2O + CO_2 \leftrightarrow H_2CO_3$$

Carbon dioxide experiences increased solubility at lower temperatures. Carbonated beverages are packed at very low temperatures, thereby increasing the solubility of both CO_2 and H_2CO_3 in the container. When the container is opened, pressure is released, freeing trapped carbonic acid as bubbles of CO_2.

Phosphoric Acid (Inorganic)

Phosphoric acid is an inorganic acid that has antimicrobial properties, the ability to buffer pH, and is also able to stabilize flavor. Colas contain phosphoric acid and typically have a pH of 2.8 to 3.2 [8], imparting a tart taste at the cost of potential negative effects on tooth enamel. Diets containing high amounts of phosphate and low amounts of calcium can theoretically lead to decalcification of bones [9]. However, there is no evidence that the casual consumption of colas leads to decreased bone density in humans [10, 11]. Further, it has been suggested that the amount of phosphoric acid present in cola is not sufficient for decalcification of bones to occur [9]. The association between phosphoric acid and bone loss remains controversial [10].

Salts

Salts are added to beverages to perform multiple functions, including enhancing or providing flavor, acting as a buffering agent to organic acids, and preserving perishable beverage contents.

Electrolytes

Magnesium chloride, calcium chloride, sodium citrate, and potassium citrate are salts that enhance beverage taste. These ions function as electrolytes in the body and stimulate glucose and water absorption in the small intestine. This is discussed further in the chapter by Maughan and Shirreffs on sports drinks. This process helps maintain extracellular fluid volume and stimulates thirst so that a person stays hydrated in order to keep plasma osmolality high [12].

Preservatives

Sodium and potassium benzoate are commonly used as preservatives in the beverage industry, and they can also function as flavor enhancers. Benzoates exert their preservative functions best in acidic environments. The most common benzoates are sodium benzoate and benzoic acid. Sodium benzoate is considered a non-antimicrobial salt that can turn into an antimicrobial, known as benzoic acid, if it is dissolved in water. Because ultra-high temperature (UHT) sterilization can degrade acidic products, lower temperature sterilization must be performed to maintain the preservative function of the benzoates. Benzoates are effective in protecting against yeasts, bacteria, and molds that are not destroyed during this lower temperature process [1]. These preservatives are most commonly associated with diet soft drinks. Sodium and potassium benzoate may be clastogenic, mutagenic, and cytotoxic to human lymphocytes at high concentrations [13]. However, studies must be conducted to determine the minimum threshold at which these complications may occur.

Sodium hexametaphosphate (SMHP) is most commonly used as a preservative and as an *emulsifier*, creating a continuous mixture from immiscible phases. It is used by the beverage industry to maintain consistency and clarity in beverages. SMHP is a chelating agent that prevents the precipitation of metals and minerals such as magnesium, iron, and calcium, whose precipitates can result in an unsightly appearance or altered taste [14].

Potassium sorbate is mainly used as a preservative because of its antimicrobial properties. It works to inhibit the growth of bacteria and molds, allowing it to protect the taste in some non-carbonated and juice-containing drinks. It is most commonly used in wines [15].

Fatty Acids

Fatty acids are sometimes added to beverages to serve as emulsifiers. In order for a stable emulsion to form, processing that applies force and creates an appropriate chemical environment is required. The integration of lipid-soluble additives that provide flavoring and coloring are made possible by emulsifiers.

An effective emulsifying compound used by industry is brominated vegetable oil (BVO), the product of the reaction between unsaturated vegetables oils and high-density Br_2. The use of BVO prevents oil from rising to the surface, maintaining the desirable uniformity qualities of the beverage. Some beverage companies are experiencing consumer pressure to discontinue the use of BVO due to concerns that bromine may accumulate in the fatty tissue of consumers [16]. A successful petition for Gatorade to end the use of BVO gained over 200,000 signatures from the public. Past studies demonstrated that feeding rats a diet containing 1.0 % BVO resulted in severe reproductive interference, high postnatal mortality, and severe behavioral impairment [17]. Even at a level of 0.1 % in the diet, rats exhibited a significant increase in triglyceride content in heart and soleus muscle and an increase in total and esterified cholesterol in the heart muscle [18]. Human clinical trials are difficult to perform due to potential health risks. Therefore, definitive understanding of the risk that BVO poses to humans remains controversial.

Coconut oil/medium-chain triglycerides (MCT) are composed of a mixture of saturated fatty acids with chain lengths of six to ten carbons. MCT may have beneficial effects on weight control and glucose and lipid metabolism when consumed in moderate amounts [19]. Compared to long-chain triglycerides, MCT are easily digested, absorbed, and used for energy by the body. Due to their ability to be quickly metabolized, digestive system stress is minimized [20]. Consequently, MCT are commonly included in sports drinks.

Hydrocolloids

Starches

Two kinds of starch are used as thickeners in the beverage industry: unmodified starch and modified starch. The selection of the kind of starch to use is dependent on the pH of the product. For example, in milk products, unmodified starch is often used as a *thickener*, increasing the viscosity of the product and creating a smooth mouthfeel. In low pH products, such as juices and soft drinks, unmodified starch breaks down and a modified food starch must be used. Starch can be modified by enzymatic, chemical, or physical processes, including bleaching, oxidation, acid and alkali treatment, acetylation, and roasting [21]. Modified food starch can originate from corn, wheat, rice, tapioca, or potato; however, FDA-regulated products must specify the source of the starch (potato starch, wheat starch, etc.), and unspecified "starch" is assumed to be derived from corn. Those who have celiac disease or wish to follow a gluten-free diet should be mindful of modified food starch and remain aware that wheat contamination is possible.

Gums and Pectins

Water-soluble gums are often used to stabilize and thicken beverages, aiding in the suspension of oils in water [21]. A wide range of plant-based gums are used in the beverage industry. Gum acacia (gum arabic) originates from the hardened sap of the acacia tree. Natural gum arabic is comprised of the mixed salts of arabic acid, carbohydrates, and some protein [22]. Glycerol ester of wood rosin (ester gum) is created by the reaction of glycerin with refined wood rosin. It is often used as a weighting agent that stabilizes liquid flavor emulsions with essential oils. Cellulose gum (sodium carboxymethyl cellulose) is derived from the natural polysaccharide cellulose that is found in plants, particularly from the cell walls of woody plants such as trees and cotton. Guar gum is extracted from guar beans. While gums are primarily used as beverage thickeners, they may also have other benefits. For instance, human studies have shown the potential of guar gum to curb diabetes and cardiovascular risk and aid in weight loss [23, 24].

Some gums originate as bacterial fermentation products. Xanthan gum is the polysaccharide product of the fermentation of sugars by strains of the bacterium *Xanthomonas*. These polysaccharides are then precipitated with isopropyl alcohol, dried, and ground to a powder [25]. The same process is used to produce gellan gum from the bacterium *Sphingomonas elodea*. Gellan gum can be found in alternative milk drinks, such as almond milk; in fortified drinks to suspend vitamins, minerals, and proteins; and in coffee drinks.

Pectin is a natural polysaccharide that is present in the cell wall of plants. Citrus fruits are commonly used as a source of pectin for food applications. Pectin acts as an emulsifier and stabilizer, aiding in the suspension of pulp, and also provides viscosity as well as texture to juices. Carrageenan is a natural carbohydrate that is extracted from red seaweed. λ, κ, and ι are the most common carrageenans that combine with milk proteins to improve the solubility and texture of products, thereby functioning as a thickener and stabilizer. Carrageenan is often added to milk, where it combines with milk proteins to suspend cocoa solids in chocolate milk, and in low-calorie products due to its ability to be substituted for fat. Undegraded carrageenan, the form of carrageenan used in food products due to its thickening properties, has been approved for human consumption. The use of carrageenan is complicated by the potential contamination of degraded carrageenan (or poligeenan), which has been shown in animal studies to have potentially negative effects on health such as the promotion of intestinal neoplasms and ulcerations [26].

Sweeteners

Caloric Sweeteners

There are multiple sources of caloric sweeteners, and many are natural. Caloric sweeteners include sucrose (table sugar), honey, molasses, agave, and high fructose corn syrup (HFCS). Other sweeteners include monosaccharides such as glucose and fructose (fruit sugar) and disaccharides such as lactose (milk sugar). Like most carbohydrates, caloric sweeteners provide 4 calories (17 kilojoules) per gram. The primary purpose of sweeteners is to preserve and/or enhance flavor.

Sucrose is a disaccharide composed of glucose and fructose molecules linked together by a relatively weak glycosidic bond. HFCS is produced by processing cornstarch to produce a nearly 100 % pure glucose product that is enzymatically converted to fructose. The result of this conversion is a syrup containing approximately 42 % fructose, aptly named HFCS 42. HFCS 42 can be further purified into a 90 % fructose syrup (HFCS 90). To make HFCS 55, the HFCS 90 is mixed with HFCS 42. The process of forming HFCS is more thoroughly described in the chapter by White and Nicklas. For many companies, HFCS has become one of the cheapest forms of sweeteners, prompting companies to switch from sucrose to HFCS.

Low and No Calorie Sweeteners

Low- and no-calorie sweeteners (nonnutritive sweeteners (NNS)) provide a sweet taste with less or without calories. Sweeteners that fall under this category include sucralose, acesulfame potassium, aspartame, and various plant-derived sweeteners such as stevia and monk fruit that are rapidly gaining popularity [27, 28]. These NNS are hundreds of times sweeter than their caloric brethren, which means that a smaller amount of NNS can be used to replace a large amount of sucrose or HFCS.

The Academy of Nutrition and Dietetics has provided an excellent review of the relative properties of NNS [27]. Aspartame is considered approximately 200 times sweeter than sucrose. It is composed of two naturally occurring amino acids, phenylalanine and aspartic acid. Aspartame is not considered stable when heated, so it is not suggested for use in thermally processed beverages. Sucralose (sold under the brand name Splenda©) is about 600 times sweeter than sucrose. Acesulfame potassium (Ace-K) is a heat-stable sweetener that is 200 times sweeter than sucrose. However, Ace-K is usually combined with other sweeteners, particularly sucralose, because alone it does not possess an adequate sweetness profile for many beverages.

Plant-derived NNS are also becoming popular for beverage applications. Steviol glycosides (Stevia) are extracted from the leaves of *Stevia rebaudiana*, a plant that is native to South America. Stevia is 200 to 400 times sweeter than sucrose. Stevia appeals to consumers due to its natural plant-based origin. *Monk Fruit* (*Siraitia grosvenorii*) is a gourd that is native to southern China and northern Thailand. The monk fruit contains varying levels of mogrosides I–V, of which mogroside V is incredibly sweet and is consequently used as a standard to measure the relative quality of the monk fruit sweetener product. Sweeteners derived from monk fruit are between 150 and 500 times sweeter than sucrose. Monk fruit has gained attention due to its use in chocolate milk that is sold as part of some school lunches in an initiative to reduce the amount of added sugar to flavored milks.

The ability of the average consumer to identify NNS from food labels based on either chemical (e.g., Sucralose) or trade name (e.g., Splenda®) is arguably weak. A survey was administered to 1,630 university freshman and sophomore students who were taking courses in biology, chemistry, or health sciences. The survey evaluated the ability of the 720 respondents to name NNS from memory [28]. Approximately two-thirds of respondents were unable to name two NNS by chemical or trade name, and only 12 % could name three or more NNS (Fig. 22.3). The poor ability of participants to know which chemicals are NNS may be partly responsible for consumer fears about NNS.

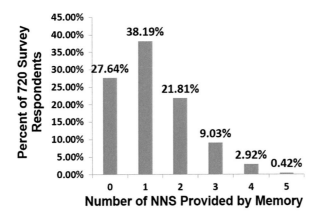

Fig. 22.3 College freshman and sophomore science students were asked to name NNS (trade or chemical name) from memory. Of the 720 respondents, 38 % could name just one NNS and less than 3 % of respondents could name four examples of NNS [30]

A recent concern associated with no- and low-calorie sweeteners is their potential association with negative health outcomes. Metabolic syndrome, weight gain, hypertension, and cardiovascular disease, as well as the possibility that the sweeteners are not associated with weight loss or even maintenance have been examined [29–31]. However, further investigation to explore the long-term effects of the overconsumption of soft drinks that use NNS on consumer health must take place to draw more definitive conclusions on their health effects.

Dyes and Coloring

Color is associated with our perception of taste. Most dyes are water-soluble and exist in many forms including liquid, powder, or granule. Dyes and coloring are used to provide color to beverages in order to influence the consumer to perceive the product in a particular way. This topic is more thoroughly described in the chapter by Spence.

Coloring substances can be extracted from a variety of sources—animal, vegetable, or mineral. There are a number of naturally derived colors used in the beverage industry. Juice made from elderberry fruit is an example of a natural dye that imparts a dark coloring. Other common natural colorings include annatto, saffron, paprika, grape skins, beetroot, cochineal, and beta-carotene. Sugar can be burned to produce a caramel coloring.

With some color additives, hypersensitivity and allergies can result from ingestion, making proper labeling important. The FDA requires that manufacturers of coloring substances provide sufficient evidence that the substance is safe for human consumption and requires that labels list all dyes that are present. The majority of dyes that are used in beverages are synthetically produced, such as blue dyes 1 and 2, and red dyes 3 and 40. The ingestion of some synthetic dyes has been implicated in the increased hyperactivity of some children [32]; however, there is no conclusive evidence existing that this is a cause of ADHD [33]. Consumers often perceive natural dyes as safer than artificial dyes, but this may be a false assumption as the relative safety of natural and artificial dyes cannot be unequivocally established.

Many different artificial colorants are used in the food and beverage industry. To impart a cherry pink color, red dye #3, also known as erythrosine, is used. It has a maximum accepted daily intake (ADI) of 0.1 mg/kg. Red dye #40 lends an orange-red color, is known as allura red, and has a maximum ADI of 7 mg/kg. To achieve an orange coloring, yellow dye #6, commonly known as sunset yellow, can be added. It has an ADI of 7.5 mg/kg. Yellow dye #5 conveys a lemon-yellow coloring, has a maximum ADI of 7.5 mg/kg, and is known as tartrazine. Blue dye #1 provides a bright blue hue, is aptly called brilliant blue, and has a maximum ADI of 12.5 mg/kg. To achieve a royal blue or indigo color, blue dye #2, or indigotine, can be added and has a maximum ADI of 5 mg/kg [34].

Negative public perceptions about the safety and palatability of dyes and colorings can lead to changes in product formulation. Consumer displeasure can lead to

Table 22.1 Amounts of caffeine in common beverages

Beverage type	Serving size (oz)	Caffeine count (mg)
Brewed coffee	8	95–200
Black tea	8	40–70
Green tea	8	24–45
Diet cola	12	23–47
Regular cola	12	23–39

reductions in sales and a consequential need for reformulation. For example, cochineal red (or carmine red) is a pigment obtained from an insect that lives on a cactus. It has been used in foods and beverages for several hundred years but was only recently linked with the promotion of allergic hypersensitivity [35]. Moreover, some consumers would probably not feel comfortable consuming a dye that is derived from an insect. Cochineal red was removed from Starbucks coffee products in 2012 [36], and there is presently pressure on Dannon to remove it from their yogurt.

Caffeine

Caffeine is a nitrogenous organic compound with stimulant effects that is found naturally in coffee and tea beverages. It is used as an additive in various beverages. Kola nuts are a commonly used source of caffeine. The typical caffeine content of various beverages is summarized in Table 22.1 [37]. Caffeine is considered GRAS (generally recognized as safe) in quantities of up to 400 mg for adults in the USA [38]. The FDA requires beverage labels to state that the product contains caffeine but does not require that manufacturers indicate the actual amount. Public pressure is increasing for the FDA to require specific caffeine content labeling, and some beverage manufacturers are now doing this in their products [39]. Labeling of the actual caffeine content can help improve marketability or for consumer education about potential risk (e.g., of energy drinks).

Conclusion

Beverages contain a diverse array of compounds that work to enhance flavor, color, composition, and overall quality of a drink. Organic acids impart a tart taste, antioxidant properties, and preservative qualities. Fatty acids serve as emulsifiers and may provide nutritional qualities. Starches, gums, and pectins provide thickness to a beverage. Salts provide electrolytes and act as preservatives. Caloric and noncaloric sweeteners modify beverage sweetness and, by extension, overall palatability. Manufacturers create the signature taste and qualities of the beverages that they market using these ingredients.

Beverage ingredients must follow regulations to ensure that consumers receive a safe and consistent product. Consumers have a growing desire to have more information regarding the function, source, and health outcomes of the ingredients that are listed on the labels of the products that they consume. Unfortunately, we do not as yet have conclusive evidence regarding the health effects, either positive or negative, of some ingredients.

References

1. American Beverage Association (ABA). History. 2015. http://www.ameribev.org/about-aba/history/. Accessed 3 Mar 2015.
2. Flores P, Hellin P, Fenoll J. Determination of organic acids in fruits and vegetables by liquid chromatography with tandem-mass spectrometry. Food Chem. 2011;132:1049–54.
3. Attin T, Weiss K, Becker K, Buchalla W, Wiegand A. Impact of modified acidic soft drinks on enamel erosion. Oral Dis. 2005;11:7–12.
4. Quitmann H, Fan R, Czermak P. Acidic organic compounds in beverage, food, and feed production. Adv Biochem Eng Biotechnol. 2014;143:91–141.
5. Shorr E, Almy T, Sloan M, Taussky H, Toscani V. The relation between the urinary excretion of citric acid and calcium; its implications for urinary calcium stone formation. Science. 1942;96:587–8.
6. MedlinePlus. Vitamin C. 2013. http://www.nlm.nih.gov/medlineplus/ency/article/002404.htm. Accessed 7 Feb 2015.
7. Food and Drug Administration (FDA). Data on benzene in soft drinks and other beverages. 2015. http://www.fda.gov/Food/FoodborneIllnessContaminants/ChemicalContaminants/ucm055815.htm. Accessed 7 Feb 2015.
8. Aghili HA, Hoseini SM, Yassaei S, Meybodi SAF, Zaeim MHT, Moghadam MG. Effects of carbonated soft drink consumption on orthodontic tooth movements in rats. J Dent (Tehran). 2014;11:123–30.
9. Brown SE, Jaffe R. Acid-alkaline balance and its effect on bone health. Int J Integrative Med. 2000;2(6).
10. Tucker KL, Morita K, Qiao N, Hannan M, Cupples AL, Kiel DP. Colas, but not other carbonated beverages, are associated with low bone mineral density in older women: the Framingham Osteoporosis Study. Am J Clin Nutr. 2006;84:936–42.
11. McGartland C, Robson PJ, Murray L, et al. Carbonated soft drink consumption and bone mineral density in adolescence: the Northern Ireland Young Hearts Project. J Bone Miner Res. 2003;18:1563–9.
12. Shirreffs SM. Hydration in sport and exercise: water, sports drinks and other drinks. Nutr Bull. 2009;34:374–9.
13. Zengin N, Yüzbaşıoğlu D, Unal F, Yılmaz S, Askoy H. The evaluation of the genotoxicity of two food preservatives: sodium benzoate and potassium benzoate. Food Chem Toxicol. 2010;49:763–9.
14. FDA. 2010. Generally Recognized as Safe (GRAS) notification for the use of sodium potassium hexametaphosphate as a food ingredient. http://www.fda.gov/ucm/groups/fdagov-public/@fdagov-foods-gen/documents/document/ucm269487.pdf. Accessed 30 Mar 2015.
15. Center for Science in the Public Interest (CSPI). Chemical cuisine. 2014. http://www.cspinet.org/reports/chemcuisine.htm#sorbicacid. Accessed 30 Mar 2015.
16. Mayo Clinic. Should I be worried that my favorite soda contains brominated vegetable oil? What is it? 2013. http://www.mayoclinic.org/healthy-living/nutrition-and-healthy-eating/expert-answers/bvo/faq-20058236. Accessed 30 Mar 2015.

17. Vorhees CV, Butcher RE, Wootten V, Brunner RL. Behavioral and reproductive effects of chronic developmental exposure to brominated vegetable oil in rats. Arch Latinoam Nutr. 1986;36:432–42.
18. Bernal C, Basilico MZ, Lombardo YB. Toxicological effects induced by the chronic intake of brominated vegetable oils. Teratology. 1983;28:309–18.
19. Marten B, Pfeuffer M, Schrezenmeir J. Medium-chain triglycerides. Int Dairy J. 2006;16: 1374–82.
20. Jiang Z, Zhang S, Wang X, Yang N, Zhu Y, Wilmore D. A comparison of medium-chain and long-chain triglycerides in surgical patients. Ann Surgery. 1993;217:175–84.
21. Codex Alimentarius. Food and Agriculture Organization of the United Nations and the World Health Organization. 2014. CODEX STAN 192-1995
22. Islam AM, Phillips GO, Sljivo A, Snowden MJ, Williams PA. A review of recent developments on the regulatory, structural and functional aspects of gum arabic. Food Hydrocoll. 1997;11:493–505.
23. Butt MS, Shahzadi N, Sharif MK, Nasir M. Guar gum: a miracle therapy for hypercholesterolemia, hyperglycemia and obesity. Crit Rev Food Sci Nutr. 2007;47:389–96.
24. Krotkiewski M. Effect of guar gum on body-weight, hunger ratings and metabolism in obese subjects. Br J Nutr. 1984;52:97–105.
25. Garcia-Ochoa F, Santos VE, Casas JA, Gomez E. Xanthan gum: production, recovery, and properties. Biotechnol Adv. 2000;18:549–79.
26. Tobacman JK. Review of harmful gastrointestinal effects of carrageenan in animal experiments. Environ Health Perspect. 2001;109:983–4.
27. Fitch C, Keim KS. Position of the academy of nutrition and dietetics: use of nutritive and non-nutritive sweeteners. J Acad Nutr Diet. 2012;112:739–58.
28. Pawar RS, Krynitsky AJ, Rader JI. Sweeteners from plants--with emphasis on Stevia rebaudiana (Bertoni) and Siraitia grosvenorii (Swingle). Anal Bioanal Chem. 2013;405:4397–407.
29. Hickman Mills C-1 School District-School Nutrition and Fitness. http://hmc1food.org/?page=cupg. Accessed April 2015.
30. Roemer CJ, Ausenhus BC, Pientok AT, Roelofs TM, Wilson T. Consumer knowledge of non-nutritive sweeteners. FASEB J. 2014;28:1020–6.
31. Swithers SE. Artificial sweeteners produce the counterintuitive effect of inducing metabolic derangements. Trends Endocrinol Metab. 2013;24:431–41.
32. Pereira MA. Diet beverages and the risk of obesity, diabetes, and cardiovascular disease: a review of the evidence. Nutr Rev. 2013;71:433–40.
33. Aune D. Soft drinks, aspartame, and the risk of cancer and cardiovascular disease. Am J Clin Nutr. 2012;96:1249–51.
34. Arnold LE, Lofthouse N, Hurt E. Artificial food colors and attention-deficit/hyperactivity symptoms: conclusions to dye for. Neurotherapeutics. 2012;9:599–609.
35. Voltolini S, Pellegrini S, Contatore M, Bignardi D, Minale P. New risks from ancient food dyes: cochineal red allergy. Eur Ann Allergy Clin Immunol. 2014;46:232–3.
36. National Public Radio (NPR). Is that a crushed bug in your frothy starbucks drink? 2012. http://www.npr.org/blogs/thesalt/2012/03/30/149700341/food-coloring-made-from-insects-irks-some-starbucks-patrons. Accessed 30 Mar 2015.
37. Wilson T, Temple NJ, editors. Beverages in health and nutrition. Totowa: Humana; 2005.
38. Code of Federal Regulations (CFR). Stimulant drug products for over the counter human use. 2014. http://www.accessdata.fda.gov/scripts/cdrh/cfdocs/cfcfr/CFRSearch.cfm?fr=340.50. Accessed 30 Mar 2015.
39. Kole J, Barnhill A. Caffeine content labeling: a missed opportunity for promoting personal and public health. J Caffeine Res. 2013;3:108–13.

Chapter 23
Labeling Requirements for Beverages in the USA

Leslie T. Krasny

Key Points

1. The beverage industry is facing a significant increase in enforcement actions brought by regulatory agencies for labeling and advertising claim violations and in class action lawsuits for false, misleading, or deceptive claims brought by private plaintiffs under state consumer protection laws.
2. The FDA considers product name, composition, packaging, serving size, recommended daily intake, marketing practices, and other factors in determining whether a liquid product should be regulated as a conventional beverage or as a dietary supplement.
3. Structure/function claims for conventional beverages and liquid dietary supplements must be substantiated by competent and reliable scientific evidence.
4. The FDA is focusing on the safety of novel substances being added to conventional foods, including beverages, because there may be higher levels than used traditionally or the substances may be added to different types of products than in the past.
5. Fermented beverages such as kombucha tea are regulated as alcoholic beverages if they contain more than 0.5 % alcohol by volume.

Keywords The Food and Drug Administration • The Federal Trade Commission • Alcohol and Tobacco Tax and Trade Bureau • Generally recognized as safe • Reference amount customarily consumed • Daily Reference Values established for macronutrients • Reference Daily Intakes established for micronutrients

L.T. Krasny, M.A., J.D. (✉)
Keller and Heckman LLP, Three Embarcadero Center,
Suite 1420, San Francisco, CA 94111, USA
e-mail: krasny@khlaw.com

© Springer International Publishing Switzerland 2016
T. Wilson, N.J. Temple (eds.), *Beverage Impacts on Health and Nutrition*,
Nutrition and Health, DOI 10.1007/978-3-319-23672-8_23

Abbreviations

FDA   The Food and Drug Administration
FTC   The Federal Trade Commission
TTB   Alcohol and Tobacco Tax and Trade Bureau
GRAS   Generally recognized as safe
RACC   Reference amount customarily consumed
DRVs   Daily Reference Values established for macronutrients
RDIs   Reference Daily Intakes established for micronutrients

Introduction

Food labeling requirements specify the product information that is mandated by law and provide the criteria for furnishing additional information, including eligibility, form, placement, disclosures, and substantiation. Claims that promote the nutritional value, ingredient quality, and health-related benefits of food have increased significantly in recent years because of consumer interest and competitive pressure. This has resulted in more enforcement actions by regulatory agencies and public prosecutors, challenges raised through industry self-regulatory bodies, and a flood of class action lawsuits for false, misleading, or deceptive claims brought by private plaintiffs under state consumer protection laws. In many instances, litigation follows enforcement actions by regulatory agencies. Therefore, a legal review of a company's labeling is critical and should have broader scope than in the past, taking into account both regulatory and litigation developments.

The labeling of nonalcoholic beverages in the USA is regulated by the Food and Drug Administration (FDA), pursuant to the Federal Food, Drug, and Cosmetic Act (FD&C Act).[1] The Federal Trade Commission (FTC) has primary jurisdiction over the advertising of nonalcoholic beverages, under the Federal Trade Commission Act (FTC Act).[2] The labeling and advertising of alcoholic beverages are regulated primarily by the Alcohol and Tobacco Tax and Trade Bureau (TTB), pursuant to the Federal Alcohol Administration Act (FAA Act).[3]

Labeling of Nonalcoholic Beverages

The term "label" means "a display of written, printed, or graphic matter upon the immediate container of any article…".[4] "Labeling" is a broader term, encompassing labels and other written, printed, or graphic matter on a product, its container or

---

[1] 21 U.S.C. §§ 331 *et seq.*
[2] 15 U.S.C. §§ 41 *et seq.*
[3] 27 U.S.C. §§ 201 *et seq.*
[4] 21 U.S.C. § 321 and 21 C.F.R. § 1.3

accompanying the product. The phrase "accompanying" is interpreted broadly and does not require physical attachment. Thus, promotional materials available with a product at the point of sale are often considered to be labeling.

Promotional materials other than labeling are regulated as advertising. The distinction between labeling and advertising can be important because the FDA examines both content and form in reviewing labeling, whereas the FTC focuses primarily on content in reviewing advertising.

The FD&C Act prohibits false or misleading labeling, and the FTC Act prohibits false or deceptive advertising. The omission of a material fact, or an implication of a material fact that is untrue, can constitute a violation of the law even if the information declared is technically true. A claim is material if it would likely influence consumers' purchasing decisions, and it is unnecessary to establish that the manufacturer had any intent to deceive or that anyone was actually misled. Both FDA and the FTC use a reasonable person standard in assessing whether marketing claims are false, misleading, or deceptive.

There is jurisdictional overlap with respect to websites. FDA takes the position that information on a company's website may be regulated as labeling, particularly when the website address appears on the label and when consumers can purchase products through the website. In fact, many FDA Warning Letters cite, as the basis for a finding of violations, information provided on a company's website as well as on product labels. And the FTC clearly has jurisdiction over product-related information on websites, as advertising.

Since 2009, the FDA and the FTC have increased their collaborative efforts with respect to enforcement actions for website claims, including references in FDA Warning Letters to violations of both the FD&C Act and the FTC Act, and Warning Letters signed jointly by the FDA and the FTC.

Both agencies have been scrutinizing social media sites. The extent to which a company could be held liable for violative product claims communicated in posts by third parties is unclear, but company actions that might be considered endorsements are potentially risky, such as retweeting statements on Twitter or "liking" a statement on Facebook.

Required Label Information

The label of a nonalcoholic beverage must declare the product identity, net quantity of contents, ingredient statement, nutrition information, and name and address of the manufacturer, packer, or distributor (signature line). The nutrition information, ingredient statement, and signature line must appear in one place without other intervening material.

For imported beverages, a country of origin declaration may be required. Under the Tariff Act of 1930, which is enforced by US Customs and Border Protection (CBP), imported articles must inform the "ultimate purchaser" of any foreign country of origin.[5] The ultimate purchaser is the last US person to receive the article in the form imported. For products imported into the USA from the other North American Free Trade Agreement (NAFTA) countries—Canada and Mexico—CBP determines whether there is change in the tariff classification. For products imported from non-NAFTA countries, the test is whether there has been a "substantial transformation."

Product Identity Statement

The product identity statement, describing the nature of the product, is required to be displayed on the principal display panel (PDP).[6] The product identity statement must be a name required by law (such as a standard of identity), or if there is no required name, the "common or usual" name of the food, or in the absence of a required name or a common or usual name, an appropriately descriptive term or a fanciful name used by the public.

When a product is deemed to have a "characterizing flavor," a statement consistent with the FDA's flavor labeling regulation must be prominently displayed as part of the product identity statement. A flavor is deemed to be characterizing if a product's label, by word, vignette, or design, makes a prominent representation with respect to a primary recognizable flavor. The form of the declaration depends on many factors, including whether a flavor is natural or artificial, and whether it is derived from the expected source or from other substances which simulate, resemble, or reinforce the characterizing flavor.[7]

There is a regulation covering the common or usual name for beverages that contain fruit or vegetable juice.[8] The product identity statement for a beverage containing less than 100 % juice must include a qualifying term such as "beverage," "cocktail," or "drink." For multiple juice beverages, any juices named in the product identity statement must be listed in descending order of predominance by weight, unless a characterizing juice listed out of order is declared as a flavor or a percentage range is included. There is also a mandatory percentage juice declaration requirement, based on minimum Brix levels listed for 53 juices in the regulation, or if there is no minimum Brix level set by FDA, the labeled percentage is calculated based on the soluble solid content of expressed juice used to make the concentrated juice.[9] And when a beverage is made from concentrate, the product identity statement must indicate that fact.

---

[5] 19 U.S.C. §§ 1304
[6] 21 C.F.R. § 101.3
[7] 21 C.F.R. § 101.22
[8] 21 C.F.R. § 102.33
[9] 21 C.F.R. § 101.30

Ingredient Statement

The ingredient statement may appear on the PDP or on the information panel (IP). The statement must list all ingredients by common or usual name, in descending order of predominance by weight, unless an exemption applies.[10]

A common or usual name must not be false or misleading. For example, the FDA issued draft guidance in 2009 that stated its view that the term "evaporated cane juice" is not an appropriate common or usual name for sweeteners derived from sugar cane syrup because the name fails to reveal the basic nature of the ingredient and its characterizing properties and because an extract of sugar cane is not the juice of a plant that consumers are accustomed to eating as a fruit or vegetable.[11] But the FDA reopened the comment period in March 2014.

Special allergen labeling requirements apply to products that contain a "major food allergen," defined as milk, eggs, fish, Crustacean shellfish, tree nuts, wheat, peanuts, and soybeans, or an ingredient that contains protein derived from a major food allergen. The label must include either (1) the common or usual name of the major food allergen in the ingredient statement followed by the name of the food source from which the major food allergen is derived, if different from the common or usual name, such as "whey (milk)," or (2) the word "contains" on a separate line, followed by the names of all major food allergens in the product, such as "contains milk and soy."

There are no regulatory requirements for "advisory" allergen labeling, which is the use of statements to indicate the possible presence of major food allergens through cross contact, such as "May contain," or "Produced in a plant that processes." The FDA permits voluntary advisory statements if they are not false or misleading, but expects companies to follow current good manufacturing practices designed to prevent or reduce the possibility of major food allergens accidentally becoming incorporated into products.

Incidental additives, including processing aids, are substances that are present in a food at insignificant levels and that have no technical or functional effect in the product.[12] They are generally exempt from the ingredient listing requirement, but if a major food allergen or derivative is present in an amount that might cause an allergic reaction, FDA would not consider the level to be "insignificant," and the substance would have to be declared as an ingredient.

Net Quantity of Contents Declaration

The net quantity of contents must accurately reflect the contents in terms of weight, measure, or numerical count.[13] Metric labeling is required, in addition to traditional units used in the USA. The accuracy of the net quantity of contents declaration is determined by the FDA or states under compliance sampling criteria.

---

[10] 21 C.F.R. § 101.4
[11] Draft Guidance for Industry: Ingredients Declared as Evaporated Cane Juice, October 2009
[12] 21 C.F.R. § 101.100(a)(3)
[13] 21 C.F.R. § 101.105

Nutrition Labeling

Nutrition labeling is required for most packaged foods.[14] Exemptions that may be applicable to beverages include small businesses, restaurant and other institution foods, ready-to-eat foods packaged on-site and not for immediate consumption, foods with no nutritional value, and small packages. Some exemptions are negated if there is a nutrition claim or any other nutrition information on the label or in labeling or advertising.

In order to facilitate nutritional comparisons between products, the FDA established "reference amounts customarily consumed" (RACCs) for most categories of food.[15] The appropriate RACC is converted to a serving size, expressed as a common household measure.

The RACC for all beverages has been 240 ml (8 fl oz) since nutrition labeling regulations were implemented in 1994. But the FDA published proposed rules, in March 2014, that would increase the RACC for certain beverages. For carbonated and noncarbonated beverages, water, coffee, and tea, the proposed rule would increase the RACC to 360 ml (12 fl oz), although the RACC for juices would remain the same under the proposal. If the proposed change is finalized, the new requirements would be effective two years after publication of the final rule. Other changes to labeling requirements were also proposed, including a separate declaration for added sugars.

Nutrition labeling is mandatory for the following nutrients: calories, calories from fat, total fat, saturated fat, trans fat, cholesterol, sodium, total carbohydrate, dietary fiber, sugars, protein, vitamin A, vitamin C, calcium, and iron. Nutrition labeling is voluntary for the following nutrients: calories from saturated fat, polyunsaturated fat, monounsaturated fat, potassium, soluble fiber, insoluble fiber, sugar alcohols, other carbohydrates, vitamin D, vitamin E, vitamin K, thiamin, riboflavin, niacin, vitamin B_6, folate, vitamin B_{12}, biotin, pantothenic acid, phosphorus, iodine, magnesium, zinc, selenium, copper, manganese, chromium, molybdenum, and chloride. The declaration of a "voluntary" nutrient becomes mandatory, however, if the nutrient is the subject of a nutrient content claim or is added to a food as a nutrient supplement. There is a standard format, and if labeling space is limited, alternative formats may be used. A simplified format is permitted, regardless of labeling space, when a product contains "insignificant" amounts of eight or more specified nutrients.

The FDA has established Reference Daily Intakes (RDIs) for vitamins and minerals and Daily Reference Values (DRVs) for fat, saturated fat, cholesterol, total carbohydrates, fiber, sodium, potassium, and protein. The Percent Daily Value (% DV) must be provided in nutrition labeling for each declared nutrient other than sugars and trans fat, except that a declaration for protein is not required unless a protein claim is made or the protein content of the product is of low quality.

The FDA's compliance policy for determining the accuracy of nutrition information distinguishes between two classes of nutrients. Class I nutrients are added to

---

[14] 21 C.F.R. § 101.9
[15] 21 C.F.R. § 101.12(b)

fortified foods, and Class II nutrients are naturally present. For Class I nutrients, the content must at least equal the declared value. For Class II nutrients that are considered to be beneficial, the content must be at least 80 % of the declared value. For other Class II nutrients, the content must not be more than 20 % above the declared value.

Regulatory Categories

There are complex rules governing health and nutrition-related claims for food, which may vary according to the regulatory category. Thus, a product that meets the regulatory criteria for more than one category of food may be able to bear different claims, depending upon the category selected and the manner in which the product is marketed.

Dietary supplements are regulated as a class of food, pursuant to the Dietary Supplement Health and Education Act (DSHEA) with some different requirements. A dietary supplement is a product that is intended to supplement the diet through ingestion, which contains one or more "dietary ingredients," that is not represented for use as a conventional food or sole item of a meal or the diet, and that is labeled as a dietary supplement.[16] Dietary ingredients include one or more of the following: a vitamin, mineral, herb or other botanical, amino acid, or other substance intended to supplement the diet by increasing the total dietary intake of that substance or a concentrate, metabolite, constituent part, extract, or combination of dietary ingredients.

The FDA issued final guidance, in 2014, to assist manufacturers in determining whether a liquid product may be marketed as a dietary supplement.[17] The FDA takes the position that terms such as "drink," "beverage," "juice," and "water" suggest that liquid products are represented for use as conventional beverages. It was noted, however, that if a term is not associated exclusively with conventional foods, such as products described as teas, the use of such a term in the product name would not necessarily indicate use as a conventional beverage. Other factors to be considered by the FDA in evaluating regulatory status, if the product name is not determinative, include packaging graphics, serving size, recommended conditions of use, and other representations about the product. In the past, the FDA challenged the regulatory status of a number of energy drinks that were marketed as dietary supplements, and now virtually all brands are labeled as conventional beverages.

Medical food is defined as "food which is formulated to be consumed or administered enterally under the supervision of a physician and which is intended for the specific dietary management of a disease or condition for which distinctive nutritional requirements, based on recognized scientific principles, are established by

---

[16] 21 C.F.R. § 321 (ff)

[17] Guidance for Industry: Distinguishing Liquid Dietary Supplements from Beverages (January 2014)

medical evaluation".[18] Medical foods are exempted from nutrition labeling, nutrient content claim, and health claim requirements. The FDA has been concerned that some products marketed as medical foods may not meet the relevant statutory and regulatory criteria and issued revised draft guidance in 2013 to emphasize its position that the definition of medical foods narrowly limits the types of products that fall within this category.[19]

Foods for special dietary use supply particular dietary needs which exist due to a physical, physiological, pathological, or other condition or age (including infancy and childhood) or supplement the ordinary or usual diet with any vitamin, mineral, or other dietary property. The FDA has issued regulations requiring additional labeling information on certain foods marketed for special dietary use, such as weight loss/maintenance and hypoallergenic foods.[20]

Allowable Ingredients

The definition of "food" encompasses raw materials and any component of a food. A food additive is a substance, "the intended use of which results or may reasonably be expected to result, directly or indirectly, in its becoming a component or otherwise affecting the characteristics of any food," and is deemed to be unsafe unless used in accordance with a food additive regulation.[21] However, substances generally recognized as safe (GRAS) for their intended use, "prior sanctioned" substances (permitted informally by the FDA before enactment of the Food Additives Amendment to the FD&C Act in 1958), and dietary ingredients used in a dietary supplement, are excluded from the definition of food additives. All ingredients of a conventional beverage must be either approved food additives, GRAS substances, or prior sanctioned substances.

With respect to the GRAS status of a beverage ingredient, manufacturers may submit a GRAS notification to the FDA or may rely on a self-determined GRAS position that is not submitted (at the risk of challenge by the FDA in the future). Information to be submitted as part of a GRAS notification includes the conditions of use (foods, levels, and purposes), the basis for the GRAS determination (scientific procedures or experience based on common use in foods prior to 1958), and detailed information about the identity of the substance. The notification must state the justification for concluding there is a reasonable certainty that the substance is not harmful under the intended conditions of use, based on consensus among qualified experts. A successful notification will result in a letter stating that the FDA has no questions regarding the GRAS assessment.

---

[18] 21 C.F.R. § 101.9(j)(8)

[19] Draft Guidance for Industry: Frequently Asked Questions About Medical Foods; Second Edition, August 2013

[20] 21 C.F.R. Part 105

[21] 21 U.S.C. § 348

Guidance issued by the FDA in January 2014 states that "We are concerned that some of the novel substances that are being added to conventional foods, including beverages, may cause the food to be adulterated because these added substances may not be GRAS for their intended use and are not being used in accordance with a food additive regulation prescribing conditions of safe use. In addition, some substances that have been present in the food supply for many years are now being added to conventional foods at levels in excess of their traditional use levels or in new types of conventional foods. This trend raises questions as to whether these higher levels and other new conditions of use are safe."[22]

The FDA has a fortification policy which establishes "a uniform set of principles that will serve as a model for the rational addition of nutrients to foods".[23] The policy states that the FDA does not consider it appropriate to fortify snack foods such as carbonated beverages. The fortification policy itself does not have the force and effect of law, but has been incorporated by reference in certain regulations covering labeling claims.

The FDA has sent Warning Letters to beverage companies based on fortification that is not in accordance with the policy, and class action lawsuits have been filed on the ground that fortification resulted in misleading marketing claims. For example, a 2008 Warning Letter to the Coca-Cola Company included the following alleged violation: "Your product Diet Coke Plus is a carbonated beverage. The policy on fortification in 21 CFR 104.20(a) states that the FDA does not consider it appropriate to fortify snack foods such as carbonated beverages."[24]

And the complaint in a class action lawsuit brought by the Center for Science in the Public Interest (CSPI) against the Dr Pepper Snapple Group, regarding 7UP "antioxidant" soft drinks, stated: "Because Defendant fortifies the Products, which are all carbonated beverages, with vitamin E, Defendant has engaged in actions that the FDA does not consider appropriate."[25] In 2013, as part of the settlement of the lawsuit, the company agreed to stop fortifying these soft drinks.

Nutrient Content Claims

"Nutrient content claims" expressly or impliedly characterize the level of a nutrient in a food and must be authorized by regulation or by notification to the FDA based on a published authoritative statement by a scientific body of the USA. The FDA permits nutrient content claims only if there is an established DRV or RDI for the nutrient and if claims are consistent with regulatory definitions.[26]

---

[22] Guidance for Industry: Considerations Regarding Substances Added to Foods, Including Beverages and Dietary Supplements (January 2014)

[23] 21 C.F.R. § 104.20

[24] http://www.fda.gov/ICECI/EnforcementActions/WarningLetters/2008/ucm1048050.htm

[25] http://cspinet.org/new/pdf/complaint-7up.pdf

[26] 21 C.F.R. § 101.13(b)

Absolute claims refer only to the nutrient content of the food bearing the claim, such as "excellent source of vitamin C." Products do not meet the requirements for a "no sugar added" claim if they contain juice concentrate that is not reconstituted back to single strength or a greater degree of dilution, because concentrates functionally substitute for added sugars.

Relative claims compare the level of a nutrient in one food to the level of that nutrient in another food, such as "reduced sugar." To ensure that comparisons are consistent and not misleading, the FDA has established two types of reference foods that may be used as a basis for comparison: similar foods and dissimilar foods within a product category, and for some claims, only similar reference foods may be used. The label must bear a "related information statement," adjacent to the claim, that identifies the reference food and the percentage or fraction by which the nutrient content has been changed. The label must also declare quantitative information comparing the level of the nutrient in the product with the level of the nutrient in the reference food.

There are special rules for antioxidant nutrient content claims. In addition to having an established RDI, the nutrient must have scientifically recognized antioxidant activity: absorption from the gastrointestinal tract and participation in physiological, biochemical, or cellular processes that inactivate free radicals or prevent free radical-initiated chemical reactions. Examples of nutrients recognized by the FDA as having antioxidant activity are vitamins A, C, and E. The specific antioxidants must be named as part of the claim. The term "antioxidant" may also be used to describe nutrients without an established RDI if the claim does not characterize the level of the nutrient and just declares the quantity of an antioxidant with no established RDI, such as flavonoids. But the FDA has taken the position, in Warning Letters, that even the term "a source of antioxidants" characterizes the level of the substance and is a nutrient content claim.

Health Claims

A health claim expressly or by implication, including third party references, written statements, symbols, or vignettes, characterizes the relationship of any substance to a disease or health-related condition.[27] For purposes of health claim requirements, a "substance" is defined as a specific food or a component of food. "Disease or health-related condition" means damage to an organ, part, structure, or system of the body such that it does not function properly or a state of health leading to such dysfunctioning.

If a health claim for a conventional food is based on the presence of a substance at other than decreased levels, the substance must serve a traditional food purpose at levels necessary to justify the claim and must be safe and lawful at the level at which it will be used in the food and the level at which it is expected to be consumed.

---

[27] 21 C.F.R. § 101.14

Traditional food purposes include taste, aroma, nutritive value, or any other technical effect in food recognized by the FDA. "Nutritive value" means having a value in sustaining human existence by such processes as promoting growth, replacing loss of essential nutrients, or providing energy. The technical effects in food recognized by the FDA include antimicrobial agents, antioxidants, colors, enzymes, flavors, formulation aids, nonnutritive sweeteners, nutrient supplements, nutritive sweeteners, oxidizing/reducing agents, pH control agents, and processing aids. Another requirement, the so-called Jelly Bean Rule, is that a conventional food bearing a health claim approved by regulation must generally contain, prior to any fortification, one or more of the following six nutrients at a level of at least 10 % of the Daily Value: vitamin A, vitamin C, calcium, iron, protein, or fiber per serving. And unless an exception applies, a health claim may not be made for a conventional food that exceeds specified levels of fat, saturated fat, cholesterol, and sodium.

Health claims require prior FDA approval or notification to the FDA based on an authoritative statement of a federal scientific agency responsible for human health or nutrition. The FD&C Act requires "significant scientific agreement" (SSA) among qualified experts that the claim is supported by the "totality of publicly available scientific evidence".[28] Some manufacturers successfully challenged SSA as the sole health claim standard on First Amendment grounds. As the result of court decisions, if there is a preponderance of evidence to support a health claim at a lower standard, the FDA must consider whether the use of an appropriate disclaimer would communicate the level of scientific support for the claim. But although "qualified" health claims are permitted now, the disclaimer language mandated by the FDA, such as "the FDA has determined that this evidence is limited and not conclusive," has made such claims generally unappealing to manufacturers.

The FDA may also permit a health claim based on a published, authoritative statement of a federal agency that has responsibility for the protection of the public health or research directly relating to human nutrition. The authoritative statement must be provided to the FDA at least 120 days prior to its use on the label or in the labeling of the food. If the FDA does not take steps, within the 120-day period, to prohibit the proposed claim, the claim may be used on appropriate products.

Structure/Function Claims

Structure/function claims describe the effect of a food or nutrient on the structure or function of the body, such as "helps maintain proper joint function," but may not suggest that a food is useful in the diagnosis, cure, treatment, prevention, or mitigation of a disease.[29] In contrast to nutrient content claims and health claims, structure/function claims do not require prior authorization from the FDA, although the manufacturer must have substantiation that the claim is truthful and not misleading.

---

[28] 21 U.S.C. § 343(r)(3)

[29] 21 U.S.C. § 343 (r)(6)

An FDA guidance document addresses the substantiation of structure/function claims for dietary supplements, and the FDA uses the same criteria to evaluate the substantiation of structure/function claims for conventional foods.[30] The FDA takes the position, however, that structure/function claims for conventional foods, but not dietary supplements, must be based on effects derived from nutritive value rather than pharmacological or physiological effects.

Popular claims such as "energy," "relaxation," and "alertness" may raise substantiation questions and may have implications regarding the regulatory status of the product, depending on the ingredients that allegedly provide the effects.

The risk of regulatory challenge is often greater for imported products because the CBP and the FDA may check websites referenced on the packaging of imports presented for entry, as well as labels. If violative claims are found, products are likely to be detained. If the only problem is website claims, typically the product will not be released until changes are made online and the FDA has reviewed and approved the revisions.

For dietary supplements bearing structure/function claims, the following disclaimer must appear on the same label panel as the claim: "This statement has not been evaluated by the Food and Drug Administration. This product is not intended to diagnose, treat, cure or prevent any disease."[31] This disclaimer requirement is not applicable to conventional foods.

Healthy Claims

The term "HEALTHY" and related terms such as "healthier," "healthful," and "health" may be used to describe beverages which are low in fat and saturated fat, do not exceed established levels for sodium and cholesterol, and are a "good" source of at least one of six nutrients (vitamin A, vitamin C, calcium, iron, fiber, and protein).[32]

Fresh Claims

The FDA's regulation on "fresh" claims is applicable whenever the term suggests that a food is unprocessed or unpreserved.[33] Thus, "fresh" is generally limited to use on foods that have not been subject to freezing, thermal processing, or any kind of chemical processing, but refrigeration does not preclude the use of the term. The regulation specifically states that a "fresh" claim may be made for pasteurized milk,

---

[30] Guidance for Industry: Substantiation for Dietary Supplement Claims Made Under Section 403(r)(6) of the Federal Food, Drug, and Cosmetic Act, December 2008

[31] 21 C.F.R. §101.93

[32] 21 C.F.R. § 101.65(d)

[33] 21 C.F.R. § 101.95

noting that such use is outside the scope of the restrictions "because the term does not imply that the food is unprocessed (consumers commonly understand that milk is nearly always pasteurized)."

Natural Claims

The FDA

The FDA has not issued a regulation defining the term "natural" for food (other than a regulation defining "natural flavors"), but adopted an informal enforcement policy many years ago which defines "natural" to mean that "nothing artificial or synthetic (including all color additives regardless of source) has been included in, or has been added to, a food that would not normally be expected to be in the food".[34] Thus, any added color is considered to be artificial, even if the source of the color is natural, such as beet juice. The FDA's policy does not limit use of the term "natural" based on the degree of processing.

Class Action Lawsuits

Private plaintiffs have brought numerous class action lawsuits, under state consumer protection laws that broadly prohibit unfair and deceptive trade practices, based on "natural" claims, alleging that ingredients are artificial or synthetic and also applying an additional criterion that the product and its ingredients are more than minimally processed (unnaturally processed). Plaintiffs have challenged many ingredients in "natural" products, including ascorbic acid, citric acid, refined sugar, corn syrup, maltodextrin, and xanthan gum. Private plaintiffs also contend that any ingredient derived from a genetically engineered crop is not natural. Many courts have rejected the defense of federal preemption in cases challenging "natural" claims on the ground that the FDA does not have a regulation defining "natural," only a policy. And the referrals of "natural" claim issues from courts to the FDA, based on primary jurisdiction, have been unsuccessful because the FDA declined to decide the issues.

Directions for Use and Warnings

The manufacturer of a beverage must provide adequate directions for use or warnings, as appropriate. Usually, directions or warnings are found on dietary supplements and medical foods, although conventional foods may also have warnings,

---

[34] 58 *Fed. Reg.* 2407 (Jan. 6, 1993)

either as determined by the manufacturer or as required by regulation. For example, diet drinks which contain aspartame must state: PHENYLKETONURICS: CONTAINS PHENYLALANINE.[35] Another example is that the label of any pre-packaged fresh (nonpasteurized) juice offered for sale at retail must bear a warning unless the processors can meet a specified pathogen reduction standard: "WARNING: This product has not been pasteurized and, therefore, may contain harmful bacteria that can cause serious illness in children, the elderly, and persons with weakened immune systems."[36]

There are currently no labeling requirements concerning caffeine, but a number of companies that are producing products with added caffeine, including energy drinks, are including a cautionary statement, on a voluntary basis, such as "Not recommended for children, teenagers, pregnant women, and others who are sensitive to caffeine." And some companies are voluntarily stating the amount of added caffeine on the label. Generally, when companies declare the amount of added caffeine, they are not including caffeine that is a naturally occurring constituent of an ingredient such as coffee, tea, or cocoa/chocolate. But there are no regulations yet on this subject, and therefore companies may not have consistent definitions of "added" caffeine.

The FDA is concerned about the fact that caffeine is currently being added to many products and issued the following statement in April 2013:

> The only time that FDA explicitly approved the added use of caffeine in a food was for cola and that was in the 1950s. Today, the environment has changed. Children and adolescents may be exposed to caffeine beyond those foods in which caffeine is naturally found and beyond anything the FDA envisioned when it made the determination regarding caffeine in cola. For that reason, the FDA is taking a fresh look at the potential impact that the totality of new and easy sources of caffeine may have on health, particularly vulnerable populations such as children and youth, and if necessary, will take appropriate action.

For additional information about energy drinks, please see Chap. 16.

Biotechnology Claims

The labeling of genetically engineered food remains a highly controversial issue in the USA. The FDA issued draft guidance in 2001 with criteria to ensure that voluntary claims concerning biotechnology are not false or misleading.[37] The guidance notes that acronyms such as "GMO" and "GM" are not generally understood by consumers and should be avoided, that "genetically modified" includes conventional breeding and therefore applies to virtually all cultivated food crops, and that "NON-GMO" and "GMO-FREE" should not be used unless there is testing

---

[35] 21 C.F.R. § 172.804

[36] 21 C.F.R. § 101.17(g)

[37] Draft Guidance for Industry: Voluntary Labeling Indicating whether Foods Have or Have Not Been Developed Using Bioengineering, January 2001

performed, using accepted analytical methods and thresholds. The following is an example of a statement suggested by the FDA that would be considered appropriate (provided that it is accurate): "We do not use ingredients that were produced using biotechnology."

Organic Claims

The Organic Foods Production Act of 1990 (OFPA) authorizes national standards for the marketing of raw and processed organic agricultural products in the USA, as implemented by the National Organic Program (NOP).[38]

There are four categories of products covered by NOP labeling regulations, based on organic content: 100 %, 95 % or more, 70 to 95 %, and less than 70 % (excluding water and salt). Beverages labeled as "100 % ORGANIC" must be composed entirely of organically produced ingredients (including processing aids). Beverages labeled as "ORGANIC" must contain at least 95 % organically produced ingredients; the additional ingredients may be permitted nonorganic substances if permitted under the NOP and not "commercially available" in organic form. Beverages labeled as "MADE WITH ORGANIC (specified ingredients or food groups)" must contain between 70 and 95 % organically produced ingredients. Beverages containing less than 70 % organic ingredients may use the term "organic" only on the information panel, to identify organic ingredients. No ingredients in the first three categories may be produced using biotechnology.

California Proposition 65 Warnings

The California Safe Drinking Water and Toxic Enforcement Act of 1986 (Proposition 65) requires California to maintain a list of chemicals known to the state to cause cancer or reproductive toxicity and provides that "no person in the course of doing business shall knowingly and intentionally expose any individual" to a listed chemical without first giving clear and reasonable warning.[39] There are currently over 900 chemicals listed.

The statute covers consumer, environmental, and occupational exposures in California. Proposition 65 permits private citizens to bring enforcement actions if officials do not file suit within 60 days after receiving notice of alleged violations.

The warning requirement for consumer products does not apply to an exposure for which the person responsible can demonstrate that there is no significant risk, assuming lifetime exposure at the level in question (for carcinogens), or that there will be no observable effect assuming exposure at 1000 times the level in question

---

[38] 7 U.S.C. § 6501 *et seq.*

[39] CA Health and Safety Code §§ 25249.5 *et seq.*

(for reproductive toxins). The required statement is "WARNING: This product contains a chemical known to the State of California to cause (cancer)/(birth defects and other reproductive harm)." There is a very limited exemption for listed chemicals that are "naturally occurring" in food, such as lead and arsenic, but it is difficult to collect sufficient evidence to prevail on that defense as the presence of the chemical cannot be due to any known human activity.

Labeling of Alcoholic Beverages

The Alcohol and Tobacco Tax and Trade Bureau (TTB) has jurisdiction over beverages in liquid form, intended for human consumption, that contain 0.5 % or more alcohol by volume.[40] The TTB regulates the labeling and advertising of wine, beer, and spirits, except that if an alcoholic beverage is not covered by the labeling provisions of the FAA Act, the product is subject to labeling requirements under the FD&C Act and the Fair Packaging and Labeling Act (FPLA), administered by the FDA, such as wine-derived beverages containing less than 7 % alcohol.

A current regulatory concern, at the TTB and the FDA, involves "kombucha" tea, which is generally a fermented beverage produced using a mixture of steeped tea and sugar, combined with a culture of yeast strains and bacteria. If these products contain 0.5 % or more alcohol by volume, they are considered to be alcoholic beverages subject to regulation by the TTB. Kombucha products will be classified as alcoholic beverages even if they contain less than 0.5 % alcohol by volume at the time of production, but the alcohol content increases to 0.5 % or more due to continued fermentation in the bottle.[41]

The label of an alcoholic beverage must include the brand name, the class and type, the alcoholic content, and the net contents. The percentage of neutral spirits and the name of the commodity from which it was distilled must also be declared. The TTB has authorized voluntary nutrient content statements to be used in the labeling and advertising of wines, distilled spirits, and malt beverages, including calorie and carbohydrate content.[42] A Certificate of Label Approval (COLA) or exemption must be obtained from the TTB prior to marketing an alcoholic beverage subject to the FAA Act.

The label of any alcoholic beverage container sold in the USA must contain a health warning statement separate from all other information: "GOVERNMENT WARNING: (see footnote 1) According to the Surgeon General, women should not drink alcoholic beverages during pregnancy because of the risk of birth defects (see footnote 2). Consumption of alcoholic beverages impairs your ability to drive a car or operate machinery, and may cause health problems."[43]

---

[40] 27 U.S.C. § 214

[41] http://www.ttb.gov/faqs/kombucha-faqs.shtml

[42] Voluntary Nutrient Content Statements in the Labeling and Advertising of Wines, Distilled Spirits, and Malt Beverages. May 2013.

[43] 27 C.F.R. § 16.21

The TTB regulations define "advertisement" as any written or verbal statement, illustration, or depiction which is in, or calculated to induce sales in, interstate or foreign commerce or is disseminated by mail. The definition includes websites and other Internet-based advertising. The FAA Act does not require prior approval of advertisements for alcoholic beverage, but the TTB offers the opportunity for a free pre-clearance review.

Regulations promulgated under the FAA Act generally prohibit statements that are false or misleading or that disparage a competitor's product. Health-related advertisements which include statements of a curative or therapeutic nature that, expressly or by implication, suggest a relationship between the consumption of alcohol and health benefits or effects on health may not contain any health-related statement that is untrue in any particular or tends to create a misleading impression. The TTB will evaluate such messages on a case-by-case basis and may require a disclaimer or other qualifying statement to correct any misleading impression. In this regard, a specific health claim will not be considered misleading if it is truthful and adequately substantiated by scientific or medical evidence, discloses the health risks associated with alcohol consumption, and summarizes the categories of individuals for whom alcohol consumption may cause health risks.

A statement that directs consumers to a third party or other source for information regarding the health effects of alcohol is presumed to be misleading unless it directs consumers, in a non-misleading manner, to a third party or other source for balanced information regarding the effects on health of alcohol consumption and includes the following statement: "This statement should not encourage you to drink or increase your alcohol consumption for health reasons" or another statement determined by the TTB to dispel any misleading impression.

Conclusion

Labeling and advertising claims are an important source of nutrition and health-related information and a driving force in the marketing of beverages. In light of the growing number of class action lawsuits in the USA for allegedly false, misleading, or deceptive food marketing claims, many companies are making more conservative risk management decisions and are phasing out claims that have been found to be violative or fall within unsettled areas of the law. To assess the likelihood of challenge, it is important to understand the regulatory requirements, policies, and interpretations, to track FDA and FTC enforcement actions, and to monitor decisions and settlements in class action lawsuits.

Part VIII
What Is the Future of What We Will Chose to Drink?

Chapter 24
Beverage Trends Affect Future Nutritional Health Impact

Ted Wilson, Rachel Dahl, and Norman Temple

Key Points

1. Beverage trends have been part of human nutrition for millennia and will be here for millennia into the future.
2. Consumer choice is perhaps the most important determinate of what effect a beverage has on our nutritional health.
3. Beverage trends can originate for a variety of reasons including perceived physiological effects, tradition, government regulation, changing affluence, and even global warming.
4. Predicting trends is an undeniable part of determining beverage impacts on nutritional health and product profitability.

Keywords Beverage trend • Energy drink • Diet Coke • Coffee house • Smoothie • Lactose intolerance

Introduction: What Is a Beverage Trend?

"Trend": a general direction in which something is developing or changing (www. oxforddictionaries.com). Understanding the direction of vectoral change in beverage consumption in the current context is important for predicting where beverage products will be in the future. Trends and changes in our direction apply to the

T. Wilson, Ph.D. (✉) • R. Dahl
Department of Biology, Winona State University,
232 Pasteur Hall, Winona, MN 54603, USA
e-mail: twilson@winona.edu

N. Temple
Centre for Science, Athabasca University, Athabasca, AB, Canada

© Springer International Publishing Switzerland 2016
T. Wilson, N.J. Temple (eds.), *Beverage Impacts on Health and Nutrition*,
Nutrition and Health, DOI 10.1007/978-3-319-23672-8_24

choices we make for clothes we choose to wear, our politics, the cars we buy, and of course the beverages we choose to consume. One cannot understand the future without being mindful of the past.

Simply put, a beverage is water, usually with added substances. It may include flavors, alcohol, colors, vitamins, minerals, alcohol, etc., which are mixed into the water. Beverages are highly variable and trends for preferred beverages have been changing for millennia. Our changing preferences for these variations are part of what create beverage trends. In his *History*, Herodotus (440 BCE) gave mention of a rumor of the fountain of youth, a fine description of an ancient beverage trend: "If the account of this fountain be true, it would be their constant use of the water from it which makes them so long-lived." [1] Is it surprising that 2,500 years later we are still seeking the fountain of youth?

This book has discussed many beverages and the peer-reviewed literature we use to make nutritional, clinical, and marketing recommendations about them. Trends are generally based on a range of factors including product availability, price, anticipated health effects, taste, effect on the body (such as stimulation by caffeine), and peer perceptions of drinking habits. Trends are the bellwether of what we are consuming now, what we are likely to consume in the future, and therefore what nutritional changes we can expect. But trends do not necessarily take place for scientific reasons.

This short final chapter asks more questions about how beverages will impact our lives in the future than it provides answers. In this respect the chapter serves as only a rough guide to some of the beverage trends that may be important in the future and the resulting influence that beverages will have on our nutritional status.

Trends for the Young: The Energy Drink

The boom in energy drinks is driven by a combination of simple, sleek labels with colorful applications of glitter or animé which are as eye-catching as the popular marketing advertisements that sell them. One notable example is the notorious Red Bull television commercials that display extreme sports that often result in violent crashes and death among these same athletes; these same images are often considered heroic by the Red Bull consumer. Along with the claim of a quick fix of energy, it is not surprising that these highly caffeinated and highly supplemented drinks attract a large audience of college students and 20-something professionals, particularly young males. The rise in sales of energy drinks illustrates how trends with beverages often have a huge economic impact. US energy drink sales were reported to be up to $9.7 billion in the year to May 2013 [2].

The popularity of these beverages suggests that they are not departing from the market any time soon. At the same time, the products that represent this trend have been repeatedly dogged by potential negative health effects related to their contents but also to their consumption in combination with alcohol, as reviewed in the chapter by Ragsdale. How this trend will evolve, grow, or dissipate, only time will tell. What energy drinks do represent is a model for creating a new product and a new direction for beverage consumption on a global scale.

Trends for Soda Sweetener Preference: Coca-Cola

Coca-Cola first began to use noncaloric sweeteners, such as aspartame, in the early 1980s in a new formulation called Diet Coke. They thereby created a beverage associated with weight control, a product that soon became extremely popular. The *FDA has approved* six high-intensity sweeteners for use in beverages such as Diet Coke [3]. Yet much has changed in 25 years, with growing consumer concerns over the safety of artificial sweeteners. A recent study of 60,000 postmenopausal women reveals the possible importance of this issue [4]. The consumption of two or more servings per day of diet soda was linked with a 30 % adjusted increase of cardiovascular events and a 50 % increased likelihood of dying from a related disease.

Although soda sales globally reign as "king," sales of diet soda beverages fell 7 % in 2012 in comparison to a drop of 2 % for regular soda, in part due to the growth of competing non-artificially sweetened low-calorie alternatives [5]. Aware of consumers' growing leeriness, Coca-Cola and Cargill have both applied for patents in order to obtain approval for go-ahead with stevia as an all-natural sweetening additive [6]. Today's thinking concerning the effect of sweeteners on health was evaluated in the chapters by Temple and Alps and by White and Nicklas.

Iconic brands such as Coca-Cola and Pepsi will likely remain internationally popular so as long as the companies behind the brands continue to adapt to meet consumer concerns. Predictions of this trend were undoubtedly the key factor that induced Coca-Cola, PepsiCo, and others to announce a voluntary commitment to reduce total caloric intake in their products by 20 % by 2025 [7]. It would not be the first time that these companies have had to change their ingredients and market focus so as to stay in sync with changing trends in beverage consumption, and it will not be the last time our nutrition changes as a result.

Trends in Government Beverage Regulation to Alter Nutritional Patterns

Trends apply to the political ideas that feed into government policy and the industries that governments attempt to regulate. The aims of governments are to promote improved nutritional health and sometimes growth in the beverage industry.

Fear of obesity is a major reason that explains why US consumers have cut their consumption of regular soda. But there are other health concerns at work: for example, 90% of doctors in the USA, the UK, and Asia link high sugar consumption and sweetened beverages with type 2 diabetes [8]. The chapter by Maher and Kobs outlines the current state of understanding of the relationship between beverage consumption and diseases related to caloric balance. Such trends in the views of the general population and of the medical and scientific community can be translated into government policy.

The link between high consumption of soda and obesity has prompted several governments to take action to curtail consumption. Most notoriously, New York

City Mayor Michael Bloomberg's 2012 proposal for a legal limit on the size of soda drinks has since been struck down as unconstitutional and is now in appeal in the New York court system [9]. A more recent proposal in the state of California to mandate warning labels on sugary drinks, Bill SB 203, stalled in the state senate Health Committee in April 2015, yet may be resurrected for debate in upcoming years [10]. Because this type of legislation tends to come from the Democratic Party, and because political candidates and their parties seek funding support from corporations, beverage trends can result in political influence that can change our nutritional outcomes for years to come. The preceding chapter by Krasny outlines many of the legal implications for the marketing of beverages to improve nutritional health.

Trends in Beverage Choices and the Preferred Drinking Environment

Starbucks is arguably the best example of a beverage company successfully responding to changing trends in consumer preferences. The original conversion of Americans to a "traditional" European coffee menu and then to the everyday lives of US consumers made Starbucks a beverage icon. At first, the novelty of buying a specialty coffee drink attracted consumers, because at the time there was no other alternative—your choice at any other cafe was either weak, bland coffee or weaker, blander coffee (black or cream and sugar). As the "coffee house" style developed, Starbucks began to cater to the new Generation Y's preference for personalized choice by offering a broader variety of options in order to individualize one's selection—not to mention the added benefit of free Wi-Fi. As part of this trend, 38 % of the 18–24-year-old group report drinking iced coffee, compared to 20 % of US consumers overall, and 77 % of the iced-coffee drinkers think it makes them feel more productive at work [11].

The accessibility of cell phone and Wi-Fi signals have become key factors by which many people evaluate the quality of coffee houses. Recent developments of apps for cell phones, such as myfitnesspal.com [12] and a plethora of others, have given consumers the tools for the evaluation of the nutritional quality of beverage choices. This trend could eventually lead to changes in the waistline for customers in coffee houses and other establishments that sell beverages.

Smoothies and Juice Bars

Smoothies developed likely as a convenience item alongside the beverage formulas for infants, senior citizens, and dieters (formula, Ensure, and Slim-Fast, as examples).

Commercially available smoothies are cocktails of fruit and vegetable juices that often also contain added nutritional supplements. They may include some of the components that are commonly found in energy drinks, such as protein, creatine, or taurine [13]. They are usually expensive and are sold at juice bars, athletic clubs, convenience stores, and a variety of other outlets.

Hundreds of juice bars have appeared across North America in recent years. For example, the Naked label of juices and smoothies [14] sell for almost $5 each, about the price of a fast-food sandwich. Similar to the Starbucks example, smoothie producers cater to the Generation Y customer base by promoting individualization with a product label for every mood or need. Need energy? Need focus? Need strength? Need fiber? Other beverage companies, such as SmartWater, market water similarly, offering many choices, but with little to no peer-reviewed literature to support their claims. The consumer appeal is strengthened by products that are labeled as "natural" or the use of sweetening by natural fruit juices.

Trends in Alternative Beverages for Lactose Intolerance

Food allergy and intolerance are other factors that drive consumer beverage choices which then create trends. The association between milk and lactose intolerance is reasonably well known among consumers; this drives new trends in the sales of cow's milk and soy alternatives, whose current status was described in the chapters by Armas, Fry, and Heaney and by Woodside, Brennan, and Cantwell. Consumption of cow's milk in the USA has dropped 30 % since 1975. Over the same period, sales of soy milk have boomed. Soy milk has migrated from dusty shelves in a corner of an organic food co-op to supermarkets. However, sales may have hit their peak [15]. The American Soybean Association reported $1.33 billion in sales of soy milk in 2011 [16], but this figure fell by 2.9 % in 2012 as demand steadily grew for new alternative beverage selections with ingredients such as coconut, hemp, almond, hazelnut, rice, and oat [15, 16].

Trends in Beverage Choice due to Changes in Purchasing Power

Trends also occur because of changes in consumer purchasing power. The choice of a beverage or other commodity may symbolize economic status and affluence among one's peers. The 1970s saw the end of Mao's communism in China and the start of phenomenal double-digit growth in GDP and increased consumer affluence. Nixon and Mao shared rice wine together and would have been quite surprised to find that as of 2013, China had become the fourth largest customer for Burgundy red wines after Japan, Britain, and the USA. Also in 2013, Chinese investors purchased more Bordeaux vineyard properties than any other foreign country [17]. With regard to projecting affluence among one's peers, image is very important, and Burgundy wine is one way to project status in China. Clearly, changes in consumer affluence can generate trends in beverage consumption which can then have a nutritional impact.

Trends Resulting from Global Climate Change and Regional Drought

Trends in beverage consumption can also be influenced indirectly by environmental changes, such as global warming. Continued climate change may make it extremely difficult for winemakers in traditional viticultural areas to continue to produce the same quality or type of wine as before [18]. Preferences in grape varietals may also change based on adaptability to climate which is a controlling factor in acidity and sweetness levels. It is far from clear what impact these changes will have on consumer taste preference, product pricing, and the availability of different types of wine.

Beverage trends can also originate from government regulation and related consumer backlash. We see this in the case of the politics of *regional* the drought in California. Sales of bottled water still command a good percentage of the beverage market. Companies such as Nestlé Waters (a subsidiary of Nestlé, one of the world's largest food corporations) have generated trouble with the state government of California over the use of water [19]. Water is not only used for bottling but also for the production of plastic packaging. These factors are likely to generate trends in beverage packaging.

In his famous poem "The Rime of the Ancient Mariner" (1834), Samuel Coleridge wrote the words "Water, water, everywhere, Nor any drop to drink." [20] This eloquently reminds us of the long-standing problems we have with securing access to the right kind of water. Trends in how we obtain this water are in rapid flux. For example, plans are sometimes mooted for dragging icebergs from the Antarctic to parched regions such as Saudi Arabia [21]. How do we ensure safe drinking water to the 7 billion people on this planet who require it, and how will these needs and delivery systems change in response to environmental change?

Conclusion

This book paints a picture of the remarkable diversity in beverages that are available and that will be available in the near future. As with solid food, beverages run the spectrum from the nutritious, safe, and economic through to the unhealthy, undesirable, and overpriced. What ties all beverages together is that we need to consume pure water or water in a beverage to survive.

In the world of beverages, we face a series of multifaceted clashes that complicate nutritional recommendations. We see a clash between good science telling us what is most healthy; at the same time there is marketing hype telling us that we should drink for simple enjoyment. We see a clash because of different levels of credibility of the supporting scientific evidence that feed into our opinions. We see a clash between the accurate presentation of information and information that is distorted by journalists (usually resulting from a poor understanding of science) or by commercial interests (usually due to scientific ignorance or the need for profitability). Finally, we see a clash between government policies aimed at improving the public health and marketing and product development focused only on improving economic issues.

Anyone looking for simple answers to the relative health value of different beverages and how to achieve the ideal balance between health, personal freedom, and responsible economics will be disappointed. We can perhaps be forgiven for being pessimistically optimistic. The tremendous progress in research related to the health effects of beverages, combined with technological developments, leads one to expect that new beverages will steadily appear that combine the best of the present with new discoveries soon to be made. Perhaps this will all be revealed in another ten years in a third edition of *Beverage Impacts on Health and Nutrition*!

References

1. Herodotus. The Histories Book 1. Translated G Rawlinson. Digireads.com 2009; p 112.
2. Wong, V. Overcaffeination concerns haven't dented energy drinks. 2013 http://www.businessweek.com/articles/2013-06-06/overcaffeination-concerns-havent-dented-energy-drinks. Accessed 1 June 2015.
3. Food and Drug Administration. High-intensity sweeteners. http://www.fda.gov/Food/IngredientsPackagingLabeling/FoodAdditivesIngredients/ucm397716.htm. Accessed 19 June 2015.
4. Vyas A, Rubenstein L, Robinson J, Seguin RA, Vitolins MZ, Kazlauskaite R, Shikany JM, Johnson KC, Snetselaar L, Wallace R. Diet drink consumption and the risk of cardiovascular events: a report from the Women's Health Initiative. J Gen Intern Med. 2015;30:462–8.
5. Gray E. Sugar crush: why diet soda sales have crashed. Time, Business & Money. 2013. http://business.time.com/2013/12/10/why-diet-soda-sales-have-crashed/. Accessed 1 May 2015.
6. Steele L. A sweet deal: Coke and Cargill pave the way for an all-natural, calorie-free sugar substitute. QSR magazine. 2014. http://www2.qsrmagazine.com/articles/features/108/sugar-free-1.phtml. Accessed 1 May 2015.
7. Francella K. Consumers make lower-calorie choices. BeverageWorld. http://www.beverageworld.com/blog/entry/25531/consumers-make-lower-calorie-choices. Accessed 9 June 2015.
8. Voight J. Coke and Pepsi Face Diabetes Backlash: Study shows 90% of doctors link disease with sugar. AdWeek. 2013. http://www.adweek.com/news/advertising-branding/coke-and-pepsi-face-diabetes-backlash-153613. Accessed 1 May 2015.
9. Ax J. Bloomberg's ban on big sodas is unconstitutional: appeals court. Reuters press. 2013. http://www.reuters.com/article/2013/07/30/us-sodaban-lawsuit-idUSBRE96T0UT20130730. Accessed 3 May 2015.
10. California Center for Public Advocacy. Warning Labels on Sugary Drinks Bill SB 203 (Monning). http://sodawarninglabels.org/. Accessed 1 May 2015.
11. Mintel Research Group. Americans enter the ice age – iced coffee goes beyond summer-only appeal. http://www.prnewswire.com/news-releases/americans-enter-the-ice-age---iced-coffee-goes-beyond-summer-only-appeal-218688151.html. Accessed 7 Aug 2013.
12. Lose Weight with MyFitnessPal. https://www.myfitnesspal.com/. Accessed 9 June 2015.
13. Customize your blend. http://www.smoothieking.com/menu/enhancers. Accessed 20 June 2015.
14. If you can't eat 'em, drink 'em! http://www.nakedjuice.com. Accessed 20 June 2015.
15. Fottrell, Q. Soy milk sales sour along with dairy. The Wall Street Journal, Market Watch. 2012. http://www.marketwatch.com/story/soy-milk-sales-sour-along-with-dairy-2012-12-11. Accessed 1 May 2015.

16. American Soybean Association. Soymilk a booming $1.3 billion business. 2012. http://westernfarmpress.com/markets/soymilk-booming-13-billion-business. Accessed 1 May 2015.
17. Doward J. Chinese move on from snapping up fine wines, to buying the whole vineyards: Christie's auction house sets up world's first estate agency for Chinese to buy wine estates. The Observer. http://www.theguardian.com/lifeandstyle/2013/may/12/bordeaux-wine-vineyards-christies-chinese. Accessed 11 May 2015.
18. Mozell MR, Thach L. The impact of climate change on the global wine industry: challenges & solutions. Wine Econ Policy. 2014;3:81–9.
19. Nestlé Waters North America Water Management Statement. http://www.nestle-watersna.com/en/nestle-water-news/statements/nestle-waters-north-america-water-management-statement. Accessed 9 June 2015.
20. Coleridge S. The rhyme of the ancient mariner. 1834. http://www.poetryfoundation.org/poem/173253. Accessed 18 June 2015.
21. Madrigal AC. The many failures and few successes of zany iceberg towing schemes. Atlantic Monthly. http://www.theatlantic.com/technology/archive/2011/08/the-many-failures-and-few-successes-of-zany-iceberg-towing-schemes/243364/ Accessed 10 June 2015.

Index

A

AAP. *See* American Academy of Pediatrics
 (AAP)
Academy of Nutrition and Dietetics, 197, 325
Acidity regulators, 318
ACSM. *See* American College of Sports
 Medicine (ACSM)
Activities of daily living (ADLs), 214
Acute myocardial infarction (AMI), 35
Additives
 beverages, 327
 color, 326
 lipid-soluble, 322
ADLs. *See* Activities of daily living (ADLs)
Advertising, 269–273, 275
Alcohol consumption, 72–75
 accidents, violence and suicide, 70
 drinking patterns, 76
 drunkenness and chronic alcohol abuse, 70
 FAS, 71
 mortality, 76
 obesity, 72
 protective effects
  CHD, 72, 73
  diabetes, 75
  impotence, 74
 quantity, 70
Alcoholic beverages labeling
 advertisement, 347
 COLA/exemption, 346
 GOVERNMENT WARNING, 346
 "kombucha" tea, 346
 TTB regulation, 346
American Academy of Pediatrics (AAP), 164

American College of Sports Medicine
 (ACSM), 228
American cranberry (*Vaccinium
 macrocarpon*), 102
 antioxidant activity, 107
 beverage formulations, consumer, 109–110
 on cancer, 108–109
 in CVD, 108
 genetic diversity, 102
 Native New Englanders, 102
 nutrients, 105
 nutrients phytochemicals and
  pharmacokinetics, 107
 phytochemicals and pharmacokinetics,
  105–107
 UTIs (*see* Urinary tract infections (UTIs))
American Heart Association, 197
AMI. *See* Acute myocardial infarction (AMI)
Anthocyanins, 107
Anticancer activity
 EGCG, 55
 theaflavin and theaflavin digallate, 56
Antioxidants, 171, 319, 320, 327
Appetite, 196
Artificially sweetened beverages (ASBs)
 advantame, 195
 appetite, 196
 calorie intake, 197
 consumption, 196
 diet drinks, 195
 epidemiological research, 196
 intervention studies, 196
 nonalcoholic beverages, 195
 observational studies, 196

© Springer International Publishing Switzerland 2016
T. Wilson, N.J. Temple (eds.), *Beverage Impacts on Health and Nutrition*,
Nutrition and Health, DOI 10.1007/978-3-319-23672-8

Artificially sweetened beverages (ASBs) (*cont.*)
   protective effect, 196
   randomized trials, 196
   sugar-sweetened products, 196
   table sugar (sucrose), 195
ASCVD. *See* Atherosclerotic cardiovascular
      disease (ASCVD)
Atherogenesis, 83
Atherosclerotic cardiovascular disease (ASCVD)
   description, 84 (*see also* Gut microbiota)
   inflammation, 89
   mortality rate, 84
   pathology, 84
Athletes
   efficacy, 226
   postexercise recovery, 234–235
   sports and hydration, 21–22

B
Benign prostatic hyperplasia, 75
Beverage consumption, 14–20
   bacteria/toxins, 12
   Cancalon, 13
   culture
      alcoholism, 18
      hospitality, 18–19
      legion, 18
      rites of Passage & Rituals, 18
   fermented beverages
      alcohol, 14
      alcoholism, 15
      social attitudes, 15
      trade and commerce, 14
   milking, 13, 14
   nonalcoholic beverages
      cacao, 16
      coffee, 16
      kola, 16
      tea, 17
   primarily water, 12
   religions
      Christianity, 19–20
      Islam, 20
      Judaism, 19
   social conflict & war, 20–21
   space flight, 22, 23
   sports, and hydration, 21, 22
   trees, crotch/natural depressions, 12
   water, 13
Beverage ingredients
   caffeine, 327
   dyes and coloring, 326–327, (*see also*
      Fatty acids)

   GRAS, 318 (*see also* Hydrocolloids)
   nonalcoholic beverages, 318 (*see also*
      Organic acids; Salts; Sweeteners)
Beverage trend
   consumer purchasing power, 355
   description, 351
   energy drink, 352
   global climate change and regional
      drought, 356
   Government beverage regulation, 353–354
   Herodotus (440 BCE), 352
   lactose intolerance, 355
   preferred drinking environment, 354
   smoothies and juice bars, 354–355
   soda sweetener preference, 353
Beverages, 182
   catechins/caffeine, 187–188
   cognition, 188
   energy balance, 183
   gastric emptying, 189
   gastrointestinal transit, 189
   hormonal response, 189
   macronutrient content and satiation/satiety,
      183–184
   macronutrients, 187
   oral processing, 188
Beverages impact on health and nutrition
   alcoholic fermentation, 5
   athletes, 6
   coffee/tea, 4, 5
   diabetes, 6
   energy drinks and bottled water, 6–7
   HFCS, 7
   ingredient Functions, 8
   juices, 5
   marketing, 7
   metabolic syndrome, 6
   milks and milk products, 5
   older persons, 6
   satiety, 6
   sugar, 7
Bioactive compounds, 169–170
Black tea
   bladder cancer, 62
   blood pressure, 59
   caffeine, 51
   components, 52
   endometrial cancer, 53
   enzymatic oxidation, 51
   stroke, 59
   T2D, 59
BMD. *See* Bone mineral density (BMD)
Body weight, 57, 139, 140, 184, 185, 209, 279
Bone health, 122

Bone mineral density (BMD)
  skeletal sites, 156
  soy isoflavone, 156
Bottled water, 260, 261
  cholera, 260
  flouride, 263
  food, 259
  industry, 260
  labeling laws and regulation
    categories, EU, 261
    purified water, 260
    sparkling, 261
    types, 261
    vitamins/electrolytes, 261
  mineral content, 261–262
  safety, drinking water, 263
  tap water, 260
  water-related diseases, 260
Brain health and cognition, 121–122
Breast cancer
  cell lines, 155
  soy food intake, 154
Breast-feeding
  advantages, 173
  childhood deaths, 173
  economics, 173–174
  politics, 174
Brominated vegetable oil (BVO), 322
BVO. *See* Brominated vegetable oil (BVO)

C
Cacao, 16
Caffeine, 187–188, 248, 249, 327
Caloric sweeteners, 324
Camellia sinensis (Theaceae) plant, 50
Cancer, 54–56
  animal models, 55
  anticancer (*see* Anticancer activity)
  anti-metastatic effect, 56–57
  atypia, 155
  breast cancer, 154
  cow's milk on human health, 138
  endometrial and ovarian, 155
  epidemiological studies, 52, 54, 154, 155
  health benefits, citrus juices, 122
  intervention studies
    chemopreventive effects, 54
    Polyphenon®, 54
  isoflavones, 155
  pre/postmenopausal women, 155
  soy milk/protein, 154
Carbohydrates, 185
  advantages, 229–230

dehydration, 230
dilute glucose–electrolyte solutions, 230
drinks, 234
electrolyte composition and concentration, 232–233
flavoring components, 233
optimum concentration, 230
osmolality, 231
types, 230
Cardiac arrhythmias, 36
Cardiovascular diseases (CVDs), 33–35, 88–89
  arterial health evaluation, 88
  ASCVD, 84
  blood lipid levels, 157
  blood pressure, 59, 157
  caffeine intake, 58
  carotid IMT and atherosclerotic burden, 158
  CHD, 156
  CLA and sphingolipids, 135
  cohort studies, 136
  coffee
    blood pressure, 33
    diabetes, 34
    serum lipids, 34
    stroke, 35
  diet rich, 156
  epidemiological studies, 85
  ethanol consumption, 85
  flavonoid and nonflavonoid phytochemicals, 85, 87
  French paradox (*see* French paradox)
  green and oolong tea, 58
  heart and blood vessels, 84
  "Heart-smart" health claims, 158
  inflammatory markers, 157
  isoflavones, 157
  isoflavones/soy protein, 157
  LDL and HDL cholesterol, 157
  LDL, in vitro oxidative damage, 85
  nonlipid risk factors, 136
  phenolic compounds, 85
  saturated fats, 135
  stroke, 36, 58
  "Western diet", 84
Cardiovascular health, 120–121
Catechins, 187–188
  animal experiments, 56
  chemopreventive effects, 54
  green tea, 54
  inhalation therapy, 62
  MCF-7 breast cancer, 58
Certificate of Label Approval (COLA), 346

CFBAI. *See* Children's Food and Beverage
    Advertising Initiative (CFBAI)
CHD. *See* Coronary heart disease (CHD)
Chelating agents, 319
Children's Food and Beverage Advertising
    Initiative (CFBAI), 272
Chocolate milk, 16, 142, 144, 146, 186,
    324, 325
Chronic alcohol abuse, 70–71
Chronic obstructive pulmonary disease
    (COPD), 75
Citrus juices flavanones
    bone health, 122
    brain health and cognition, 121–122
    cancer, 122
    cardiovascular health, 120–121
    grapefruit–drug interaction, 123–124
    juices, modified juices and drink
        blends, 117
    juices, modified juices and drink
        blendsyears, 117
    minerals and vitamins, 116, (*see also*
        Phytochemicals)
    phytochemicals and polyphenols, 116
    sugar metabolism and insulin resistance,
        122–123
CMA. *See* Cow's milk allergy (CMA)
Coca-Cola, 353
Code of Federal Regulations, 288
Coffee consumption, 31–33, 36–42, 44
    bioactive compounds, 30
    bladder cancer, 44
    caffeine, 30, 31
    cancer
        bladder, 40, 41
        colorectum, 37
        endometrium, 39, 40
        fatal cases, 41
        liver, 38
        mortality, 36
        oral cavity & pharynx, 37
        pancreas, 39
        prostate cancer, 41
    mortality
        cancer/cardiovascular disease, 33
        chronic diseases, 33
        coffee, 32, 33
        hazard ratios (HR), 31
        risk, 33
        tobacco, 31
    neurologic diseases
        dose–exposure, 42
        Parkinson's disease, 42
        types, 41

osteoporosis, 42
pregnancy
    preterm delivery, 42
    trimester, 42
stroke, 44
COLA. *See* Certificate of Label Approval
    (COLA)
Color in beverages perception
    cross-cultural differences, 310–311
    description, 308
    flavor identification responses, 307
    food choices and consumption
        behaviors, 306
    laboratory-based research, 313
    odor intensity, 307
    off colors, 310
    orange- and blackcurrant-flavored
        solutions, 308, 309
    orthonasal and retronasal olfaction, 307
    product-extrinsic color, 311–313
    researchers, 306
    sensory incongruency, 309–310
    supertasters and nontasters, 308
    taste sensitivity, 306
Condensed tannins, 106
COPD. *See* Chronic obstructive pulmonary
    disease (COPD)
Coronary heart disease (CHD), 72, 73, 278
    soy milk/soy protein, 156
Cow's milk allergy (CMA), 165
    IgE-mediated, 154
    infants and children, 154
Cow's milk on human health
    cancer, 138
    carbohydrates, 133
    consumption of, 142
    CVD, 135–136
    diabetes and insulin resistance, 140
    economic researchers, 143
    fat, 133, 134
    hypertension and stroke, 136–137
    industry efforts to increase milk
        consumption, 144–146, (*see also*
        Kidney stones)
    lactose intolerance, 141
    nomadic pastoralists, 131
    nonfat/reduced-fat milk, 135
    nutrient density, 132, 133
    osteoporosis, 137
    per capita total milk consumption (gallons)
        in USA, 141
    proteins, 133
    surrogate markers of disease, 135
    US per capita sales, 143

weight control, 138–139
younger generations of Americans, 144
C-reactive proteins (CRP), 280
CRP. *See* C-reactive proteins (CRP)
Culture
　beverage consumption
　　alcoholism, 18
　　hospitality, 18–19
　　legion, 18
　　rites of Passage & Rituals, 18
　human, 5
CVDs. *See* Cardiovascular diseases (CVD)

D
Daily Reference Values (DRVs), 336
DASH. *See* Dietary Approaches to Stop
　　Hypertension (DASH) study
Dehydration
　carbohydrate (CHO), 226
　fatigue, 238
　hyperthermia and hypernatremia,
　　226, 232
Dental caries, 277, 280–282
Deoxypyridinoline (DPD), 156
Diabetes, 75, 280
　and insulin resistance, 140
Diabetes mellitus (DM), 198–200
　alcohol-containing beverages, 200–201
　carbohydrates and caloric intake, 194
　carbonated beverages and sodium, 201
　cmmercial beverage preparations, 202
　CVD, 194
　dairy and dairy substitute beverages
　　breast milk, 199
　　calcium consumption, 199
　　cow's milk consumption, 198
　　gut microbiome, 199
　　health-promoting benefits, 200
　　hormonal and behavioral factors, 199
　　natural and artificial milks, 199
　　pasteurization destroys, 199
　　phosphorus, 200
　　potassium, 200
　　vegetable beverages, 199
　　vitamin D, 199
　diet, 194
　fruit and vegetable juices, 197, 198
　functional beverage phytochemicals,
　　201–202
　macronutrient intake, 194
　obesity, 194
　risk factors and diagnosis, 194
　sweetened beverages, 195

Diet and microbiome
　immune dysfunction, 92
　metabolite profiles, 93
　metagenomes, 93
　optimal health outcomes, 93
Diet Coke, 353
Dietary Approaches to Stop Hypertension
　　(DASH) study, 136
Dietary fiber, 116
Dietary reference intakes (DRIs), 164
Direct antioxidant theory, 118–119
Disconfirmed expectation, 305
DPD. *See* Deoxypyridinoline (DPD)
DRIs. *See* Dietary reference intakes (DRIs)
DRVs. *See* Daily Reference Values (DRVs)
Dyslipidemia, 194

E
EGCG. *See* (−)-Epigallocatechin gallate
　　(EGCG)
Emulsifiers, 322, 323, 327
Energy drinks (ED), 245–247, 352
　adverse effects, 252–253
　caffeine, 248, 249
　food safety, 244
　Governmental Oversight, 253–254
　herbal ingredients, 251
　Lucozade aids recovery, 244
　manufacturers' market strategy and
　　audience
　　beverage industry, 247
　　caffeine consumption, 246
　　energy supplements, 245
　　labeling requirements, 247
　　methyl xanthines, 247
　　organic and fair-trade products, 246
　　sales, 246
　　sports events, 245
　　theophylline and theobromine, 247
　　US and European markets, 246
　　vague nature, 247
　　weight-conscious consumers, 246
　medicine show syrups, 244
　"replace lost energy", 244
　sugar, 249
　sweetened beverages, 245
　taurine, 250
　vitamins, 250–251
Enzymes, 170–171
(−)-Epigallocatechin gallate (EGCG)
　apoptosis, 56
　Fas, 55
　microRNA, 55

(−)-Epigallocatechin gallate (EGCG) (*cont.*)
    nonmelanoma skin cancer, 56
    peroral administratio, 55
    polyphenol theasinensin, 56
    tea components, 56
    theaflavin and theaflavin digallate, 56
Estrogen replacement therapy, 156
European Food Safety Authority (EFSA), 254
Exercise performance, 230, 239

F
FAA. *See* Federal Alcohol Administration Act
    (FAA Act)
FAE. *See* Fetal alcohol effects (FAE)
FAS. *See* Fetal lcohol syndrome (FAS)
Fatty acids
    brominated vegetable oil (BVO), 322
    emulsifiers, 322
    MCT, 322
FCs. *See* Furanocoumarins (FCs)
FD&C. *See* Federal Food, Drug, and Cosmetic
    Act (FD&C Act)
FDA. *See* Food and Drug Administration
    (FDA)
Federal Alcohol Administration Act
    (FAA Act), 332
Federal Food, Drug, and Cosmetic Act
    (FD&C Act), 332
Federal Trade Commission (FTC), 332
Fermentation, 5, 13, 14, 85, 140, 186, 202,
    318, 320, 323, 346
Ferric reducing ability of plasma (FRAP)
    assay, 107
Fetal alcohol effects (FAE), 71
Fetal alcohol syndrome (FAS), 71
Fiber, 186–187
Flavored milk, 142–145, 147, 325
Flouride, 263
Food and Drug Administration (FDA), 332
Food Chemicals Codex, 288
Food labelling requirements, 343–344
    allowable ingredients, 338–339
    biotechnology claims, 344–345
    California Proposition 65 Warnings,
        345–346
    fresh claims, 342–343
    health claims, 340–342
    ingredient statement, 335
    NAFTA countries, 334
    natural claims
        class action lawsuits, 343
        FDA, 343

    use and warnings, 343–344
    net quantity, contents declaration, 335
    nonalcoholic beverages, 332–346
    nutrition information, ingredient statement
        and signature line, 333
    nutrition labeling, 336–337
    organic claims, 345
    product identity statement, 334
    product information, 332
    regulatory categories, 337–338
    structure/function claims, 341–342
FRAP. *See* Ferric reducing ability of plasma
    (FRAP) assay
French paradox
    ASCVD and NAC, 88
    diet and microbiome, 92–93
    gut microbiota, 90
    hypothesized mechanisms, 88
    inflammation sources, 89
    microbiome, 89
    polyphenol bioavailability, 88–89
    saturated fat, red meat and ASCVD redux,
        90–92
    wine and gut microbiota, 93–95
Fruit juice, 101, 110, 115, 117, 118, 122, 123,
    141, 197, 198, 202, 281
FTC. *See* Federal Trade Commission (FTC)
Furanocoumarins (FCs), 117, 123

G
Generally recognised as safe (GRAS), 166
Genomics epigenetics, 119–120
GHSPx. *See* Glutathione peroxidase (GHSPx)
Ginkgo, 251
Ginkgo biloba, 251
Ginseng, 251
Glutathione peroxidase (GHSPx), 171
Governmental oversight, 253–254
Government regulation, 269, 273–275, 356
Grapefruit–drug interaction, 123–124
GRAS. *See* Generally recognised as safe
    (GRAS)
Green tea
    antidiabetic effects, 59
    blood pressure, 59
    catechins, 55
    components, 52
    EGCG, 56
    interferon/ribavirin, 61–62
    metachronous colorectal adenomas, 54
    MetS, 57
    mRNA level, 60

obesity and arteriosclerosis, 58
ovarian cancer, 53
Polyphenon®, 54
powder capsules, 54
steaming fresh tea leaves, 51
TNF-α, 61
water-soluble polyphenols, 51
Gut microbiota, 93–95
    description, 90
    dysregulated cross talk, 90
    microbiota-derived factors, 90
    and wine
        microbial metabolites, 94
        microbiome-gut-brain axis, 94
        pharmacologic doses, 95
        phytochemicals, 93

H
Heart disease
    CHD, 72
    and coffee, 35–36
    and diabetes, 116
Hepatoprotective effects
    galactosamine, 60
    hypertensive nonalcoholic
        steatohepatitis, 61
    obese, 61
HFCS. *See* High-fructose corn syrup (HFCS)
High-fructose corn syrup (HFCS), 7, 278,
        289–290, 294–297
    cell metabolism, 286
    food and beverage industry, 286
    fructose level in, 288, 289
    health effects
        added sugars, 297
        experimental designs, 296
        foods and beverages, 295
        metabolic/endocrine responses, 295
        metabolism site, 296
        overconsumption of, 294
        RCTs, 297
        regulatory control, 296
        sugars absorption, 296
    vs. sucrose, 286–288, (*see also* Sucrose
        manufacture)
Human milk and infant formula
    adequate intake (AI), 164
    antioxidants, 171
    bioactive compounds, 169–170
    breast-fed infants, 172
    breast-feeding, 164
    cholesterol, 166

CMA, 165
cognitive development, 172–173
colic and constipation, 166
developing countries, 166
enzymes, 170–171
formula manufacturers, 165
growth, 164, 172
health benefits, 172
maternal influences, 169
metabolism, 166
microbiome, 171
milk food, 164, 165
minerals, 167–168
North America, 165
nutrient requirements, 166
polyunsaturated fatty acids, 165
protein, lipids, and carbohydrate, 167
supplements, 168
uniquely superior, 165
vitamins, 168
Hydrocolloids
    gums and pectins, 323–324
    starches, 323
Hyperglycemia, 200
Hyperhydration, 238–239
Hypertension, 195, 196
Hypertension and stroke, 136–137
Hypohydration, 225, 227, 232, 239

I
Infant formula, 163–175
Inflammation signaling theory, 119
Ingredient label, 8, 23
Ingredient statement, 335
In-school marketing, 269, 275
International Society of Beverage
        Technologists (ISBT), 289
ISBT. *See* International Society of Beverage
        Technologists (ISBT)
Isoflavones
    bone health, 156
    CHD risk, 157
    CVD, 157
    mammary tumors, 155
    soy milk, 152

J
Juice
    citrus (*see* Citrus juices flavanones)
    cranberry (*see* Cranberry juice)
    fruit and vegetable, 197–198

K

Kidney stones
    disorders with low calcium intakes, 140
    high calcium intake, 140
Kola, 16–17, 327

L

Labeling requirements
    Dietary Supplement Health and Education
        Act of 1994, 247
    food (see Food labeling requirements)
    industry-published values and satisfies
        government regulatory, 289
Lactase nonpersistence, 141
Lactose intolerance, 141, 355
    CMA, 154
    glucose and galactose, 154
Liquid nutritional supplements, 216
Low and no calorie sweeteners
    Academy of Nutrition and Dietetics, 325
    negative health outcomes, 326
    plant-derived, 324, 325
    trade/chemical name, 325

M

Malnutrition, 71, 173, 207–215, 219
Marketing
    aggressive, 165
    beverage sugar and high-fructose corn
        syrup, 7
    EDs, 244
    International Code of Marketing of
        Breast-milk Substitutes, 166
    neonate/infant formula, 5
    safe water, 7
    SSBs (see Sugar-sweetened beverages
        (SSBs))
MCT. See Medium-chain triglycerides (MCT)
Medium-chain triglycerides (MCT), 322
Menopausal symptoms
    phytoestrogen supplements, 158
Metabolic syndrome (MetS), 280
    BMI, 57
    CVD and T2D, 57 (see also Diabetes
        mellitus (DM))
    diastolic blood pressure, 57
    green tea, 57
MetS. See Metabolic syndrome (MetS)
Microbiome, 171
Microbiota, 83, 89, 90, 93–95, 107
Milk consumption, 5, 14, 131, 133, 135, 137,
    138, 141–146

Milk Processor Education Program
    (MilkPEP), 145
MilkPEP. See Milk Processor Education
    Program (MilkPEP)
Mineral water, 260–262
Minerals, 167–168
miRNA, 55, 120, 124
Monk Fruit (Siraitia grosvenorii), 325
'Monster' drink, 245–249, 254
Multisensory integration, 307

N

NAFTA. See North American Free Trade
    Agreement (NAFTA) countries
National Dairy Promotion and Research Board
    and milk processors, 145
National Longitudinal Survey of Youth
    (NLSY), 172
National Organic Program (NOP), 345
NLSY. See National Longitudinal Survey of
    Youth (NLSY)
Nondairy milks
    almond, 159
    coconut, 159
    grain, 158
    oat, 159
    oat milk, 159
Nonnutritive sweeteners (NNS). See Low and
    no calorie sweeteners
NOP. See National Organic
    Program (NOP)
North American Free Trade Agreement
    (NAFTA) countries, 334
Nutrient content claims
    antioxidant, 340
    description, 339
    "excellent source of vitamin C", 340
    "reduced sugar", 340
Nutrition labeling
    FDA's compliance policy, 336
    ingredients, 336
    packaged foods, 336
    RACCs, 336
    RDIs, 336
Nutrition Labeling and Education
    Act, 247

O

Obesity, 58, 181
    epidemiological studies, 57–58
    in vitro and animal experiments
        catechin-free fraction, 58

pancreatic lipase, 58
intervention studies, 57–58
OFPA. *See* Organic Foods Production Act of
1990 (OFPA)
Older adults
clinical benefits, 214–219
community, 209–210
comprehensive assessment, 210
energy intake, 214
malnutrition, 208
medicare-certified nursing homes, 209
ONS, 211–214
oral nutritional beverage, 208–209
support programs, 210–211
treatment plan, 209
Olympics, 247, 271
Oolong tea
bladder cancer, 54
monomeric catechins, 51
ovarian cancer, 53
polyphenol theasinensin, 56
T2D, 59
theaflavins, 51
thearubigins, 51
ORAC. *See* Oxygen radical absorbance
capacity (ORAC)
Orange, 23, 115–118, 122, 307
Organic acids
acidity regulators/buffers, 318
antioxidants, 319
ascorbic acid (vitamin C), 319
calcium disodium EDTA, 320
carbonated water, 320
chemical structures, 319
citric acid, 319
description, 318
erythorbic acid, 320
fumaric and malic acid, 319
phosphoric acid (inorganic), 321
preservatives, 319
sequestrants/chelating agents, 319
stereoisomers, 320
tartaric acid, 320
Organic Foods Production Act of 1990
(OFPA), 345
Orthonasal olfaction, 307
Osmolality, 231
Osteoporosis, 137
BMD, 156
DPD, 156
estrogen replacement therapy, 156
spine, 156
Oxygen radical absorbance capacity
(ORAC), 107

P
PAC. *See* Proanthocyanidins (PAC)
Panax ginseng, 251
Paullinia cupana, 251
Pectin, 323
Phosphoric acid, inorganic, 321
Physical form, 182
Phytochemicals
bioavailability and metabolic
transformations in vivo, 118
direct antioxidant theory,
118–119
FCs, 117
genomics epigenetics, 119–120
inflammation signaling
theory, 119
research, 117
Phytoestrogens
isoflavones, 153
soy milk/protein, 153
Polyphenol
Fasn gene, 58
oolong tea, 56
Potassium sorbate, 322
Preservative, 317–319, 321–322, 327
Proanthocyanidins (PAC), 104, 106
Procyanidins, 106
Product identity statement, 334
Protein, 186
Pulse-wave velocity (PWV), 108
PWV. *See* Pulse-wave velocity
(PWV)

R
RACCs. *See* Reference amounts customarily
consumed (RACCs)
Randomized controlled trials
(RCTs), 279
RCTs. *See* Randomized controlled
trials (RCTs)
Red Bull, 245
Austria, 244
B vitamins, 250
monster, 245
Reference amounts customarily consumed
(RACCs), 336
Reference Daily Intakes (RDIs) established
for micronutrients, 336
Religion
Christianity, 19–20
Islam, 20
Judaism, 19
Retronasal olfaction, 307

S
Salts
    description, 321
    electrolytes, 321
    preservatives, 321–322
Satiation, 184
    appetite control and food intake, 182
    eating or drinking behavior, 183
    energy balance, 182
Satiety
    appetite control and food intake, 182
    carbohydrates, 185
    eating or drinking behavior, 183
    energy balance, 182
    fiber, 186–187
    protein, 186
Self-regulation
    by food industry, 272–273
    vs. government regulation, 273–275
Sequestrants, 319
Signaling pathways
Sip feeds, 211, 215
SMHP. *See* Sodium hexametaphosphate
        (SMHP)
Smoothies and juice bars, 354–355
Sodium hexametaphosphate (SMHP), 322
Soft drinks
    carbonated, 288
    sales, 292
Soy milk products
    cancer, 154–155
    vs. cow's milk, 152
    CVD, 157, 158
    isoflavones, 152
    lactose intolerance, 154
    menopausal symptoms, 158
    nondairy milks, 158–159
    osteoporosis, 156
    phytoestrogens, 153
    plant-based milks, 152
Soy protein
    allergy, 154
    animal protein, 158
    blood pressure, 157
    bone health, 156
    CHD, 156
    IgE-mediated CMA, 154
    infant milk formulas, 153
    inflammatory markers, 157
    phytoestrogens, 153
Space flight, 22–23
Sports beverages
    diet, 226
    factors, 225

fatigue, brain, 238
    fluid and electrolyte balance, 235–236
    fluid ingestion, 228
    hydration and performance, 227–228
    hyperhydration, 238–239
    limitations, endurance performance,
            226–227
    muscle glycogen resynthesis, 236–237
    postexercise recovery, 234–235
    protein synthesis and tissue remodeling, 237
    water, 226
Sports drinks, 3, 16, 226–232, 234, 238, 239,
        272, 317, 321
SSBs. *See* Sugar-sweetened beverages (SSBs)
Stabilizer, 165, 323, 324
Stroke, 33–36, 73, 75, 84, 120, 136–137
Sucrose manufacture
    acid stability, 291–292
    comparison of, 290
    flavor enhancement, 291
    high-fructose *corn* syrup, 289
    physical and functional properties, 290
    physical form, 292
    sweetness, 291
    US per capita availability, 292, 293
    worldwide comparison, 293, 294
Sucrose *vs.* HFCS
    carbohydrate sugars (saccharides), 286
    chemical structures, 286, 287
    Corn Refiners Association, 288
    pre- and post-digestion, 287, 288
Sugar, 249
    CHD, 278
    diet quality, 281
    dietary recommendations, 281–282
    HFCS, 278
    soda/cola drinks, 278
    SSBs, 278
    sucrose, 278
Sugar metabolism and insulin resistance,
        122–123
Sugar-sweetened beverages (SSBs), 184,
        273–275, 278
    beverage marketing, schools, 272
    cardiometabolic risk factors and
            CHD, 280
    dental caries, 280–281
    marketing and expenditure, 270–271
    metabolic syndrome and diabetes, 280
    public health challenge, 282
    research methods, 278–279
    self-regulation *vs.* government regulation
            food industry, 273, 274
            healthy products, 273

television, 273
tobacco, alcohol and foods, 274
unhealthy foods, 275
self-regulation, food industry, 272–273
weight gain and obesity, 279–280
Sweat loss, 232, 233, 235–237
Sweeteners
caloric, 324
low and no calorie, 324–326
Synergists, 319

T
T2D. *See* Type 2 diabetes (T2D)
TAP. *See* Total antioxidant performance
(TAP) assays
Tap water, 260–264
Taste perception, 4, 7, 12
Taurine, 250
Tea consumption, 59
black tea, 51
caffeine, 51
Camellia sinensis (Theaceae) plant, 50
cancer, 52–57
CVD, 58–59
green tea, 51
hepatoprotective effects, 60–62
MetS, 57
obesity, 57–58
oolong tea, 51
type 2 diabetes (*see* Type 2 diabetes (T2D))
Thickeners, 323
TMA. *See* Trimethylamine (TMA)
Tobacco Tax and Trade Bureau (TTB),
332, 346
Total antioxidant performance (TAP)
assays, 107
Trimethylamine (TMA), 90
Trp. *See* Tryptophan (Trp)
Tryptophan (Trp), 238
TTB. *See* Tobacco Tax and Trade Bureau
(TTB)
Type 2 diabetes (T2D), 60, 280
black/oolong teas, 59

cellular and animal experiments
α-amylase activity, 60
gluconeogenesis, 60
glucose intake, 60
insulin sensitivity, 60
tea catechins, 60
hemoglobin A1c levels, 59

U
UHT. *See* Ultra-high temperature (UHT)
sterilization
Ultra-high temperature (UHT) sterilization, 321
Undegraded carrageenan, 324
Undernutrition, 208, 209
Urinary tract infections (UTIs)
bacterial interactions with cranberry
juice, 104
clinical evidence, 103
cranberries and prevention, 103–104
cystitis and pyelonephritis, 102
double-blind human clinical trial, 103
Escherichia coli, 102
health-care system, 103
in free-living adults, 103
p-fimbriae, 102
US Food and Drug Administration
(FDA), 195

V
Vaccinium macrocarpon (*see* American
cranberry (*Vaccinium
macrocarpon*))
Vasodilation, 108
Visual dominance, 313
Vitamins, 168, 250–251

W
War, 11, 21
Water-soluble gums, 323
Wine consumption. *See* Gut microbiota
World Health Organization (WHO), 274

Printed in the United States
By Bookmasters